PREGNANCY WITH TYPE 1 DIABETES

YOUR MONTH-TO-MONTH GUIDE TO BLOOD SUGAR MANAGEMENT

PREGNANCY WITH TYPE 1 DIABETES

YOUR MONTH-TO-MONTH GUIDE TO BLOOD SUGAR MANAGEMENT

Ginger Vieira, CHC, CPT
Jennifer C. Smith, RD, CDE

Foreword by Nat Strand, MD

FOR
OSKAR AND LUCY,
CONAN AND VIOLET,
YOU'RE WORTH IT.

THANK YOU
TO OUR DEDICATED MFM/OB HEALTHCARE TEAMS
FOR TAKING SUCH GREAT CARE OF US
AS MOTHERS WITH DIABETES—AND OUR BABIES—
DURING OUR PREGNANCIES.
WE ARE FOREVER GRATEFUL!

RECOMMENDED READING

- ☐ *Think Like a Pancreas* by Gary Scheiner
- ☐ *The Ultimate Guide to Accurate Carb-Counting* by Gary Scheiner
- ☐ *Pumping Insulin* by John Walsh and Ruth Roberts
- ☐ *Emotional Eating with Diabetes* by Ginger Vieira
- ☐ *Dealing with Diabetes Burnout* by Ginger Vieira
- ☐ *Balancing Pregnancy with Pre-Existing Diabetes* by Cheryl Alkon
- ☐ *A Woman's Guide to Diabetes* by Brandy Barnes & Natalie Strand
- ☐ *100 Healthiest Foods to Eat During Pregnancy* by Jonny Bowden & Allison Tannis
- ☐ *What to Expect When You're Expecting* by Heidi Murkoff

MONTH-TO-MONTH GUIDE

MONTH 1

- MAMA'S MENTAL HEALTH
- NUTRITION
- BLOOD SUGAR MANAGEMENT
- AT THE DOCTOR'S OFFICE
- GINGER'S PREGNANCY DIARY

MONTH 2

- MAMA'S MENTAL HEALTH
- NUTRITION
- BLOOD SUGAR MANAGEMENT
- AT THE DOCTOR'S OFFICE
- GINGER'S PREGNANCY DIARY

MONTH 3

- MAMA'S MENTAL HEALTH
- NUTRITION
- BLOOD SUGAR MANAGEMENT
- AT THE DOCTOR'S OFFICE
- GINGER'S PREGNANCY DIARY

MONTH 4

- MAMA'S MENTAL HEALTH
- NUTRITION
- BLOOD SUGAR MANAGEMENT
- AT THE DOCTOR'S OFFICE
- GINGER'S PREGNANCY DIARY

MONTH 5

- MAMA'S MENTAL HEALTH
- NUTRITION
- BLOOD SUGAR MANAGEMENT
- AT THE DOCTOR'S OFFICE
- GINGER'S PREGNANCY DIARY

MONTH 6

- MAMA'S MENTAL HEALTH
- NUTRITION
- BLOOD SUGAR MANAGEMENT
- AT THE DOCTOR'S OFFICE
- GINGER'S PREGNANCY DIARY

MONTH 7

- MAMA'S MENTAL HEALTH
- NUTRITION
- BLOOD SUGAR MANAGEMENT
- AT THE DOCTOR'S OFFICE
- GINGER'S PREGNANCY DIARY

MONTH 8

- MAMA'S MENTAL HEALTH
- NUTRITION
- BLOOD SUGAR MANAGEMENT
- AT THE DOCTOR'S OFFICE
- GINGER'S PREGNANCY DIARY

MONTH 9

- MAMA'S MENTAL HEALTH
- NUTRITION
- BLOOD SUGAR MANAGEMENT
- AT THE DOCTOR'S OFFICE
- GINGER'S PREGNANCY DIARY

DELIVERING YOUR BABY

- YOUR BIRTH PLAN
- NATURAL BIRTH
- C-SECTION
- INDUCTION
- POST-DELIVERY

BY NAT STRAND, M.D.,

Nat was diagnosed with type 1 diabetes at age 12, was the 2010 winner of The Amazing Race, and is a mother of two healthy, beautiful children!

There is perhaps nothing more emotional in life with type 1 diabetes for a woman than thinking about having a baby and managing her diabetes at the same time. If you are reading this right now, chances are you are pregnant or you are thinking about becoming pregnant.

Let me just take a guess at the thoughts that have been going through your mind:

"I wonder if I can have kids. Oh, I know I probably CAN have kids, but should I? I'm afraid to have kids. I am afraid I can't do what it takes to manage diabetes while I'm pregnant. I don't know what I need to to have a healthy pregnancy. Should I adopt? Should I consider a surrogate? Am I going to be OK? Is my baby going to be OK?"

The questions, doubts and fears go on and on. I know. I just had two babies in the past two years, after having had type 1 diabetes for over 25 years.

At first I didn't know if I could even have kids. I mean, I knew it was possible, for other people, but I knew my diabetes was not perfect. I had lots of highs. I traveled a lot. I went out to dinner. I had an erratic work schedule. I liked to exercise and go on adventures, which usually left me in some sort of blood sugar flux. I had been told to get my A1C as close to normal as possible prior to conception. That seemed impossible!

I have to credit my type 1 ladies here—it's only through conversations with other mamas in the same position that I worked up the courage to give it a go. I personally worked with Jenny Smith, co-author of this book, for both of my pregnancies. Being a type 1, a CDE, and a mama herself, she had endless support for every single micro-detail of diabetes management. And there so many micro-details to consider!

I honestly want to say, ladies, if I can do it, you can do it. It's amazing how great diabetes management can be when it's the 1st, 2nd, and 3rd priority in your life. During your pregnancy, blood sugar management is going to be the focus of your attention. You will be the best at managing your diabetes than you ever have been. You will amaze yourself with the lengths you'll go to all to protect the life growing inside you. You will feel like a diabetes super hero. And you will be right!

It's not easy. I think having a great diabetes care team is so important. For me, this was Dr. Anne Peters who graciously managed me from a distance, Dr. Karrie Francois, my high-risk OB who really didn't think that my diabetes placed me at high risk (bless her!), and Jenny Smith, my nutrition and blood glucose guru. Social support is also really important. When you are counting out blueberries and logging everything you put in your mouth while all you really want is to polish-off a gigantic rice krispie treat while lying on the couch; you are going to need girlfriends/family/spouses who understand. If you are lucky, you have someone nearby.

For the rest of us, we need to find books like this, online groups, Facebook groups, Instagram feeds—whatever it takes to find a voice that understands and says, "Keep up the work, you are doing great!".

I happily can say that with very hard (but realistic) work, my A1C was in the 5's for the only time in my life with both pregnancies. Not the entire time, but I got there, and for that I am beyond proud.

For me the prize has been two healthy babies. Both of my babies were born via planned C-section. My first had no complications at all. My second had mildly low blood sugars at birth, and was fine after her first meal.

I am so happy that Ginger and Jenny are putting this out there. They are two of the sweetest, smartest, and "super hero"-est mamas that I know. I hope their words motivate and guide you the way their friendships have motivated and guided me.

You can do this!

With love and respect to all the type 1 mamas and mamas-to-be,

～ NATALIE H. STRAND, MD

OH, UM...I'VE TOTALLY CHANGED MY MIND!

Within three weeks of dating Roger, I knew I had to tell him that I wasn't really sure if I wanted kids. In fact, I think I was much more clear on the subject: "I know this seems too soon to talk about, but I have to tell you now because I know you love kids..." I stammered, still wondering if this was going to be a deal-breaker for him. I'd actually been stressing about this topic since our first date, because I'd known Roger for several years prior to that date, and it was very clear that he adored his four nieces and would love to have children of his own.

But I continued: "You need to know that I don't think I want to have children. At least, I don't think I want to give birth to my own."

There, I said it.

I knew he loved kids. I knew he wanted kids. But, being 14 years older than I was, he'd also passed the typical age when a man might traditionally start his family. He was 40 and I was 26 when we started dating. So, maybe, this wouldn't be a deal-breaker after all?

(Honestly, I knew after two weeks that I wanted to marry him. It was an overwhelming feeling I'd never ever felt before that made me think, "Ohhhh! This is what everyone is talking about! I love this man! I am going to marry him." But I was smart enough to know I should probably wait a while before revealing that to him!)

Roger's response to my I-don't-want-any-babies-confession was simple.

"You're sure?" he asked.

"Yes, I'm sure," I answered.

"Okay, that's okay," he said.

But I knew he was disappointed—it was obvious. Over the next few months I realized that he really didn't actually believe me—or at least didn't want to believe me. Instead, he had convinced himself I'd change my mind some day. He later on admitted that he was also in denial over the fact that pregnancy and type 1 diabetes are not an easy combination.

I was diagnosed with type 1 diabetes at age 13, and diagnosed with celiac disease when I was 14 years old. Many years later, after nearly four years of increasing muscle spasms throughout my entire body and other variations of bizarre pain, I was diagnosed with fibromyalgia at the age of 29, just a few months before I began trying to get pregnant and thinking about writing this book.

If you had asked me when I was 18 years old if I wanted babies, I would've said, "No way. Absolutely not." I'd felt that way for as long as I could remember. I never saw other people's babies and thought, "I want one of my own!" Instead, I usually thought, "What a cutie...but not for me!" And I always dismissed that damn biological clock theory. I was sure that I didn't want kids.

Looking back, I realize now that I saw babies and pregnancy as a threat to my own well-being and health. I realize that I saw my diabetes as a threat to babies and pregnancy.

Looking back, I realize that my feelings around pregnancy were actually fueled by fear.

While I definitely don't live in fear on a daily basis, and certainly don't think about my fears around diabetes regularly—for they have never stopped me from pursuing other adventures, dreams, and challenges—those fears are still there, lurking in the back of my mind. And I would guess that may be true for many of the people I know with type 1 diabetes. No matter how diligent we are, how many marathons we run, powerlifting competitions we win, or promotions we get at work...no matter what our A1C is, there is still always that fearful little voice somewhere in there that's saying, "My body doesn't function properly."

I realize now that that subtle fear for my own lifelong health was so overwhelming that I didn't even allow myself to dream or imagine what life would be like as a mother, to have a baby, to raise a child, to make Roger a daddy.

I rationalized with myself that a woman with type 1 diabetes doesn't need or deserve to endure that stress of pregnancy or raising an infant while trying to maintain healthy blood sugar levels. At one point, I'm embarrassed to admit that I even thought maybe women with type 1 diabetes shouldn't put themselves or a baby through that kind of stress. Balancing blood sugars is hard enough, even without adding a growing fetus to the mix! Maintaining an A1C around 6.0 percent? Ah! I've never done that before, how would I possibly figure out how to do it with a flood of hormones and a growing fetus in my body?

And I told myself that my career was too important—a baby would get in the way. One afternoon, I even told Roger I wanted to get my tubes tied so I could ensure that I'd never become pregnant by accident. I honestly don't know what had gotten into me that week. I think it was more of a way to stubbornly say, "You cannot guilt-trip me into having a baby!"

But he had never guilt-tripped me. Not once.

He never begged. Or demanded. He never asked me to change my mind. Instead, he just left conversations open-ended, gently implying, "You know, it's okay to change your mind in a little while," or "It's okay if you don't want a baby, but we don't have to decide that right now."

But I didn't like that pressure of knowing he was hoping I might change my mind. It annoyed me. It made me feel tremendously guilty even if that wasn't his intention.

And every time he said, "It's okay if we don't have babies," I never believed he really meant it, because I've seen this man hanging out with my friends' children. Not only is he a natural with kids, it's just always so obvious that he just enjoys every second of it. Instead of sitting at the dining room table with a glass of wine, Roger will be in the living room playing with trains and cars with your kids, having pretend conversations on plastic telephones.

And then, for some reason—well, a variety of reasons, but I'll get into that in a moment—I suddenly found my brain thinking about babies.

BABIES.

The thoughts surprised me, because they were absolutely nothing I'd ever found myself thinking about before—at least not like this. These were thoughts of wanting and wondering what it would be like to have a baby. Wanting. While I'm not good at containing any of my own secrets, I actually didn't tell anyone about these babymaking thoughts, not even Roger, for several months, and the thoughts kept on coming. It was almost as though the thoughts had been working hard all these years to bash down that fearful wall...and they had finally gotten through.

I remember it was Father's Day of 2013, when Roger and I went out for dinner, just the two of us. Our waiter asked Roger if he was a father, and instead we were wishing the waiter a Happy Father's Day because he had several children at home. After the waiter left the table, I couldn't help myself, I said to Roger, "If I did want to have a child, I know you'd be an amazing father."

He smiled, thanked me, and said, "I'll be happy with you either way, my love," because as far as he knew, there was nothing in me that wanted to have a baby.

But this time his "I'll be happy either way" sentiment felt genuine—in a way that his statements in the past never did. He truly meant it: he'd be happy even if we didn't have children. The pressure was off. He wasn't waiting for me to change my mind anymore. There was just something about the expression on his face, the look in his eye, that I knew he really meant it. However, I did not go on to tell him that I had been overwhelmingly full of thoughts about making him a daddy, but I knew it was no longer being expected or demanded of me.

It was okay, whatever I decided. No guilt. My shoulders, my heart—whatever part of the body holds on to guilt—felt lighter after that evening.

And still, I kept my baby-wanting-thoughts to myself for a few more weeks as they became stronger and stronger.

But I still worried.

How would I work as much as I do now and raise a baby? How would I make sure I had plenty of time during the pregnancy to dedicate to every blood sugar reading, every meal, every insulin dose? Yes, there are mothers working full-time who do it all and endure pregnancy with type 1 diabetes successfully, but that doesn't look easy. I wanted to know I would be able to find the time and mental energy to give towards every morsel of food I ate, every insulin dose, every workout at the gym, every walk with my dogs, and get all the rest I'd need considering my newly diagnosed fibromyalgia.

And then, I'm not sure what changed...but I started to realize I could do it. I could handle the immense amount of extra work that a woman with type 1 diabetes is going to face during pregnancy, and everything that comes after. I was finding my rhythm and personal needs to keep my fibromyalgia symptoms at a dull roar. I realized I could do it...and I suddenly believed fully and completely in my ability to do it well.

Believe me, I was scared, too. But I kept reading the stories from other women's pregnancies with type 1 diabetes. I thought of the amazing women to whom I am so grateful because they shared their adventures in pregnancy with type 1 diabetes publicly in the diabetes online community: Jenny, Sarah, Alejandra, Kerri, Lindsay, Kim, Shannon, Amylia, Elizabeth, Cheryl, Sysy, Dalice, Christel, Brandy, Anna, Jen, Jess, Shannon, and Gina. And so many more.

And I thought, "They did it. I can do it."

I can do it. I can totally do this.

(At this point, by the way, Roger and I had bought a house together and had a wedding date approaching quickly on the calendar. Sure, you're supposed to get married first, but we couldn't not buy a house when interest rates were at 3.5 percent! C'mon!)

And so, one afternoon, after visiting my friend Laura's newborn baby, I confessed one of the only secrets of my own that I've ever managed to keep. We were driving home, and I said, "Lover, I've gotta tell you about something I've been thinking about a lot lately."

"Okay," he said. Knowing me well, I wouldn't have shocked Roger if I'd said I wanted to paint the house lime green, rescue 5 stray dogs, or start my own strawberry farm. The last thing he would've ever expected to come out of my mouth was what I actually said.

"Well…," I began. "For the past couple of months I've been thinking about babies a lot. And how I'd like to spend the next year preparing my diabetes and my body for pregnancy."

As you can see, I am never subtle. I say exactly what I mean.

Fortunately, his level of shock and surprise was contained enough that he did not drive right off the highway.

"Really?" he asked, in totally blissful shock. His eyebrows practically flew off the top of his head, his smile went from ear to ear, and the sparkle in the whites of his eyes was shimmering like somebody just plugged in the lights on a Christmas tree.

"Yup," I said blushing with a bright smile. "I've got major baby on the brain."

"Wow." He couldn't think of much more to say. While I know he would love me forever even if I didn't want to have a baby, I knew without a doubt that no news could've made him happier. Not a single thing I might ever say or do in our marriage would probably be as unexpected as this—and that's saying a lot, because I'm known for making big decisions quickly and he's learned to embrace this fact.

(The last surprise I'd planted on him was that we were adopting a third dog. He wasn't a big fan of the idea—in fact, he loathed the idea especially because it was more like I didn't really ask before falling irreversibly in love with the dog—and then Roger actually met little Petey Pete the next day and fell in love with him, too. And the surprise before that was when I adopted our second dog, Einstein. I told him about it over the phone while driving home from the shelter with this 10 year old mutt in the back of my car. Einstein quickly became his favorite dog, by the way. And don't worry, I finally have enough dogs, but it was about time I surprised him with something that wouldn't make him roll his eyes and groan at first. Instead this surprise went directly straight to happiness).

The next day, he said, "I'm still trying to process what you told me yesterday," he said.

For the next week, he'd just walk up to me several times a day with a giant smile on his face and nothing to say. Eventually he found words, and he'd say things like, "I can't believe you're going to do this" and "I know this is a really big decision for you."

Throughout the next few months, I would spontaneously announce things like, "I wanna have your baby!" with a goofy smile on my face, or "When we have a baby, we should keep his toys over here. And here." Or I'd point to various aspects of Roger's face, or his broad shoulders, and say, "If we have a boy, I hope he has shoulders like yours when he grows up."

(I also regularly hoped out loud that the baby would be born with Roger's ability to obey speed limits while driving and his remarkably patient temperament. These are both qualities I lack.)

Once, the cat was out of the bag, getting pregnant was all I could think about. (Unfortunately, I still had to wait for that damn wedding part to get over with!)

But my brain was also flooded with things like:

Ok, so I'm gonna have to eat more than my usual 50 to 75 grams of carbs a day when I'm pregnant...that'll be weird. I wonder if I'll feed the baby gluten when it's born even though I don't eat gluten? Since I won't be eating gluten throughout my entire pregnancy, does that mean the baby will be really sensitive to gluten when he/she eats it on their own? Maybe the baby shouldn't have gluten. If I don't give the baby gluten, he/she is gonna have to be the weird kid at friends' birthday parties. Maybe by then, more people will have stopped feeding their kids gluten. Or maybe I should feed him gluten every now and then unless told otherwise by a doctor. I really hope my baby doesn't ever develop type 1 diabetes. I really, really hope. No one else in my family has type 1 diabetes. But I don't wanna think about that right now. I don't think I want my baby to eat gluten.

Geez. Gah. Oy. Eeee!

8 months before our wedding, I decided I was going to start learning more about the blood sugar standards for a pregnant woman with type 1 diabetes. 6 months out from our wedding, I decided I was going to start managing my blood sugar like a pregnant woman with type 1 diabetes.

By the end of that 6 months, I wasn't afraid anymore.

I didn't just believe in my ability to manage my diabetes tightly during pregnancy, I knew I could do it. I'd shown myself that I could do it. Sure, I can't prepare myself for every challenge or hormone fluctuation of pregnancy, but I knew that no matter what came my way and how it impacted my blood sugars, I could handle it. I could feel safe and responsible while undertaking one of the most incredible things my body can do: create a little munchkin.

If you're reading this, and your mind is flooded with questions, concerns and worries, I want you to know that that is why we wrote this book. For you. Jenny and I not only understand those fears because we both live with type 1 diabetes, but we have felt that fear, felt the immense pressure of trying to maintain near-perfect blood sugars for the sake of a growing fetus, and we know that managing type 1 diabetes is exhausting enough all on its own. We've been there.

And we've learned as much as possible (well, I learned it all from Jenny) about our diabetic bodies so we can push aside the fears, and instead, embrace the challenges that come with type 1 diabetes and pregnancy.

You can do this. To support you on your journey, the pages in this book are filled with education, experience, and encouragement, because it won't be easy, but it will definitely be worth it.

As Jenny says, "Managing type 1 diabetes during pregnancy is a labor of love."

Never give up!

~ GINGER VIEIRA

YOUR DIABETES PREGNANCY COACH

(AND A TYPE 1 MAMA, TOO!)

I have always known I wanted to have children, or at least one child. I loved my baby dolls as a child, my first job was as a babysitter and I was really good at it, too! Many of the kids I watched asked for their parents to call me instead of their other sitters—that must mean I was meant to be a mom, right?

I also knew soon after my husband and I started dating that he would be an outstanding father. This actually says a lot considering we started dating when we were 17—yes, we were high-school sweethearts. The way I saw him interact with kids and the fact that he was (and still is) a big kid inside an adult body told me he'd be fantastic as a daddy some day. We've been together for a long time, and Nathan has only known me as a person with diabetes. I was diagnosed before high school at age 13, so when we met our freshman year in high school I had been living with type 1 for about 1.5 years already.

I knew there was something different and wonderful about Nathan as soon as we started dating too. He never expressed worry or looked uneasy when I tested my blood sugar in front of him and when we went to prom (which was before our first official date) he actually pinched the back of my arm so I could take my injection in the parking lot before we went into the restaurant to eat! Now that's a keeper in my book!

Babies were of course not on my mind as I went off to college and Nathan joined the Marine Corp, but I still knew I'd one day like a child of my own. We had a lot of adventures together before we got married—a long distance relationship, at times across the country from each other, but we made it to the same city eventually and that's when we decided it was time to talk marriage. Still, we had no plans for kids at this point although we knew we'd be ready at some point. We were young and just out of college when we got married and we had a lot we wanted to do yet before we really settled down the way we felt would be needed when kids were in the picture. We moved around the country and enjoyed learning about new cities, spaces and traffic patterns—Wisconsin, Colorado, Florida, Washington DC/Northern Virginia and finally back to Wisconsin.

During all of this moving, growing up and change, I was making changes to my diabetes management plan. I went from using multiple daily injections (MDI) to using an insulin pump. I started using a continuous glucose monitor (CGM) so I could track any fluctuation in my blood sugar—especially during my monthly cycle and exercise. Once we moved to Wisconsin, we decided it was time to add to our family. I had my A1C in a healthy range 5.7%, I was eating well and exercising and got my brain into "I'm going to have a baby" mode!

It felt a bit like I was watching someone else when I took the pregnancy test that gave a positive result. I couldn't believe it was a big ol' + on that stick that I peed on! Was it real? Nathan and I were excited to say the least and then I thought—"Oh my goodness, I really need to make sure I keep things in check now!" I was a bit starry-eyed in the weeks between finding the positive result and my first visit with our OB to check things out. I was more on top of clicking that little button on my CGM to follow my trends after meals, after exercise…I just didn't want to mess anything up.

Nathan and I went to the first visit with our OB together—a long visit where they do initial testing, look at an ultrasound to confirm the fetal age based on my last period, and with diabetes, discuss all the things I needed to do to ensure a successful pregnancy.

I debated sharing this next part of my initial experience with pregnancy because it can be frightening—we hear about all the issues that can happen in pregnancy with a pre-existing condition like type 1 diabetes. But, I included this because I want to share that it had nothing to do with diabetes:

At about 9 weeks of pregnancy I had a miscarriage—this happened about a week after my initial visit during which the pregnancy was confirmed. My high risk OB assured me that I couldn't have been any healthier or done anything differently. She noted, "The body knows when something isn't quite right—a spontaneous miscarriage is the body's way of saying it isn't the right time." While I understood this from a medical standpoint, I didn't get it from a personal point of view. I had done everything I was supposed to do: I kept my blood sugar in target pre-conception, ate good food, I took prenatal vitamins for one year before starting to try to conceive, exercised daily, etc.— what could be not right about the environment for a baby to grow!?

We were disappointed, sad, and at a loss. A loss is always hard, regardless of when it happens or why it happens...and with diabetes in the background it made me question my health again.

We waited about 5 months to start trying again—we needed time to make sure we could be fully happy about another positive result if and when it came.

We thankfully didn't have to wait long—our first try led to a positive result. We were so excited, but a bit cautious. We waited to tell family and friends until we were 14 weeks pregnant—by which time it was exciting to show ultrasound photos of a growing baby that actually looked like a baby!

We enjoyed the days of the pregnancy as we planned what we needed, arranged the baby's room, chose names and watched as I changed and grew. My sister-in-law had a "Mother's Blessing" gathering for me—a bit different than a baby shower. It focused on me becoming a Mother for the first time—a major change in life for a woman. She likened becoming a mother to that of a caterpillar becoming a butterfly. As I thought further about my walk through pregnancy with diabetes this description really made sense to me—all the changes and adjustments made it my pregnancy experience. I would never be a single, unattached female after our baby arrived. There would always be someone else to consider in all my daily decisions—even in my diabetes decisions.

Several days before our official due-date, we had our last ultrasound—the last in-utero view of our baby before meeting face-to-face. Another angle was thrown into the mix when our OB doctor said our baby was going to be big—like 10 lbs 8 oz big! Nathan and I looked at each other and thought, "Really? How is that possible?" Our baby had been measuring in the 75% for the whole pregnancy—the previous ultrasound in no way predicted that our baby would be large.

My blood sugars hadn't changed to allow for rapid growth of the baby in those last weeks. We were so confused. As our OB told us what this would mean for delivery, she very strongly encouraged us to have a C-section. She noted my smaller body size wasn't likely to successfully deliver a large child and would most likely end in C-section anyway.

We were disappointed to say the least. Crying in the consultation room as we scheduled our C-section birth, I again wondered, "What did I do wrong?" Our OB assured us there was nothing that I could have done differently—she said I was a star example of what a pregnancy with diabetes should look like. Really? Then how is it that we were to have a big baby after all I did to prevent it!?

My husband has a faith-filled attitude towards many things: "It happens as it was meant to happen." While he knew how much I wanted a natural childbirth, he also helped me to see that in the end we would have a healthy baby, and that was what we worked for from the start of the pregnancy. The birth-day happens as it will—whether it's via natural childbirth, induced labor, or C-section, the ultimate goal was to have a healthy child

We arrived at the hospital, got settled into the prep room where we met all those who would assist with the C-section delivery. I went through all the diabetes management strategies we wanted in place for the delivery—including my continued use of my pump and CGM during the delivery.

Our son, Oskar, arrived on December 20th, 2012—on the last day of fall, in the middle of a blizzard! Really—20 inches of snow fell from early morning through the night of the day he arrived. And interestingly, his weight was not a whopping 10 lbs! Instead, he was 8lb 10oz and had no issues with low blood sugars after delivery. No need for the NICU or supplemental feeding—thankfully he started nursing very well from the beginning...

So, then there were three...at last. A long journey. A labor of love. A love of myself to ensure a healthy child. We are blessed!

I wish there had been a resource that included all of the information through my pregnancy that I so painstakingly looked up, researched, noted and applied. The information is out there, but it isn't all in one definitive place. And most of what is available isn't actually catered specifically to type 1 diabetes, and it's usually written in very clinical language that doesn't make it easy for patients to understand and apply to real life with this disease.

As a Certified Diabetes Educator at Integrated Diabetes Services, I have the ability to work with clients from "pre-conception" through to "post-partum." My goal with each of my patients, and all of you reading, is to provide you with as much of the information as possible that you'll need for healthy diabetes management during pregnancy. You deserve and need that information. Yes, your pregnancy isn't going to be the same as the pregnancies you've watched your non-diabetic friends go through, but you do still deserve to enjoy your pregnancy, to glow, to be that cute lady in the grocery store with that cute little bump. It isn't all about your diabetes. It's also about becoming a mother and growing your family!

We truly hope that this book serves as an inspiring and informative tool and resource for every woman pursuing pregnancy with type 1 diabetes. We also hope it provides you with the support you need when communicating with your own healthcare team, and empowers you during each day of your pregnancy.

Wishing you strength and joy on your pregnancy journey!

~ JENNY SMITH

PREPARING FOR PREGNANCY

IT'S NEVER TOO EARLY!

Congratulations! If you're reading this book then you're at least considering taking on one of the most life-changing and awesome endeavors of your life: pregnancy...with type 1 diabetes. Thankfully this is something many women have already done before us—successfully and healthfully—but it is still a brave and courageous decision because it won't be easy and it will be challenging. But every moment of effort and hard work will definitely be worth it. We promise! (Our firstborn little ones, Oskar and Lucy, say, "See! Look at us! We're so adorable!")

Your responsibilities as a mother with type 1 diabetes actually begin long before you're officially pregnant. One of the first and most wonderful things you can do for the baby you haven't even yet conceived is spend at least 6 months preparing your diabetes (and your head) for pregnancy.

Certainly, with or without type 1 diabetes, not all pregnancies are planned, but even for those of you who learn you're pregnant unexpectedly will need to dive head-first into the same intense focus on your diabetes management as the women who try to plan their pregnancies far in advance. In the end, we're all in the same boat and type 1 diabetes is along for the ride.

As women with type 1 diabetes, we can absolutely experience healthy and successful pregnancies, but we inevitably have an extra workload on our shoulders and have to be much more diligent in certain aspects of our health than our non-diabetic friends, sisters, and mothers. This huge responsibility can feel overwhelming, but as Jenny will remind us all regularly, diabetes management during pregnancy is a "labor of love," and that hard work really needs to begin before you even start trying to become pregnant for the optimal health of everyone involved: mom and baby.

Depending on who you are and your current relationship with your diabetes, the concept of "preparing your diabetes for pregnancy" could translate as:

- building confidence in your ability to achieve lower blood sugar levels
- fine-tuning your insulin doses with tedious basal testing ('cause it's been awhile)
- re-learning the basics of diabetes management and truly applying them to your day
- continuing what you already do...but with "baby on the brain"
- searching for a new CDE or endocrinologist for the support you'll need
- finding new inspiration to make diabetes management a bigger part of your life
- overcoming habits around overeating, emotional eating, bingeing during lows, etc.
- eagerly learning as much as you can about your body and your insulin needs

Regardless, if planning for your pregnancy is a possibility, seize that opportunity because it will help you during those intensely rigorous 9 months of diabetes management.

DIABETES MANAGEMENT ACRONYMS

Here's a list of the diabetes management acronyms we'll use frequently throughout the book:

BG: blood sugar or blood glucose
A1C: glycated hemoglobin or hbA1C
EAG: estimated average glucose
MDI: multiple daily injections (via pen or syringe)
CGM: continuous glucose monitor
TDD: total daily dose (your entire daily insulin consumption)
ICR: insulin-to-carbohydrate ratio (the amount of carbohydrates you eat per 1 unit of insulin)
CF: correction factor (the number of points 1 unit of insulin reduces your blood sugar)
IOB: insulin-on-board (the amount of insulin currently working in your bloodstream)
MG/DL: milligrams per deciliter
MMOL/L: millimole per liter
OB-GYN: obstetrics and gynecology
CDE: certified diabetes educator
MFM: maternal fetal medicine (high-risk OB-GYN care)
RD: registered dietitian
NICU: neonatal intensive care unit

BEFORE WE GET ANY FURTHER, LET'S TACKLE THE BIG QUESTION THAT'S ON ALL OF OUR MINDS:
WHAT IS MY CHILD'S RISK OF DEVELOPING TYPE 1 DIABETES?

There are several factors and tests you can use to help determine if your child is at risk for developing type 1 diabetes. At the time this book was written there is no current treatment method to conclusively prevent the onset of type 1 diabetes in someone with a greater risk; however, there are many studies in progress that are proving successful in at least delaying the onset of the disease.

FIRST, THE BASIC FACTORS THAT CAN IMPACT YOUR CHILD'S RISK:

The Joslin Diabetes Center reported this study from the Harvard School of Public Health, by Dr. Warram, to determine a person's risk of developing type 1 diabetes:

If an immediate relative (parent, brother, sister, son or daughter) has type 1 diabetes, one's risk of developing type 1 diabetes is 10 to 20 times the risk of the general population; your risk can go from 1 in 100 to roughly 1 in 10 or possibly higher, depending on which family member has the diabetes and when they developed it.

If one child in a family has type 1 diabetes, their siblings have about a 1 in 10 risk of developing it by age 50.

The risk for a child of a parent with type 1 diabetes is lower if it is the mother—rather than the father—who has diabetes. "If the father has it, the risk is about 1 in 10 (10 percent) that his child will develop type 1 diabetes—the same as the risk to a sibling of an affected child," Dr. Warram says. On the other hand, if the mother has type 1 diabetes and is age 25 or younger when the child is born, the risk is reduced to 1 in 25, and if the mother is over age 25, the risk drops to 1 in 100—virtually the same as the average American.

If one of the parents developed type 1 diabetes before age 11, their child's risk of developing type 1 diabetes is somewhat higher than these figures, and it's lower if the parent was diagnosed after their 11th birthday.

About 1 in 7 people with type 1 have a condition known as type 2 polyglandular autoimmune syndrome. In addition to type 1 diabetes, these people have thyroid disease, malfunctioning adrenal glands and sometimes other immune disorders. For those with this syndrome, the child's risk of having the syndrome, including type 1 diabetes, is 1 in 2, according to the American Diabetes Association (ADA).

"Caucasians (whites) have a higher risk of type 1 diabetes than any other race," continues the report from the Joslin Diabetes Center. "Whether this is due to differences in environment or genes is unclear. Even among whites, most people who are susceptible do not develop diabetes. Therefore, scientists are studying what environmental factors may be at work. Genes influencing the function of the immune system are the most closely linked to type 1 diabetes susceptibility, regardless of race. One of those genes is HLA-DR. Most Caucasians with diabetes carry alleles (gene variants) 3 and/ or 4 of the HLA-DR gene. The HLA-DR7 allele plays a role in diabetes in blacks, while HLA-DR9 allele is important in diabetes among Japanese."

At the time this book was written, there was also some research—albeit inconclusive—based on the theory that gluten and cow's milk, both known for causing inflammation in anyone, can potentially trigger the onset of type 1 diabetes in a child. Inflammation is a known factor in the onset of autoimmune diseases so reducing the consumption of foods that are known to cause inflammation.

Some research has even demonstrated a link between gluten in the pregnant mother's diet and the incidence of type 1 diabetes in children. Simply put: gluten can trigger an "autoimmunogenic" response in the body, as if the body is under attack by a virus. While there hasn't been enough research to make any firm conclusions, it's worth taking into account.

For that reason, some people choose to keep their children gluten-free and/ or dairy-free for as long as possible. Some women choose to avoid gluten and cow's milk while nursing as well.

Children who are diagnosed with type 1 diabetes are also commonly found to have very low vitamin D levels, so supplementing a child (even as young as infant age) with liquid vitamin D drops is another precaution one can take. (Liquid drops are easy to find online and in health stores!)

And today, more and more research is finding a connection between the good bacteria (or microbiota) of the gut and type 1 diabetes. At this time, that research has pinpointed a connection, but whether that gut biome changed prior to the onset of the disease or as a direct result of having the disease is still a bit unclear. Regardless, giving a child with a higher risk of diabetes a probiotic is also a precaution one can take. (Infant probiotics are easy to find online and in health stores!)

While it is uncertain whether avoiding gluten or dairy and taking probiotics and vitamin D can actually prevent type 1 from ever occurring if someone has a genetic disposition to developing the disease, the theory is that it may at least delay the onset from occurring at an early age, like when your child is a toddler, compared to developing type 1 during adolescence or older.

GETTING YOUR CHILD'S RISK OF DIABETES TESTED

To get a much more "firm" idea of your child's impending risk of developing type 1 diabetes, you can have their blood tested for autoantibodies through TrialNet. TrialNet is an international network of researchers who are passionately dedicated to "exploring ways to prevent, delay, and reverse the progression of type 1 diabetes."

In a nutshell: autoantibodies are a protein that becomes present in the blood if the body is attacking its own tissues. An autoantibody count of 1 or 2 means your child does have a risk of developing type 1 diabetes but they may not develop it at all. An autoantibody of 3 or 4 or higher indicates that your child is very likely to develop the disease. This test can actually help predict if a person was going to develop type 1 diabetes even 10 years from when the test is taken.

HERE'S HOW TRIALNET SCREENING AND TESTING WORKS

First, visit the DiabetesTrialNet.org website to find the nearest location to you. If it's too far of a drive, call them to request the consent paperwork and testing kit be sent to you. Then you'll take that kit to the nearest medical facility that works with Quest Diagnostics, which you can find at QuestDiagnostics.com.

"Those who test positive [for autoantibodies] are eligible to enter the monitoring phase which includes a baseline monitoring visit at a TrialNet site to estimate the level of risk of developing T1D," explains the TrialNet website. "Participants are followed-up either annually or semiannually depending on their risk level."

"All participants will have repeat testing for autoantibodies and HbA1c; those with higher risk will be closely monitored with Oral Glucose Tolerance Tests (OGTT)," explains the TrialNet website. "Participants who initially receive annual monitoring will be followed with semi-annual monitoring if their risk level for developing T1D increases. Participants who develop diabetes may be invited to enroll in an early treatment study aimed at preservation of islet cell function."

You are under no obligation to continue having your child tested after the first test. If you want to have them tested every 5 years, you can do that, too! It is entirely up to you and your family.

To learn more, visit DiabetesTrialNet.org

JENNY & GINGER'S PERSONAL THOUGHTS ON SCREENING THEIR CHILDREN

GINGER: "I will always worry about my children developing type 1 diabetes. Always. Because I just know it's a possible reality, and it could happen at age 7, 14, or 29! My first child didn't eat gluten until she was 3 years old, simply because it was one thing I could easily do to minimize the risk of triggering an autoimmune response in her body when she was really young. My second child eats very little gluten, but more than her sister ever did at this age. And both drink almond milk rather than cow's milk, but both did drink dairy-based formula. At first, I hesitated on having them tested through TrialNet because it felt like, "Well, there's nothing we can do about it if the test says type 1 is developing!" But that's not true anymore -- there are studies that are delaying or altogether (so far) preventing the full development of type 1 in children whose tests come back with higher numbers of autoantibodies. That being said, if either of my children ever develop type 1 diabetes someday, I know we will face it together with courage and a deep breath."

JENNY: "It will always be something in the back of my mind. I have checked my son's blood sugar many times since he was born. Now that he is 3, he is curious and it is more of a numbers game when we check to see if he can say the numbers that pop up on the screen. But, it's also a learning tool since he is getting a general idea of what I am doing when I test my blood sugar. I chose to keep him off of gluten and dairy for about 2 years (I also nursed him for 2 years as new foods were introduced, since new research has shown the benefit of mother's breast milk is preventative for those who are at higher risk of autoimmune disorders)—and it is only occasionally now that he has something with gluten or cow's milk based dairy (we use goat's milk or sheep's milk based cheese and yogurt)."

In the end, the decision is completely yours!

And now...back to pregnancy!

ALL ABOUT YOUR A1C

Before we start talking about your A1C before and during pregnancy, let's make sure we're all on the same page when it comes to A1Cs in general.

The A1C test measures what percentage of your hemoglobin—a protein in red blood cells that carries oxygen—is coated with sugar (glycated). It is represented as a percentage that comes from a simple blood test, and it is a test you'll have done often during your pregnancy. Some practitioners may want to see your A1C results every 30 days, others may only require A1C test results every other month.

Regardless, your A1C tells the approximate range of your blood sugar control for the prior 3 months based on the amount of Advanced Glycogenated End-Products (AGEs) that have accumulated in your blood. AGEs are, in a nutshell, the result of excess glucose in your bloodstream.

The higher your blood sugar levels are, the more AGEs are present. AGEs are also responsible for the development of long-term diabetes complications such as retinopathy and neuropathy, because that accumulation will build and irritate crucial nerve-endings.

To help people with diabetes understand their A1C in real day-to-day terms, the medical world has developed the "eAG" measurement: Estimated Average Glucose. Your eAG will give your A1C reading in a blood sugar level of mg/dL or mmol/L just like you're used to seeing on your glucose meter.

The American Diabetes Association translates A1C percentages as the following eAG levels:

```
12.0% = 298 mg/dL (16.5 mmol/L)
11.5% = 283 mg/dL (15.7 mmol/L)
11.0% = 269 mg/dL (14.9 mmol/L)
10.5% = 255 mg/dL (14.1 mmol/L)
10.0% = 240 mg/dL (13.4 mmol/L)
 9.5% = 226 mg/dL (12.6 mmol/L)
 9.0% = 212 mg/dL (11.8 mmol/L)
 8.5% = 197 mg/dL (10.9 mmol/L)
 8.0% = 183 mg/dL (10.1 mmol/L)
 7.5% = 169 mg/dL (9.4 mmol/L)
 7.0% = 154 mg/dL (8.6 mmol/L)
 6.5% = 140 mg/dL (7.8 mmol/L
 6.0% = 126 mg/dL (7.0 mmol/L)
 5.5% = 111 mg/dL (6.1 mmol/L)
 5.0% = 97 mg/dL  (5.3 mmol/L)
```

During pregnancy with diabetes, an A1C lower than 6.5 percent is ideal for the healthy development of your baby, and your own long-term health. A person without diabetes has an A1C that is typically around 5.0 percent, with blood sugars running between 65 mg/dL to 130 mg/dL.

One issue to keep in mind that we'll discuss throughout the book is that a low A1C that is actually the result of repeated low blood sugars is not ideal. If achieving an A1C of 5.5 percent means that you're having multiple severe low blood sugars each day, then that is probably not an ideal A1C range for you. Yes, you could strive to determine what insulin imbalance is causing those severe lows, but the safest immediate action you should take is to aim for a slightly higher blood sugar range in order to keep you both safe from repeated low blood sugar events.

If achieving an A1C of 6.0 percent feels like a range you could maintain that feels sustainable and safe, then that would be a better choice than a lower A1C range that is causing you severe hypoglycemia, or a roller coaster of low to high on a regular basis.

For mothers who already have one or several children to care for while pregnant with their next child, severe low blood sugars are not only tedious and dangerous for the mom's safety, they are dangerous for the safety of the other children she's caring for too. On top of all that, low blood sugars are also exhausting. Recovering your energy after a severe low can sometimes take hours, and a busy mom doesn't have hours to spend lying on the couch waiting to feel better.

Think about your personal safety needs and what you can personally achieve that is best for you. Safety first. A1C goals second.

WHY & WHEN YOUR BLOOD SUGAR MATTERS MOST

There are two things you can definitely expect will be said to you by total strangers, friends, and several family members because you have diabetes:

"Doesn't that mean your baby will be huge?"

"So, is your baby probably going to get diabetes, too?"

Both questions are rather rude—sure—but both implications are also very far from accurate.

MAYBE: Persistent high blood sugars during pregnancy can lead to a larger baby—this is a simple truth. But people without diabetes can have very large babies, too. And people with diabetes have good ol' fashioned regularly sized babies, too. There is no way to assure the size of a baby at birth. Skinny women can have huge babies just like an overweight woman can give birth to a very small baby. Women who eat a lot during pregnancy can have small babies! In the end, you can manage your diabetes extremely tightly and still have a larger than average baby because blood sugar control is not the only thing that impacts the size of your baby at birth. And more importantly, a large birth-weight is not the only complication that can result from a mother's elevated blood sugar levels.

NO: Just because you have diabetes does not mean your baby will absolutely develop diabetes some day, too! There is no definitive research at present that shows you can do anything during pregnancy to prevent your baby from developing diabetes. So take a very deep breath, mama, because that is not something you can control, and your baby's risk of developing type 1 diabetes is actually only about 2 percent higher than the risk of a non-diabetic woman's baby developing type 1 diabetes. Feel free to share that little factoid with the many people who are going to ask you that question. We'll talk about those statistics more in a moment.

The simple truth is that our blood sugars will impact our baby's growth, development, and well-being (and your own well-being) in different ways at different times:

PRE-CONCEPTION: Your blood sugars prior to getting pregnant actually matter tremendously for a few reasons. First, persistently high blood sugar levels will impact your ability to conceive a child. Generally speaking, consistent A1C levels above 7.0 percent can decrease your fertility and increase the risk of very early miscarriage. Specifically, persistently high blood sugars could cause a miscarriage that actually seems like it's your period, just several days late, in that first month of waiting to find out if you're pregnant.

And the second reason that your A1C prior to getting pregnant is so important is that persistently high blood sugars—particularly during the 6 months prior to getting pregnant—can increase the risk of your baby developing a birth defect because your blood sugars impact how your body functions, too (eggs, ovulation, health of reproductive system). A healthy mama is going to increase the chances of a healthy baby. It's just that simple.

Ideally, we'd all maintain A1Cs as close to 6.0 percent (or lower) as possible prior to getting pregnant, but the general recommendation is anything below 7.0 percent will help to reduce those risks mentioned above. If you're able to get your A1C under 7.0 percent, then you could also try aiming to get below 6.5 percent.

1ST TRIMESTER: Once you're pregnant, you'll likely find the motivation to get your A1C closer to that 6.0 percent goal for the remainder of your pregnancy. Your A1C during the 1st trimester is just as important as your A1C during the 3rd trimester.

If a birth defect (in any baby with a diabetic mom or not) is going to occur, it will happen during the first 8 to 10 weeks of the embryo's life when the "body systems" are forming. Those body systems include: digestive system, endocrine system, respiratory system, reproductive system, circulatory system, skeletal system, lymphatic system, muscular system, urinary system, nervous system.

Once those systems are developed, the fetus is growing and essentially "learning" for 9 months in utero how to use all the body systems that have been established. Some systems include organs that mature over time, such as the lungs, but once they are formed in those first 8 to 10 weeks, the birth defects already exist.

Again, this means that blood sugar management during the months prior to conception and during that first trimester is vitally important for preventing the development of birth defects.

Remember, though, while aiming for that 6.0 A1C, that your goal is also to not experience frequent hypoglycemia. (Yes, you can smirk and laugh at the irony.) If you're experiencing severe low blood sugars every day, or even just multiple mild to moderate low blood sugars every day in your pursuit of a 6.0 A1C, talk to your healthcare team ASAP to help fine-tune how you're dosing your insulin. (And keep reading these prep chapters because we'll talk more about the finer details of achieving a 6.0 A1C in every section!)

2ND TRIMESTER: You know that cute little baby bump you'll find yourself impatiently waiting to appear around month 4 or 5 or 6? Well, obviously, that's your adorable little baby growing inside you! And what helps a baby grow more than normal? Sugar. As in...too much sugar in mama's bloodstream.

The higher your blood sugar levels are throughout your pregnancy, the more insulin your baby's pancreas is going to produce (pancreas starts producing insulin around 13-14 weeks gestation) in order to manage its own blood sugar levels. (It's painfully amusing to think about the fact that there will be a fully functioning pancreas, plenty of real insulin and a totally healthy immune system in your body that you have no access to!)

What does the baby do with all that extra sugar? Since insulin is an energy-storing hormone, excess levels of insulin from the mom's persistently elevated blood sugar levels means even your baby is going to be storing more body fat.

Now, having a high blood sugar here or there, or for a few hours once in awhile doesn't mean your baby is going to be huge, but high blood sugars and high A1C levels persistently throughout your pregnancy, particularly in the 2nd and 3rd trimester will likely result in a larger baby and can mean you'll likely need a cesarean section to safely birth your child. (For the record, both Jenny and I delivered our babies via C-section and the experience was just as overwhelmingly amazing!)

3RD TRIMESTER: There are two additional complications that can arise from persistent high blood sugars during the third trimester.

A) PRE-ECLAMPSIA: The first is your risk of developing pre-eclampsia. Pre-eclampsia is marked by high blood pressure, swelling in the face, and protein in the urine. (Swelling can and will normally occur in the hands and feet for most women by the end of the day in the 3rd trimester. The real tell-tale sign of pre-eclampsia is when it occurs in the face and lasts through the day. It is often accompanied by a headache.) The more severe the state of the pre-eclampsia, the more it can include dysfunction in the kidneys and your liver, disturbed vision, low blood platelet levels, low red blood cell levels, and fluid in the lungs that can cause shortness of breath.

Pre-eclampsia becomes eclampsia if or when a woman experiences a seizure—which can be life-threatening to both mom and baby. Women showing signs of pre-eclampsia will be closely monitored and sometimes hospitalized during the latter part of the pregnancy to prevent eclampsia from occurring.

Women with type 1 diabetes are at a higher risk of developing pre-eclampsia because of the added stress on our body systems due to elevated blood glucose levels. A study published in the medical journal, Diabetes Care, in November 2014 concluded that women with an A1C level higher than 6.0 percent during the 2nd and 3rd trimesters had a significantly higher risk of developing pre-eclampsia.

As a woman with type 1 diabetes, your OB-GYN team should and will ask you at every appointment during your pregnancy if you've noticed swelling in your face, hands and feet. Your blood pressure should and will be measured at every appointment. And kidney function and protein output in your urine should and will be measured prior to your pregnancy and at the start of your pregnancy in order to have something to compare to during the 3rd trimester when you're being closely watched for pre-eclampsia. Most women with type 1 diabetes will experience some protein output in their urine simply because our kidneys do have to work harder than non-diabetics', but your doctor will be looking for a drastic elevation in that output.

B) BABY'S BLOOD SUGAR AT BIRTH: The second reason your blood sugar levels matter during the 3rd trimester is because your baby's body will become accustomed to producing a certain amount of insulin to meet the amount of glucose in your bloodstream.

A healthy and "normal" blood sugar level for a newborn baby is anything above 45 mg/dL (2.5 mmol/L).

When a baby is born (in a mother whose blood sugar levels were persistently high during the last trimester, and especially if it is high through labor and delivery) the baby is quickly disconnected from that sugar supply when the umbilical cord is cut. However, the pancreas is still producing the same amount of insulin during the first few hours of life outside of the mom's body. This means that the baby's blood sugar levels will be low, possibly dangerously low, and they may need an IV of glucose immediately after birth to prevent having seizures from hypoglycemia.

You may have read or been told that all babies born to a mother with diabetes will be "whisked away" to have their blood sugar checked and given a bottle, but the reality is that all babies are "whisked away" eventually after being born for a few moments to be cleaned up. If you give birth vaginally, your baby can be immediately placed on your chest (where you can nurse immediately—this helps to prevent your baby from experiencing a low blood sugar. Eventually your baby will be taken to a table in the same room to be cleaned up and assessed.

If you give birth via C-section then your baby will first be cleaned up and assessed and then brought to you...but it's really a matter of minutes that you're waiting to meet your baby. (And often your partner is able to stand right next to them, and even hold their little hand!)

Unless your baby is showing obvious physical signs of hypoglycemia immediately after birth, your baby's blood sugar is not actually tested until approximately 1 hour later. Then 1 hour after that, and 1 hour after that. Each test is looking for a blood sugar above 45 mg/dL (2.5 mmol/L). If you plan to breastfeed, you will be able to start right after delivery to aid in helping your baby's blood sugars stabilize. If you do not plan to breastfeed, formula will be provided via bottle. If their blood sugar doesn't stabilize, then the baby may be started on an IV of glucose to bring their blood sugar up to normal.

Generally, a baby whose blood sugar levels were mildly low at birth will stabilize within a few hours of being born. This is common for women with type 1 diabetes, and it can clearly be treated, but you can help prevent it entirely with tight diabetes management throughout your entire pregnancy and especially during your 3rd trimester.

We will discuss labor and delivery and postpartum extensively in later chapters of this book!

CREATING YOUR DIABETES PREGNANCY TEAM

There's no one way you have to create your Diabetes Pregnancy Team, but no matter how you create it, it's something you want to think about as far ahead as possible.

CHOOSING AN OB-GYN: In most hospitals, there is a Maternal Fetal Medicine office specifically for women with "high-risk pregnancy." Type 1 diabetes absolutely qualifies you as "high-risk" merely because it is complicated even if everything goes smoothly, and this is likely the first place your primary care or endocrinologist will recommend you go for your OB-GYN care, but you do have options.

Perhaps you already have a great relationship with an OB-GYN who doesn't necessarily specialize in high-risk pregnancies? You and your current OB-GYN can schedule appointment with the Maternal Fetal Medicine office to assess how you're doing and support your OB-GYN's ongoing work with you. Regardless of whether or not you work primarily with the Maternal Fetal Medicine office, you will go there for two different ultrasounds during your pregnancy—this is one of the perks of being a "high-risk" pregnancy, you get extra time to see your baby!

Your OB-GYN will likely have you do some preliminary tests to get a baseline for things such as your kidney function (you'll collect your urine for 24 hours in a jug! Fun!), iron levels, etc. So it's good to give them a head's up that you're pursuing pregnancy before you're actually pregnant!

CHOOSING AN ENDOCRINOLOGIST OR CERTIFIED DIABETES EDUCATOR: Here's the thing, you don't have to work with an endocrinologist during your pregnancy, but you'd be really, really, really smart to make sure you have a CDE on your team who has a deep understanding of diabetes management during pregnancy. Don't assume every CDE has this knowledge and experience. Do your research!

DOULAS AND HOME-BIRTHS? Can a woman with type 1 diabetes have a homebirth? Technically, yes, anything is possible, but it is not the wisest or safest idea. No matter how well you "plan" your pregnancy, no matter how tough you are and intend to do an "all natural" birth, any mother will tell you: you have no control over how that birth will really go in the end.

Just one example of the millions of potential scenarios that could take place: that little bambino could get stuck halfway down the vaginal canal and you will need an emergency C-section. That's a complicated scenario enough on its own but when you add type 1 diabetes to that mix, blood sugar management, insulin dosing, keeping your blood sugar in a safe range...it's really complicated. The safest situation for both mama and baby is to have you in a hospital with everything from IVs to an operating room right around the corner.

In the end, if you opt to use a doula for laboring in the hospital, make sure your delivery team is ok with that plan. Ensure the hospital policy allows them to be in the room helping you through the labor and delivery. Do your research and find a doula who is experienced with higher risk pregnancy and delivery. A doula who is certified and doesn't feel they can give you the care you need will not even accept a "high-risk" pregnancy patient because they know all too well how essential that hospital room may be to the health and safety of everyone involved. It may take a lot of interviews to find the right person.

HOW GINGER CREATED HER DIABETES PREGNANCY TEAM: "I know I wasn't going to be working with the endocrinology office in my area—they weren't a good fit for me prior to pregnancy. I had been working with my primary care nurse practitioner, who is wonderful and always a pleasure to see (the first requirement I have for any of my healthcare team) and works on the maternity floor of the hospital in addition to her role as a primary care NP! I went to her for the sake of getting prescriptions, A1C tests, and general health care, so I continued to see her for my general diabetes management. When I became pregnant, I added Jenny to my team because I knew she had the rare combination background of being both a CDE and a woman with type 1 diabetes who had been through pregnancy and coached many other women through pregnancy! I met with Jenny regularly via Skype thru her position at IntegratedDiabetes.com, and she was always an email away between our Skype sessions!"

"During my first pregnancy, I chose to work with a small OB-GYN practice that did not specialize in diabetes, because I knew I had what I needed from Jenny. I feared that going to the high-risk Maternal Fetal Medicine office at the hospital meant they would try to micromanage my diabetes and insulin doses! I was wrong! Instead, the smaller office knew so little about type 1 diabetes that they constantly compared me to their gestational diabetes patients and treated me like I didn't know what I was doing even when my A1C was 5.1 percent! For my second pregnancy, I went to the Maternal Fetal Medicine office….and they have been wonderful! They know what educated diabetes management looks like and they haven't questioned me or my understanding of my diabetes once. They've been wonderful!"

HOW JENNY CREATED HER DIABETES PREGNANCY TEAM:
"I choose to work with my Maternal Fetal Medicine office for my management through pregnancy. My regular OB doesn't work with high risk clients and thus I was referred over to the MFM when I called to announce my positive pregnancy test. The team I worked with was comprised of two MFM doctors, both of whom had an outstanding background and experience with pregnancy with type 1 diabetes. Although I do have an Endocrinologist as well, and I met with him a few times through my pregnancy, most of my discussion was with my MFM team."

"I chose to work with the MFM clinic because I wanted the attention to detail that I knew they could provide. At my first visit, they took the time to ask about 'MY' diabetes management strategies and really listened to the goals for management I had right from the beginning. They offered suggestions for what I would expect to encounter as each trimester moved on and explained all the tests/results and upcoming appointments so I was comfortable."

"I felt that I also had a bit of a head start on my management based on what I do for a job. I did not seek an additional CDE to work with through my pregnancy—although Gary Scheiner (IntegratedDiabetes. com) offered to help me review my data as I needed for an extra set of eyes. If my general OB office would have worked with me, I would have asked to be switched to a MFM clinic. I have preference for any practitioner who lives with type 1, or has chosen to go the 'extra mile' to get the experience and education to understand what it means to take on a pregnancy with diabetes. I was absolutely happy with the care that I received from my MFM team. They listened to me (and my husband) through the whole pregnancy—even with the million questions I asked and the reasons I gave for why I did something or didn't do something. I would gladly go back to them for a future pregnancy."

DIGGING INTO THE DETAILS OF DIABETES MANAGEMENT

Okay, so now that you have a fuller understanding of just how and why your blood sugar levels before and during pregnancy are so important, you're still left with the ever so hefty task of managing type 1 diabetes day-in and day-out as "perfectly" as possible.

In the next 8 parts of this Preparing for Pregnancy chapter, we're going to cover the most important aspects of diabetes management—whether or not a person is actually pregnant. These 8 topics will give you crucial nuggets of knowledge that will hopefully have the greatest impact on your ability to reach your A1C and blood sugar goals throughout your entire pregnancy. While each month of your pregnancy will be discussed in other chapters, giving you information on what to expect in terms of blood sugar fluctuations and insulin dose adjustments, all of that information will rely heavily on your understanding of these first 8 parts of diabetes management.

For some of you, the information in some of these sections will feel like a review of diabetes management knowledge you've been putting into practice for many years. For others, this might be the first time you've heard these types of topics ever mentioned. If you've never learned much about how to assess and adjust your own insulin doses, we also recommend reading "Think Like a Pancreas" by Gary Scheiner, CDE and founder of Integrated Diabetes Services.

THESE 8 PARTS ARE:
1. Diabetes Technology: Know Your Options
2. Fine-Tuning Your Own Insulin Doses
3. New Standards for "High" and "Low" Blood Sugars
4. Preventing the Roller Coaster Ride
5. The Magically Amazing Pre-Bolus
6. Mostly "Clean" & Consistent Nutrition
7. Exercising with Diabetes
8. Supporting a Pregnant Woman with Type 1 Diabetes

Here goes nothing…and remember, in the words of type 1 mama, Kim Vlasnik: *you can do this.*

PREPARING FOR PREGNANCY
PART 1

DIABETES TECHNOLOGY: KNOW YOUR OPTIONS!

As women with type 1 diabetes in a year where even 8-year-olds have cell-phones, we are particularly fortunate because the technology we have today—albeit still far from the cure we really want—enables us to manage our diabetes in ways that were never even a possibility for pregnant women in the 1950's, 1960's, 1970s, '80s, and even in the '90s. And yet, somehow, those women persevered and became mothers with so little technology to help them come anywhere close to the non-diabetic blood sugar levels we can achieve today! We must tip our hats to them for their bravery, and thank our lucky stars we don't have to walk that same road.

Insulin pumps (with and without tubing) and continuous glucose monitors: These types of technology are certainly not required in order to experience a healthy and safe pregnancy, but if you aren't achieving the blood sugar levels and A1C levels you'd like to, and you haven't explored these forms of diabetes technology, we highly recommend them both!

CONTINUOUS GLUCOSE MONITORS

While insulin pumps have existed much longer than continuous glucose monitors, we're talking about CGMs first because we feel strongly that everyone should use an CGM for pregnancy. Using a pump during pregnancy is certainly incredibly helpful for most women, a CGM provides a level of information that is absolutely impossible to simulate with a glucose meter alone.

The best time to give a CGM a try is before you get pregnant, merely because the stress of learning a new diabetes management system on top of the stress of being pregnant is...well, a lot to take on at the same time.

HOW A CGM WORKS:

CGMs consist of a sensor, a transmitter, and a receiver. The sensor is inserted into the skin with a needle, but the needle is then immediately removed, leaving the sensor in a place that you can't actually feel (it is about the size of a toothbrush hair). The sensor stays in place with an adhesive tape. The transmitter is then clicked into place on top of the sensor, on the outside of the skin. The sensor receives blood sugar data from the interstitial fluid (where glucose is transported) and then the transmitter sends this blood sugar data to the receiver, which looks like a pager, or for some systems sends it via Bluetooth to an App on a smartphone/smart watch. You can set an alert so the system notifies you when your blood sugar is "high" and "low" and alarms are customizable. CGMs allow you

29

to see your blood sugar on the screen at all times, and the direction in which your glucose is headed. Most CGM sensors can be used for about 6 to 7 days before a new sensor will need to be applied.

THE BENEFITS OF USING A CGM:

Ask any type 1 diabetic who wears both a pump and a CGM, "Which device would you keep if you could only choose one?"

Many type 1s will answer the same way: "I would absolutely choose my CGM over my pump."

That's because CGMs offer so much more information than your ol' glucose meter. An insulin pump is another way to deliver insulin into your body, but the service of a CGM can't be matched with a glucose meter.

Even if you checked your blood sugar 14 times a day, you still wouldn't have the intense degree of information that a CGM gives you. A CGM doesn't just report your blood sugar in any given moment, it reports the direction your glucose is headed, it alerts you to potentially oncoming high values before you're even high...which means you can prevent the high or correct it sooner. This also helps you fine-tune your insulin doses for meals, because you can see how much your blood sugar is rising after eating which will help you determine if you need to wait longer between taking your insulin and eating your meal.

A CGM also warns you of potential drops in blood sugar before you're so low that you can't avoid shaking and sweating. This makes you safer in all situations but especially in pregnancy when you're trying to maintain blood sugar levels between 70 to 120 mg/dL (3.8 mmol/L to 6.6 mmol/L) all day long. You can go to sleep with a blood sugar of 90 mg/dL (5 mmol/L) and not worry about dropping low while you're sleeping without warning.

Applying a CGM is easy and takes less than 60 seconds once you get the hang of it. It only needs to be replaced every 7 to 14 days.

THE DOWNSIDE TO USING A CGM:

The only "downside" to using a CGM is that you have to wear a device in and on your skin, but the sensor itself isn't much thicker than a toothbrush hair. While sensors are approved for wear up to 7 days per sensor, most people can get at least 10 to 14 days out of one sensor before having to apply a new one. (Tip: just press "stop sensor" and "start sensor" to continue using it beyond 7 days if it is still giving you accurate blood sugar readings.)

Additionally, the first week you wear a CGM can be a little overwhelming because you'll be seeing the rising and falling of your blood sugar all day long rather than just the number on your meter when you happen to check. So keep in mind that those overwhelming feelings will pass very quickly—just take a deep breath, step back from the CGM, and give yourself time to get used to your new diabetes technology!

CURRENT CGM TECHNOLOGY

- **DEXCOM:** Without a doubt, Dexcom is the leader in CGM technology. Dexcom's CGM technology has been implemented into the Animas Vibe and Animas Ping insulin pumps, as well as Tandem's t:slim and t:flex insulin pumps.

- **MEDTRONIC ENLITE:** Medtronic's Enlite sensor has improved considerably over older models and just about meets the standards set by Dexcom. Today they are indeed practically equal in function and ability. Most people use the Enlite Sensor with the Medtronic insulin pump as a complete system (CGM data displays on the screen of the pump).

- **OUTSIDE OF THE USA:** The Abbott Navigator II and the Abbott Freestyle Libre are both CGMs available in many countries. While the Libre does not "alert" like other CGMs, it does provide the same frequent blood sugar data.

- **NO INSULIN PUMP?** Both leading CGM systems can be worn without using an insulin pump. If you choose Dexcom, it works independent of a pump. If you choose Medtronic's CGM system, you'll be using the Guardian Real Time CGM system.

GETTING A CGM

The very first step to get the ball rolling for a CGM is to call the DexCom or Medtronic. They will give you the paperwork to complete (including forms your prescribing physician will need to complete) and they will contact your insurance company to determine coverage and get all the paperwork shuffling.

Depending on the country you live in, getting coverage from your health insurance plan can be very easy or very tedious—but don't give up, CGMs are being considered more and more a necessary part of type 1 diabetes management. Regardless, your insurance company will likely make you jump through a variety of hoops, mainly to prove that you're testing blood sugar responsibly and regularly with your glucose meter.

Usually, insurance companies request three months worth of blood sugar results from your meter. You don't have to directly download these results from your meter, you can simply fill out a spreadsheet with three months' dates and four blood sugar results per day. Your insurance company is not going to require you to compare or match these results with your meter, they simply need to see that you are regularly checking your blood sugar. This paperwork, along with necessary paperwork that the CGM manufacturer (Dexcom or Medtronic) will send to your doctor, will go to your insurance company.

Be prepared that this process can take several months, so if you're planning your pregnancy, you'll want to begin the process of getting a CGM many months ahead of time, including at least a month if not several to get used to wearing it and using it as part of your diabetes management system.

* *For assistance with interpreting your CGM data, ask your healthcare team for a referral to a CDE. Many endocrinology offices have a CDE, dietician or nurse available for educational purposes. If you feel the information you've received from your current health practitioners is lacking and you need more in-depth guidance, consider working with Jenny or the other educators at Integrated Diabetes Services—available via Skype around the globe! Visit IntegratedDiabetes.com to learn more.*

INSULIN PUMPS

If you've never tried an insulin pump, the best time to give it a try is before you get pregnant, merely because the stress of learning a new diabetes management system on top of the stress of being pregnant is...well, a lot to take on at the same time. That being said, it can certainly be done if you learn that you're suddenly pregnant and want to consider using an insulin pump during pregnancy.

While there are certainly women who prefer multiple daily injections over insulin pumps, and it's absolutely possible to maintain superb blood sugar control with injections, most people tend to find pumping easier.

HOW INSULIN PUMPS WORK:

Insulin pumps only use rapid-acting insulin.

The pump drips out small amounts of insulin throughout the entire day just as your pancreas normally would, and you can program it to deliver insulin in very specific doses, such as 1.3 units or 2.7 units per hour.

This drip of insulin meets your basal (or "background") insulin needs. In addition, when you eat or correct a high blood sugar, the pump uses your insulin-to-carbohydrate ratios (ICR) and correction factors (CF) to deliver a bolus of insulin as well.

Most of today's insulin pumps look somewhat similar to a traditional pager, with a reservoir of insulin inside and thin tubing that delivers the insulin into your body through a port called a cannula. The small, flexible cannula is inserted every 3 to 4 days via a small needle. During pregnancy, the cannula may need to be changed every 2 days once insulin needs increase towards the end of the 2nd trimester and through the 3rd trimester.

Once inserted, the needle is removed and the cannula remains. This cannula is flexible and moves with your body, you shouldn't feel it as it delivers insulin, or if you lie on it in bed. The pump is worn 24 hours per day, but you can remove it temporarily for showers, intercourse, and swimming. Instead of a "peak" in the basal insulin from the long acting injection, the pump can be programed to give you more or less insulin throughout the day based on your body's needs—an option you do not have with long-acting basal insulin such as Lantus, Levemir, Toujeo and Tresiba.

HOW TUBELESS OR PATCH PUMPS WORK: These are similar to a tubed pump but the way you wear it is the biggest difference. The only tubeless pump currently on the market to give full pump control (basal and bolus) is made by Insulet: the Omnipod. This pump attaches to your skin with an adhesive and is about the length of the top two digits of your pointer finger and about the thickness of a finger as well. Each new pod is filled with insulin every 3 days just like the tubed pumps.

Unlike other pumps where you might get 3.5 or 4 days out of a reservoir, the Omnipod is programmed to expire and shut down after 3 days plus an 8 hour "grace period" in case you can't change your pod right away.

To program your pod and tell it when and how much insulin to deliver to your body, you carry an extra device with you (a PDM—personal diabetes manager) that looks like a thick cell phone.

Omnipod can be carefully fine-tuned, just like the tubed pump, which allows you to deliver the basal insulin in precise units (0.45, 1.25, etc.) based on your specific needs as well as dose for meals and to correct high blood sugar.

THE BENEFITS OF AN INSULIN PUMP:

- Improved control with less micromanagement: Statistics show that pump users have lower A1C's than those on injections. Highs and lows are less dramatic.
- Flexibility. Schedules for people differ day to day. With the ability to adjust rates to match body physiology as well as smart features that allow for adjustment based on the ups and downs of life, pumps can meet this need better.
- Precision in dosing. Injections allow a dose of 0.5 units (or ½ unit) at the smallest. An insulin pump allows for 0.025 unit adjustments.
- More options for delivery of insulin. Insulin absorption from one site and with one type of insulin can improve the body's response to insulin. Once you are pregnant you'll find that delivery of insulin needs to be adjusted to meet the changes that happen along the way. An insulin pump allows a user to deliver a bolus of insulin all at once (just like an injections), or over a specified amount of time (called an "extended bolus"). As digestion changes and insulin needs change through pregnancy, this can be a major benefit compared to injections (unless you are okay with micro-managing with multiple little injections through the day).

THE DOWNSIDE OF USING AN INSULIN PUMP:

There are two specific downsides to getting your insulin via a pump: cost and the increased risk of ketones when an infusion site is blocked/ kinked, if the pump fails (rare), or if the insulin goes bad, etc. The issue of increased cost is simple: insulin pumps require not only an upfront purchase of the pump itself but also the on-going expenses of the supplies that need to be changed out every 3 to 4 days. Compared to syringes or insulin pens, pump supplies are much more expensive, but most insurance companies today consider insulin pump technology a standard of care for people with type 1 diabetes so getting approval isn't usually difficult.

For the increased incidence of ketones, it's important to understand that this isn't necessarily DKA we're talking about but simply ketones from very sudden high blood sugars because insulin isn't able to get into the body properly through the infusion site.

For a person taking a long-acting insulin with multiple daily injections, there is always some long-acting insulin in the system, so ketones from having no insulin on board is nearly impossible. In those using insulin pumps, it can happen easily because the only insulin on board is what makes its way through that infusion site.

This can happen in any pump regardless of brand, and at any time. It's simply an aspect of pumping that one must deal with in order to enjoy the many benefits of using a pump. Having a pump emergency plan is key and it is something that should be discussed with your care team when you do decide to start using a pump. A back up plan would include how to return to use of long acting insulin and knowing what your dosing ratios are for calculating manual injections until a replacement pump can be sent to you. Most pump companies try very hard to express overnight ship a new/replacement pump so that you are not long without your pump.

CURRENT INSULIN PUMP TECHNOLOGY

Okay, so you've decided you're going to try pumping, but...how will you possibly choose from the half-dozen options out there today? Here's a breakdown of the current pump technology available (USA availability. Global availability differs from country to country).

- MEDTRONIC'S 530G: The Medtronic pump offers both a CGM (the Enlite) and insulin pump in one device, but with two different sites applied to your body (infusion site and sensor site). CGM data is seen on the pump's screen. This is the only device on the US market that currently has a low glucose suspend system that can be enabled. If glucose level goes lower than the set alert level and the user does not respond to the alert, the pump will suspend insulin delivery for a designated time until glucose rises above the low alert.

- MEDTRONIC'S 630G & 670G: The 630G has the simplest control algorithm, enabling it to suspend basal insulin delivery when the low blood sugar threshold is crossed, identical to the MiniMed 530G/Enlite. As a reminder, the 640G (available in Europe and countries outside of the USA) predictively suspends basal insulin delivery before a low blood sugar is reached. Medtronic's 670G is features additional programming that automatically increases basal rates when blood sugars are high, making it a "closed-loop" system. You still tell it when to bolus for meals and correction doses, but it adjusts your basal rates automatically based on incoming data every 5 minutes from your continuous glucose monitor.

- INSULET'S OMNIPOD: This is the only "patch" pump, or tubeless pump on the market. A CGM would function separately from this pump. Two sites - one for the pod and one for the CGM sensor.

- TANDEM'S T:SLIM G4 / T:FLEX G4: A traditional pump with tubing, the t:slim and t:flex have the sleekest appearance, looking more like an iPhone than a pump with touch screens. The t:slim G4 receives data from the G4 transmitter and displays it on the pump face instead of on a separate receiver.

   * Learn more about the pros and cons of each insulin pump at IntegratedDiabetes. com's Resources page on "Insulin Pump Comparisons."*

Each pump on the market delivers a continuous drip of insulin under the skin through a cannula as well as boluses of insulin for meals and corrections for high blood sugars. They all provide the same ability to "pump" insulin into your body. The differences between the pumps reside in the aesthetics as well as how each person's lifestyle dictates need for certain features that work a bit differently in each pump.

Some people decide on an insulin pump brand based on where they feel the company is going—upgrades, technology advancement, etc. Some patients want more of an all-in-one type of pump—one that has the CGM on the screen of the pump so they don't' have too many devices to carry around with them. Most people determine the pump they will use based on what they need it to do to improve their life. Having CGM data on the screen of the pump may limit choices, but since there are only a few on the market that provide this option, it can help narrow down your choices! All in all, they function to deliver insulin and offer flexibility that is ideal for pregnancy.

* *All pump manufacturers provide you with a qualified trainer to perform pump training sessions with patients. It may be preferable to work with a CDE who is certified as a trainer and understands the unique ins and outs of life with diabetes—including Jenny and other CDEs at IntegratedDiabetes.com—to learn how to use your pump and get your doses adjusted appropriately. No matter whom you work with, we highly recommend learning how to use your insulin pump or pod with the guidance of a qualified healthcare professional.*

NOTES

PREPARING FOR PREGNANCY
PART 2
FINE-TUNING YOUR OWN INSULIN DOSES

This section is overwhelming, merely because it's a lot of diabetes education packed into 25 pages. This section is the no-nonsense science of "diabetes math" for ensuring that your insulin doses are accurate before you even become pregnant. And then of course, you'll need this information in order to assess your insulin doses throughout your pregnancy, too.

So, if you've never done "basal testing" or never used an "insulin-to-carbohydrate ratio" before, here's a suggestion for approaching this in-depth material:

1. Just give it a skim the first time you read it.
2. Think about which part of your insulin doses need the most attention.
3. Focus on that part for a week or two.
4. When you're ready, focus on the next aspect of insulin doses that needs fine-tuning.
5. Take a deep breath! Do the best you can. This is the nuts and bolts of daily diabetes management, whether you're pregnant or not, and it's not something you learn overnight. It takes years of experience to feel truly comfortable with this knowledge. It's a non-stop learning process.

HERE WE GO...

No matter how perfectly you count your carbs and dose your insulin, your blood sugars won't stand a chance of staying within your target ranges if your insulin doses aren't accurate. Specifically, we're talking about your background/basal insulin doses, your insulin-to-carbohydrate ratio (ICR) insulin doses, and your correction factor (CF) insulin doses. The doses you were given during your last doctor's appointment three, six or nine months ago may need reassessment. Plan to test these even if your doctor already recommended adjustments.

If you've had the same basal rates set in your insulin pump for the past three years or the same dose of long-acting insulin, chances are that things need to be fine-tuned, because your insulin needs will change throughout your entire life. Stress, changes in diet, weight gain, weight loss, changes in exercise and activity levels, summertime, wintertime, summer camp, a new sport, the end of school for the year...the list goes on and on. These are all things that can change your basal rate or long-acting insulin needs drastically.

If you become more sensitive to insulin that means you'll actually need less of it on a daily basis. If you become less sensitive to insulin, you'll need more insulin on a daily basis. This applies to both your short-acting insulin doses or meal boluses, and your background insulin doses (both on MDI and on a pump).

WHAT MEDICATIONS ARE YOU TAKING?

Before we get to all the crucial insulin chatter, it's important to think about the entire list of medications and supplements you're taking before becoming pregnant. There are many medications and even natural herbs and supplements that are not safe to take during pregnancy.

NON−INSULIN DIABETES MEDICATIONS: The medications currently approved for use in pregnancy are Glucophage (metformin) and glyburide. Discuss your dosages of these medications with your doctor prior to getting pregnant or as soon as you are aware you are pregnant. All other non-insulin diabetes medications should be discussed with your doctor, because most are not approved for use during pregnancy.

All other non-insulin diabetes medications should not be taken during pregnancy. Discuss any medications and adjustments that will need to be made with your healthcare team prior to or as soon as you know you are pregnant.

OTHER MEDICATIONS: Even non-insulin diabetes injectable medications should be heavily researched and approved by your healthcare team before taking during pregnancy. Just because it's safe for you now does not mean it's safe for a growing fetus. (Even turmeric supplements or St. John's Wort, for example, are not safe for pregnancy despite being very safe for a non-pregnant diabetic woman.)

Did you recently stop taking your birth-control? Most hormonal birth-control medications tend to cause an increase in insulin needs, so when you stop taking them, you may find that your insulin doses need to be reduced as a result!

Make a thorough list of everything you take regularly and even the things you take as needed, such as medications for sleeping or pain relief or depression or other health conditions. Every single thing should go on that list.

Then you should do your own research on the internet for each of those products and their safety during pregnancy, and then confirm what you find with your healthcare team. We're suggesting you do your own research first because your healthcare team may not have an expertise on each and every supplement that exists! It's just about being extra careful.

INSULIN. INSULIN. INSULIN.

How do you know if your insulin doses need to be changed?

If your insulin doses are accurate, then you should be able to:

- ...consume no food or calorie/caffeine-containing beverages for 4 to 6 hours and still see fairly stable blood sugar levels. They really shouldn't drop or rise more than 30 mg/dl (1.6 mmol) if your background insulin dose is accurate, and this also means you're sitting stable at the blood sugar number you want: i.e. 70 to 120 mg/dL (3.8 to 6.6 mmol/L) during pregnancy. The one exception to this is in the morning between when you would normally eat breakfast and lunchtime, because skipping breakfast can often lead to a rise in blood sugar due to your body saying, "Hey, you didn't give me any fuel to break the fast! So...I'm going to dump a little glycogen from my liver, convert that to glucose, and use that as fuel! But p.s. you may need a little bolus of insulin to cover this potential rise."

- ...dose the exact amount of insulin you need for an exact amount of carbohydrates using your ICR and see your blood sugar within your target range within 2 to 3 hours of eating. Exceptions to this would of course be any high-fat, high-carb junk food meals, like Chinese food, pizza, ice cream, or a burger and fries. Even foods that are "healthy," such as a salad with lots of oil or veggies sautéed in butter/oil or large amounts of plant based fat at a meal can alter this as well.

- ...eat a balanced dinner, take the proper amount of insulin using your ICR, and wake up with your blood sugar in target range. It's often assumed that no amount of insulin can compensate for the dawn phenomenon (a part of the day between 3 to 8 a.m. in which your body begins producing more hormones that can cause your blood sugar to rise). Your background insulin doses should be adjusted to compensate for this time of day, preventing high blood sugars from occurring first thing in the morning.

- ...take a specific amount of insulin using your CF to lower a high blood sugar and see your blood sugar back in your target range within 3 to 4 hours.

These are just a few examples. The real point is that too often we are told things about diabetes management that imply you can't really keep your blood sugar in non-diabetic range in real life with diabetes. We're lead to believe it's impossible. But the truth is: with really diligent habits, proper insulin doses, and a lot of effort, it is absolutely possible to stay within your target range most of the time, helping you get your A1C in the 5s or low 6s, which is ideal and safest for both mom and baby.

Consider clearing your head of any old beliefs you have around what you can or cannot achieve in your blood sugar management, and take a closer look at what your body really needs.

First, let's take a look at what types of insulin and insulin-delivery options are available and *safe for pregnancy:*

INSULIN & INSULIN-DELIVERY OPTIONS DURING PREGNANCY

Insulin, just like other drugs, is given a drug classification for use in pregnancy. There are almost no drugs deemed 100% safe for pregnancy merely because it would be impossible to fully study all the possible risks a medication could have on a developing fetus. In pregnancy, the drug classifications that are optimal are categories "A" or "B."

BACKGROUND/BASAL INSULIN FOR PREGNANCY

The only basal-insulin brands that have been studied during pregnancy at the time this book was published are Levemir and the older intermediate acting insulin N or NPH (this is the cloudy insulin that needs to be taken two times/day). The other basal or long acting brands of insulin, Lantus, Toujeo and Tresiba, have not been studied on pregnant women, so they are rated an AU TGA pregnancy category B3, FDA pregnancy category C. Although their drug classification is not A or B, many women who have used these insulins long term prior to conception, have experienced completely successful and safe pregnancies on these unstudied insulins. For some women a change to a completely new insulin before or early on in pregnancy may cause more issue than sticking with the Lantus, Toujeo or Tresiba. Always discuss with your care team before making any changes.

NPH OR N: This type of insulin is referred to as intermediate acting. It has an action time of about 8 to 16 hours and needs to be dosed two times per day. There is a peak to its action between 4 and 8 hours, and timing of dose as well as regular intake of meals and snacks is important. This is not a preferred insulin for basal coverage in pregnancy since it does not provide much flexibility, but it is less expensive and may have benefit for times of day when insulin resistance is at its highest and a need for a peak in insulin may be necessary.

* *Some physicians have preference for intermediate acting insulin. If you are on a new basal insulin (as described below), advocate to stay on your current basal insulin even if they encourage a change to N or NPH.*

LEVEMIR: This basal insulin lasts in the body for up to 24 hours but it does tend to have a slight peak at about 6 to 8 hours, which means you are more likely to have a low blood sugar at that time. Some people might find their blood sugars drop at this 6 to 8 hour peak, especially those who have higher levels of insulin sensitivity. Levemir is generally taken twice per day, via syringe/pen. In pregnancy, the timing of the dose is very important and shouldn't be varied from day to day.

LANTUS: This basal insulin is said to last in the body 18 to 24 hours. It is said to have no peak but in those with higher levels of insulin sensitivity you may also see lower blood sugars approximately 4 to 8 hours after injecting. These lower blood sugars tend to be specific to the user and if noted, adjustment to timing and/or dose is needed. Lantus is generally taken once per day, via syringe/pen. Time of daily injection should be consistent and adjusted with assistance of your medical team if issues are noted.

TOUJEO: This new basal insulin is similar to Lantus (also made by Sanofi) but is said to cause fewer lows, doesn't burn upon injection, and stays in the body beyond 24 hours. If you'd like to try this insulin, it's best to try it long before you consider getting pregnant so you can determine its effect on you.

TRESIBA: This new basal insulin (made by Novo Nordisk) has a long action profile (up to 30 hours) and is able to be taken at any time of the day. It helps to take it at about the same time of day, but because its action profile can extend longer than 24 hours, the time of the daily dose can be a bit more flexible if you forget to take it at your usual time.

BASAGLAR: The newest of basal insulins (made by Lilly), this is also similar to Lantus—and it does burn upon injection. It stays in the body for about 24 hours, and like any of these basal insulins, some people love it, and some are reporting that they have to keep increasing their dose to get the same affect.

* *Some people experience drastically different reactions to one basal insulin option over the other. Your doctor may tell you they're the same, but if you feel as though you really have an easier time managing your blood sugars with one versus another, speak up, and demand to be on the insulin that you feel works best for you!*

RAPID-ACTING INSULIN FOR PREGNANCY

NOVOLOG, NOVORAPID, HUMALOG AND APIDRA: All of these are designed to begin working in the blood stream in as quickly as 15 minutes. They generally remain in your bloodstream for 3 to 5 hours. Some people prefer one or the other but the differences between them are fairly subtle and dosing amounts can be expected to be very close if not identical. These can be delivered either via syringe/pen, or used in insulin pumps and pods (explained below) and are taken multiple times per day for meals and correction doses.

DRUG CATEGORY:

APIDRA: AU TGA pregnancy category: B3, US FDA pregnancy category: C

NOVOLOG/NOVORAPID: FDA pregnancy category B

HUMALOG: AU TGA pregnancy category: A, US FDA pregnancy category: B

* *Short-acting insulin (R insulin) is not recommended for pregnancy because the time it takes for the insulin to begin working in the bloodstream is significantly longer than seen with the newer rapid-acting insulin. Short-acting insulin is less expensive and if needed, can be used, but the timing of doses and the components of a meal need to be more controlled to ensure optimal blood sugar control.*

To review how insulin pumps work with rapid-acting insulin please refer to Prep 1.

YOUR BACKGROUND INSULIN DOSE (BASAL)

The "basal rates" in your insulin pump or your "long-acting" insulin dose is also known as your "background insulin." Throughout your pregnancy, basal/background insulin doses will need to be changed constantly. Well, okay, maybe not constantly, but it will feel constant compared to how often we normally need to make adjustments in our background insulin. Some months you'll find you're making only one or two adjustments in your doses, but other months you'll be making adjustments once or twice in one week.

"Basal/Background insulin" is the insulin your body needs to function 24 hours a day, seven days a week, whether or not you ever even eat a meal! Even when you're exercising your body needs that background insulin! Your body always needs insulin.

Increasing or decreasing your total basal insulin dose, even by only two or three units, can have a tremendous impact on your blood sugar levels. It can be enough of a change to prevent those unwanted fluctuations, and it will make the balancing act much easier.

When your background insulin doses aren't in line with what your body really needs, you will be playing tug-of-war with your blood sugar all day long. Your background insulin dose is the foundation of your diabetes management, just like the foundation of a house: you can't build the first and second floors if you haven't built the foundation!

CHANGES IN YOUR LIFE = CHANGES IN YOUR INSULIN NEEDS

Here are 5 areas of your life that will have the biggest impact on your insulin needs:

1. **EXERCISE AND DAILY ACTIVITY LEVEL**

   Sure, exercise impacts your blood sugars during the activity and for several hours afterwards, but if you're adding exercise to your life, you're going to see an overall impact on your basal insulin needs! This is a good thing—but if you don't make gradual adjustments in your doses, you may find yourself frustrated with more frequent, unexpected low blood sugars.

2. **BODY WEIGHT**

   Weight-loss, even just a loss of 3 to 5 pounds, can mean you'll need less basal insulin. Weight-gain of even just 3 to 5 pounds can mean you'll need an increase in your basal insulin. Even just a change up or down of one unit can make all the difference in your blood sugar levels.

3. **NUTRITION HABITS**

   We often think that the only insulin we take for what we eat is our meal boluses, but if you make changes in your diet, you're going to see an impact on your overall insulin needs for meals, blood sugar levels and possibly your background insulin needs, too. It might only require a one-unit change in your total background insulin, or maybe several units.

4. **DAILY LEVEL OF STRESS**

   Just like persistent changes in your nutrition or activity level, a new regular stress in your life (something you encounter for many days in a row versus just one stressful afternoon) could mean you'll need a slight increase in your background insulin doses. Or perhaps you've removed a major stressor from your life? You may find you're experiencing more low blood sugars because of the reduction in stress hormones, and you need to decrease your insulin doses.

5. **AGE**

   Ahhh, it's just a fact of life: we all get older. Age also means our metabolism changes, we produce different levels of certain hormones, we can lose muscle mass if we don't do something to maintain it, etc. These are things that can affect your insulin needs. If you're getting older as in going from a teenager to an adult, you may find your insulin needs decrease because you're producing lower levels of growth hormone. If you're getting older as in going through menopause, you may find you need more insulin for a time followed by a decrease in need. (But don't forget: nothing helps to slow down the aging process on our bodies like regular exercise and good nutrition!)

AND OF COURSE, #6...PREGNANCY!

During pregnancy your background insulin doses are going to change because of constantly increasing hormone levels. There may be a brief period of pregnancy during which your pancreas may begin producing a bit of its own insulin again, and hormone levels shift—this happens in the first trimester and may mean you need to reduce insulin for a while. But eventually pregnancy brings an increase in hormones (progesterone for one), weight-gain, and a definite change in activity level, especially during the last trimester. This book will guide you through each trimester and help you anticipate decreases and increases in your background insulin needs.

IF THIS IS YOUR 2ND OR 3RD PREGNANCY: research has shown that a woman's insulin needs during one pregnancy do not necessarily dictate her needs for her next pregnancy. There can be a great deal of difference in insulin needs from one pregnancy to another!

If you're able to plan your pregnancy, that gives you a bit more flexibility and practice in terms of assessing and fine-tuning your current background insulin doses.

TWO METHODS TO ASSESS YOUR BASAL RATE INSULIN DOSES

1. **FASTED BASAL TESTING:** You may already be very familiar with the fasting method of testing your basal insulin needs. While it can provide great information, the very fact that this requires you to fast (i.e.: not eat) for at least five hours probably prevents many people from bothering to use this method of testing your basal rates in the first place. It's tedious and a bit inconvenient.

   While this is the recommended method from a doctor's perspective, if you are already pregnant, then this is not the method you should use merely for the fact that a pregnant woman shouldn't be fasting for any reason unless otherwise clearly directed by her OB-GYN. If you are in the First Trimester and really need to assess basal, try to basal test before you are at the 10 to 12 week mark.

   Whether or not you're pregnant, another concern with fasted testing is that when you don't eat your normal amount of calories, your body is naturally more sensitive to the insulin you take. Metabolic caloric needs will also show how much or how little basal insulin is needed. Someone who needs 1200 calories is going to require a person to need less basal insulin than a person on a diet of 2000 calories, but activity factor needs to be considered too.

Ideally, your basal rates should allow you to skip a meal during the day and have no more than a 30 mg/dL (1.6mmol) difference in blood sugar. Going all day without eating as a way to test your background insulin doses will give you an incorrect assessment of how much insulin your body needs (the liver will kick out glucose to compensate if fasting longer than 8 hours). For this reason, a fasting experiment will never last longer than 8 to 10 hours.

If you've never taken the time to perform a fasting basal insulin experiment, it is worth your time.

But this isn't your only option.

2. **OBSERVATIONAL BACKGROUND TESTING:** The word "observational" implies that you will continue your normal daily life and daily nutrition, while closely watching for the highs and lows in your blood sugar. This method requires you to pay close attention to your insulin-to-carbohydrate ratios as well, and your food choices.

If you miscount your carbohydrates or under-bolus for a meal, or eat foods that have longer lasting effect on blood sugar, it will impact your blood sugar levels in a severe or unpredictable manner (such as pizza and other high-carb/high-fat meals).

When choosing this method it's important to make careful choices around food so that you can trust the data you're seeing.

This method is really quite simple in that you are tracking your blood sugar for an extended period of time while also eating and taking your rapid-acting insulin for meals very carefully. After conducting several experiments or even just one very careful experience, you will either see blood sugars higher than normal, lower than normal, or right in your intended target. If your blood sugars are consistently higher than you'd like, while you're also counting your carbohydrates and bolusing accurately, you can conclude that you may need more background insulin.

* *This method assumes the I:Carb ratio is fairly close to accurate and carb counts are precise. If you are starting from scratch to assess all basal doses and bolus ratios, DO NOT use the observational method.*

BASAL RATE TESTING PROCEDURE

Depending on whether you wear a pump or MDI, your background insulin tests will be slightly different merely because someone using a pump of any kind can program different rates of insulin for specific times of day while someone using a long-acting insulin and MDI is going to have 1 or maybe 2 different doses they can adjust.

Regardless, the following are guidelines for your fasted background insulin tests:

* *REMINDER: fasted background insulin tests are to be used only if you are less than 12 weeks pregnant.*

1. All background insulin dose testing should be performed during a period of the day when you are not exercising (one of many things that would naturally drop your blood sugar and add an additional variable to your test). If you live an active lifestyle and have an active job then that level of activity is typical for you and your background insulin dose will naturally reflect that lifestyle, even if you aren't exercising during the test. (Balancing your blood sugar during different types of exercise is a whole different topic that we will discuss later!)

2. The time frame for a fasted test should never be longer than 8 hours (perhaps a bit longer for overnight basal tests). For fasted basal tests and observational tests, it is ideal to focus on a specific part of the day rather than the entire day at once merely because there are too many variables. The more variables you can control (i.e.: choosing foods you know the carb-counts of, etc.) the more you'll be able to pinpoint what type of adjustments you need in your basal insulin doses.

3. Especially when fasted, perform only one basal insulin test in a day. In other words, choose only one 8-hour window of time in which you will experiment. Normally, in a non-pregnant body, it can be ideal to wait about 2 to 3 days before performing another background insulin test or making additional changes, because it can take a few days to really see the full impact of any insulin dose changes you make. During your pregnancy, you're going to want to make those changes more quickly if you aren't seeing the numbers you want, because every day of high blood sugars is...well, another day of high blood sugars that your baby's body has to deal with. The more you practice while you are not pregnant, the more comfortable you'll feel making these changes when you are. In pregnancy we make adjustments after 2 days of what appears to be a trend (i.e. higher fasting blood sugar, higher between meal values, etc.).

4. When fasting for a test, it should begin 3 to 4 hours after your last meal. For example, if you ate lunch and bolused for that meal at noon, you will wait until 4 p.m. to begin an experiment. If you ate dinner at 6:30 p.m., you will wait until 10:30 p.m. to begin an experiment. This is because that bolus of insulin will still be in your system for up to 4 hours

after taking it. For those on an insulin pump, look at your active insulin time or DIA (duration of insulin action) that is set in the pump. Use this to evaluate when to start a basal test after a bolus.

5. For those on injections, adjustments in your background insulin dose will be a total of no more than 1 to 2 units at a time. For example, a Lantus insulin dose of 36 units would be increased to no more than 38 units or reduced to 34 units within one day based on the results of your test. For pumpers, remember to look at your total daily basal rate of insulin in your pump settings before making adjustments so you know how much you were taking, and therefore how much you altered the basal rates.

The important thing to note when making changes in your basal rate on a pump is that you are also still aiming to make an adjustment of approximately 1 to 3 units total at a time. It is easy to increase a basal rate from 0.8 units per hour to 1.0 unit per hour and feel as though it is a drastic change, but it might not actually add up to a significant increase in your total background dose.

For example, if I were experimenting with a window of time, from 1 p.m. to 6 p.m., and I began with a basal rate of 0.8 units per hour, what would it look like if I increased that rate to 1.2 units per hour? That may sound like a huge increase, but take a look at the numbers down below:

```
.8 units x 5 hours = 4 units (current basal rate)
1.0 units x 5 hours = 5 units (increase of only 1 unit)
1.2 units x 5 hours = 6 units (increase of 2 units)
```

So, while you're making specific changes to your basal rates, remember to pay attention to the big picture!

6. When fasting, do not take correction doses of insulin during the test. That extra dose of insulin becomes a new variable, making it impossible to truly study your basal insulin dose and assess how well that insulin is managing blood sugar on its own.

7. Be prepared for lows! Because you will be not eating for the duration of a test, you will of course run the risk of dropping low if you are getting too much basal insulin. Try to keep your choice of treatment for low blood sugars nearby! People often assume that they should and will go low if they don't eat regularly as people with type 1 diabetes, but if your basal insulin doses are accurate, you technically should be able to skip a meal and still see stable blood sugars!

BASAL RATE TESTING SCHEDULE

INJECTED BASAL/BACKGROUND INSULIN:

Typically this is tested only overnight, since most people are taking their dose of long acting basal insulin at or near bedtime. To perform this evaluation, do the following:

1. Eat a healthy dinner and take your insulin for the meal about 3 to 4 hours before you plan to go to bed. Avoid meals high in fat, restaurant food that isn't accurately counted and possibly meals that are out of the ordinary for you.

2. Take your long acting insulin at the normal time of night—do not adjust the time. If you take it with dinner, then take it at that same time. If you take it at 11 p.m., then take it at the normal time.

3. Test your blood sugar 3 to 4 hours after dinner. If blood sugar is between 80 mg/dL (4.4 mmol) and 250 mg/dL (13.9 mmol) go ahead and continue the test. Do not bolus for a high blood sugar unless it's above 250 mg/dL (13.9 mmol) and do not eat any extra food unless your blood sugar is less than 80 mg/dL (4.4 mmol). If your blood sugar is less than or greater than the noted values, eat or correct and do the test another night.

4. Check your blood sugar about 3 to 4 hours after you took the post dinner test and again when you wake up in the morning (fasting). If you have a continuous glucose monitor, you can skip the overnight finger-stick and use the trend on the CGM for reference to blood sugar trend. The middle of the night blood sugar check is very important to evaluate if your value is stable overnight, dropping and rising, or rising and dropping on its own.

HOW DO I INTERPRET THE RESULTS?

Success in a basal test happens when the blood sugar doesn't fluctuate up or down more than 30 mg/dL (1.7 mmol) from bedtime to fasting.

- For adjustment: if your blood sugar increases more than 30 mg/dL (1.7 mmol) increase your basal dose about 10%. If blood sugar decreases more than 30 mg/dL (1.7 mmol) decrease your basal dose about 10%.

- Test again if you have to adjust the dose of basal insulin to ensure the adjustment you made is appropriate.

- What about that overnight blood sugar? How does it play into adjustments? Do you know about the Somogyi Phenomenon? If you test your bedtime blood sugar and it is normal, and the next morning your blood sugar is high you might think this just means you need more basal insulin overnight. But, when testing your basal insulin you might find a low blood sugar in the middle of the night. This is commonly referred to as the Somogyi effect. Many people don't see the low blood sugar overnight, but they do see a high blood sugar upon rising in the morning—thinking this means they need more basal insulin, they add more to the bedtime dose and then have more pronounced low blood sugar overnight as well as higher blood sugars upon waking. This happens because the low blood sugar overnight can trigger a hormone response by the body that naturally raises blood sugar. If your test reveals a low blood sugar overnight, the best option is to decrease that basal dose at night and of course re-evaluate the overnight and fasting blood sugars to confirm.

BASAL RATE TESTING IN YOUR INSULIN PUMP:

Pump users should fine tune basal settings for the following periods of the day: overnight, morning, afternoon and evening.

To do a basal test in any time period, the bolus needs to be completely finished working to judge the true effectiveness of the basal and assess if an adjustment is needed.

To test each time period follow these guidelines:

HOW DO I INTERPRET THE RESULTS?

As each time period is tested and results are evaluated one important factor needs to be considered—time of the basal change. When changing basal insulin doses it's vital to understand that a change in basal insulin dose will not be "effective" in the bloodstream for about 1 to 2 hours after that adjustment is made. If you see a rise or fall in blood sugar starting at 3 a.m., then the basal adjustment needs to be made at 1 a.m. or 2 a.m. to avoid the rise or fall by 3 a.m.

It's also important to understand that a pump is trying to imitate what your own body would need physiologically. We typically see that people have one peak in insulin need through the day and one valley—essentially one point of the day where insulin needs and rate are going to be highest and one period where needs will be lowest. This can change a bit through pregnancy due to hormone shifts, but if you are testing before conception, then it's a good place to start when understanding basal settings and adjustment.

If blood sugar changes more than 30 mg/dL (1.7 mmol/L) during any portion of the basal testing time, then adjustment to the rate is needed.

You can start with basic adjustments by considering your current total daily insulin dose (reminder: TDD is basal/background dose plus the boluses you take through the day). Typically the less your blood sugar changes, the smaller the adjustment in basal rate is needed; the more the blood sugar changes, the larger the adjustment to basal rate is needed.

For example, if your TDD is about 20 units and your blood sugar rises or falls about 40 mg/dl (2.2 mmol/L), an adjustment to the basal dose in that time period of about 0.025 u/hr. up or down (or 0.05 if your pump doesn't allow for 0.025) would help to stabilize blood sugar. Likewise, for someone with a TDD of 50 units the same 40 mg/dL (2.2 mmol/L) change in blood sugar in the testing time period would require about 0.1 units/hr. in change to offset the blood sugar shift.

An estimate for adjustments shows that for every 10-unit increase in TDD above 20 units, the change in basal dose would go up about 0.025 for a blood sugar shift of 40 mg/dL (2.2 mmol/L). (A 20-unit per day TDD with a blood sugar shift of 40 mg/dL (2.2 mmol/L) would adjust basal rate up by 0.025 and a person with 30 units TDD needs would adjust their basal rate up by 0.05 for the same 40 mg/dL (2.2 mmol/L) rise in blood sugar).

OBVIOUS SIGNS THAT YOU NEED MORE BACKGROUND INSULIN

So all the guidelines in the world won't help you change your background insulin doses if you don't know what you're looking for and what the common red flags are that indicate your background insulin doses need fine-tuning.

- Remember, your background insulin dose is the foundation of your "house." If it's not accurate, the walls and the floors and the windows

TIME PERIOD	EAT AND BOLUS BY	TEST: BG	STOP TEST AND EAT/BOLUS
OVERNIGHT	7 PM	TEST BG AT 10 PM, 2 AM, 4 AM AND FASTING UPON WALKING	UPON WAKING OR IF BG IS AT >250 OR <80
MORNING	SKIP BREAKFAST	UPON WAKING AND EVERY 2HRS UNTIL LUNCH	TEST AND BOLUS FOR LUNCH. STOP TEST IF BG IS >250 OR <80
AFTERNOON	8 AM SKIP LUNCH	TEST BG AT 11 AM, 1 PM, 3 PM, AND 6 PM	TEST AND BOLUS FOR SNACK OR DINNER AT 6 PM. STOP TEST IF BG >250 OR <80
EVENING	1 PM SKIP DINNER	TEST BG AT 4 PM, 6 PM, 8 PM, 10PM	TEST AND BOLUS FOR A LATE DINNER OR SNACK BEFORE BEDTIME. STOP TEST IF BG >250 OR <80

are going to fall apart. The foundation has to be accurate in order for "everything else" to work successfully on top of it.

- "Everything Else" is considered your ICR, CF, exercise/stress/hormone adjustments, etc. You cannot expect your ICR to work well if the basal behind this isn't enough or is too much.

- If your A1C is higher than you'd like, or your blood sugars in general are running higher than you'd like (especially in a fasting state (overnight, or when a meal is skipped), you know that your body needs more insulin. It sounds so simple, and yet people with high A1Cs are often convinced they'll experience too many low blood sugars if they increase their insulin doses. The reality may actually be that they are constantly trying to correct high blood sugars and all those corrections are actually the cause of their lows, not their background insulin doses. By ensuring that the foundation of your insulin needs (your background insulin) is accurate you'll have much better luck managing your blood sugars after meals, around exercise, after correcting, etc.

- It's easy to underestimate how powerful an increase of only two or three units in background insulin can be.

- The same logic of course applies on the other end: if you experience low blood sugars on a regular basis that you can't explain, your body clearly needs less insulin.

  - It is important to evaluate when the lows are happening. Is it in a fasted state (no food or Insulin on board (IOB) from a bolus) or is it after a bolus, exercise, etc.

- If you take a correction dose of insulin for a high blood sugar, and 3 hours later your blood sugar hasn't budged and stays stable, but high, (and a high fat, high protein meal or high stress/illness isn't to blame), you may need more basal insulin. Basal test this time period without food or bolus, unless you are already pregnant.

- Lastly, if your blood sugar starts to rise specifically when it's been at least 4 hours since you last took a bolus, then your background insulin likely needs an increase. In other words: if your blood sugar is only maintaining itself because you've unknowingly gotten into a habit of taking more insulin for your meals and that insulin is actually acting as a cover for some of your background insulin needs as well...you need to increase your background doses and take a closer look at what you actually need for your meals now that your background doses are accurate.

YOUR INSULIN-TO-CARBOHYDRATE RATIOS

Your insulin-to-carbohydrate ratio (ICR) is the number of grams of carbohydrates that one unit of rapid-acting insulin can cover to transport the glucose out of the blood stream and into the body's cells.

But first...we need to make sure everyone reading this book has had a chance to learn about what carbohydrates are, why they matter so much to diabetes management, and how to count them:

Carbohydrates are the number one nutrient in food that is most easily converted into glucose ("sugar") in our bloodstream, and most easily raises our blood glucose (or blood sugar) levels.

THINGS TO KNOW ABOUT CARBOHYDRATES & TYPE 1 DIABETES:

- All forms carbohydrates, except for fiber, are broken-down and converted into sugar in our bloodstream, whether those carbohydrates came from Sour Patch Kids candy or whole grain pasta or your grandmother's freshly squeezed orange juice.

- Carbohydrates can be found in foods like: all grains (rice, quinoa, corn, flour), cereal, all fruits, some vegetables (vegetables like potatoes are high in carbohydrates, beans are medium, and green veggies like bell peppers and cucumbers are low), pasta, crackers, cookies, cereal, breads, muffins, cake, pizza, beer, cider, wine, juice, soda, popcorn, candy, etc. And in dairy products like yogurt, milk, cottage cheese, and ice cream.

- Dietary fiber is a part of some sources of carbohydrates that are not digested, and therefore not broken down into glucose. (That means, you don't have to count the grams of dietary fiber when adding up how many grams of carbohydrates are in your meal!)

- There are "simple" and "complex" carbohydrates. Simple implies that they are broken down quickly, raising your blood sugar more easily, and tend to offer less nutritional value. Complex carbohydrates have higher fiber quantities, which helps slow down the rate at which they are digested and the rate at which they raise your blood sugar. These carbs also tend to offer more vitamins, nutrients, etc.

- Using an app or website like CalorieKing.com or an app like MyFitnessPal can be a great first step to learning how many carbohydrates you are currently consuming in a day!

NOW, LET'S COUNT THE TOTAL CARBOHYDRATES OF A BOWL OF KELLOGG'S RAISIN BRAN WITH 2% MILK:

Some foods have nutrition labels printed clearly on them, while others might require you to research the nutrition information with an app or website.

What to look for on the nutrition label:

"Total Carbohydrates" are 45 grams in Raisin Bran cereal.

Beneath "Total Carbohydrates" you'll find "Dietary Fiber." Those 7 grams of dietary fiber are important to notice, because this is a form of carbohydrate your body does not even digest! Therefore, you can subtract 7 from 45, and that leaves you with 38 grams of carbohydrates.

FOR EXAMPLE: 45 total grams of carbohydrates - 7 grams of fiber = 38 grams of digestible carbohydrates that will impact your blood sugar. If you fill the bowl to the brim, with about 2 cups of cereal, that would give you a grand total of 76 grams of carbohydrates. *(And we're not even looking at just the sugar content in this supposedly "healthy" cereal!)*

Now, it's time to add 1 cup of 2% milk. There is no dietary fiber, so the "Total Carbohydrates" is listed as 12.5 grams.

Calculating the entire quantity of carbohydrates in your meal:
76 grams from cereal + 12.5 grams from the milk = 88.5 total grams of digestible carbohydrates.

Even if you only have the patience to measure you food for one week, you will improve your knowledge of how much you're consuming! While we often think we're good at "eyeballing" serving sizes, our eyes may not be as reliable as we think, and a little re-training couldn't hurt!

In pregnancy, measuring your carbohydrate servings carefully will inevitably help you more accurately assess how much insulin you need for that meal, which will inevitably help you stay in your blood sugar range goals more easily!

DETERMINING YOUR INSULIN-TO-CARBOHYDRATE RATIO:

An ICR is usually written like this:
- 1: X
- The "1" represents "1 unit of insulin."
- The "X" represents the amount of carbohydrates in grams that one unit of insulin can cover in your body at a given time.

- An ICR of "1:15" is commonly assigned to newly diagnosed children and adults. This means that one unit of insulin should be taken for every 15 grams of carbohydrates to be consumed.
- If this was my ratio, and I ate a container of yogurt with 23 grams of carbohydrates in it, I would divide 23 by 15 to tell me that I need 1.5 units of insulin with that yogurt to keep my blood sugar from going too high or too low during the hours after the meal.
  - 23 grams carbohydrates ÷ 15 (1:15 ICR) = 1.5 units of insulin

While some folks can get away with using one ICR for their entire day, more often than not, we need more than one. And we also need to change our ICR throughout our life as other parts of life change. When pregnant, you will definitely need to adjust your ICR often, so learning how to do this is crucial to managing your blood sugar.

However, how often do you find yourself high two hours after breakfast, and then still high by the end of the active insulin time 4 hours later, even though you counted your carbohydrates meticulously and took your insulin? How often do you plummet into hypoglycemia after your post-exercise meal and injection? As long as your basal insulin has been evaluated/adjusted and holds you stable in the time frame without a bolus, then, when you do bolus and your blood sugar stays high, it is a good time to test the ICR or CF.

The reality is that we don't need just one ICR; we usually need at least two, if not three, throughout the day. Often the morning or fasting ICR is lower (meaning you need more insulin to cover carbohydrates) and the afternoon and evening ratios are higher (which means you need less insulin to cover carbohydrates).

Your non-diabetic brother probably doesn't produce the same amount of insulin to cover the carbohydrates in his breakfast as he does for the carbohydrates in his lunch. You need more insulin at certain times of the day and less insulin at other times of the day, and there are very clear reasons as to why that happens.

Have you spent the past ___ number of years managing your diabetes without any insulin-to-carbohydrate ratio or perhaps you've been given that 1:15 ratio and you have been trying to use it for all meals through the day? Not only may you want to find a different healthcare team for your diabetes management, you may want to give an ICR a try!

Let's talk about a few methods to determine your ICR.

THE "500" RULE

The "500/85 Rule" is the most common method of determining your ICR. This methods should be tested for each meal time period of the day to ensure it is accurate for that meal. It is not uncommon to have an ICR that is different for each meal or one for breakfast and another for lunch and dinner.

If you currently have no knowledge of an approximate insulin-to-carbohydrate ratio for your body, then it's best to start with this "rule" or begin with 1:15. You do need a ratio in order to get started. But 1:15 is just a ratio you'll use as a starting point. There is more fine-tuning to do!

In the "500/85 Rule," you are asked to add up your TDD of insulin including your long-acting insulin dose and all of your bolus insulin doses at mealtimes. If you're using a pump, you're adding the total amount of insulin units given for your basal rates plus all of your meal boluses, and most pumps these days tally up that information for you on one screen (usually in bolus history).

Once you know your TDD, then you divide the number 500 by your TDD. For example, if your TDD is 95 units, you will divide 500 by 95 to get 5.26 units.

$$\frac{500}{95_{\text{TDD}}} = 5.26 \text{ UNITS}$$

Let's round this to 5 units.

So, for every single meal this rule suggests you use 1 unit of rapid-acting insulin to cover every 5 grams of carbohydrates. If your meal consisted of 25 grams of carbohydrates, you will divide 25 by 5 to get 5 units of insulin as your total meal dose.

Total grams of carbohydrates in meal ÷ grams of carbohydrates in ratio = total units of insulin for meal dose.

$$\frac{25 \text{ grams of carbohydrates}}{5 \text{ grams of carbohydrates in ratio (1:5)}} = 5 \text{ units of insulin for meal dose}$$

WHY DO I NEED MORE THAN ONE RATIO?

The beginning ratio may work very well for one or even 2 meals of the day. It will likely need some adjustments (increase or decrease) depending on several factors.

- Insulin resistance in the morning. Due to the increase in natural hormone production, resistance impacts both your ICR and basal/background insulin needs. The ICR in the morning is typically lower than it is for lunch and dinner—meaning you get more insulin to cover less carbs.

- Understand that while the ratio(s) works well once established, exercise and post-exercise meals require specific adjustments in the calculated bolus that uses this ratio because you are more sensitive to insulin at these times. This doesn't mean the ratio needs to be changed overall, it just means you need to learn how much to add or deduct from that calculated dose if you have been or plan to be active.

- Meals high in protein(over 25 to 30 grams) can contribute to changes in blood sugar as well, if not covered with insulin. (See "Other Factors" below.)

- Meals high in fat, over 20 grams, will blunt your insulin sensitivity, requiring more insulin to prevent high blood sugars well after the meal. (See "Other Factors" below.)

- Depending on your lifestyle and work, you may have much more active or more sedentary parts of each day and the meal bolus during that time of day should support that regular activity level.

If I were to apply the "500 rule" to my ICR and diabetes management right now, I would find an average TDD of 55 units of insulin, and the calculation would tell me I need 1 unit of insulin for every 9 grams of carbohydrate. Now, I can tell you, I would be low throughout the entire day if I applied that ICR to my body, constantly sipping juice boxes and snacks to bring it back up, and then I would gain weight from the extra calorie intake. If I only used 1:9 at breakfast, my natural hormone production would blunt the insulin's efficacy, sending my blood sugar sky high by 10:30 a.m.

While a small difference of 5 grams between two ratios may not seem like a big deal, the impact each ratio has on the amount of insulin you end up injecting at each meal is major, and truly important. It can be the difference between a plummeting low after a meal or a spiking high.

For example: a meal containing 35 grams of carbohydrates using a 1:15 ICR would tell me to take about 2.5 units. For the same meal, using a 1:9 ICR, would tell me to take about 4 units! That is an extra 1.5 units, and according to my Correction Factor, an extra 1.5 units would drop my blood sugar by almost another 150 mg/dL (8.3 mmol/L)!

It is the difference between watching my blood sugar shoot up to 250 mg/dL (13.8 mmol/L) and dropping quickly to 50 mg/dL (2.7 mmol/L). That crazy blood sugar rollercoaster leads to exhaustion, frustration, weight gain, and overall poor management. It's certainly no way to live. Establishing at least two different insulin-to-carbohydrate ratios for your day will save you a great deal of coaster-riding!

THE GLYCEMIC INDEX & YOUR MEAL BOLUS

Are all carbs created equal? For example, does 30 grams of carbohydrates from a serving of tortilla chips have the same effect as 30 grams of carbohydrates from a glass of prune juice or 30 grams from wild rice?

The answer is no. There are different kinds of carbs: some carbs are digested quickly, some slowly, and some are not digested at all! The rate at which the carbs are digested alters their effect on blood sugar. Carbs that are digested more slowly raise blood sugar over a longer period of time. This leads to less extreme after-meal blood glucose levels than carbs that are digested quickly. Slowly digested carbs also tend to contribute less to weight gain while leaving you feeling full longer.

WHAT IS THE GLYCEMIC INDEX?

To place a number on how quickly various foods are moved into the bloodstream after digestion, a measurement called the "glycemic index" (GI) is used. The GI of a food rates how much a person's blood sugar will increase over 2 hours compared to a reference, which is usually pure glucose. On the glycemic index scale, foods rank between 0 and 100 (pure glucose has a glycemic index of 100). Foods are labeled as low-GI when they have a GI value of less than 55.

LOOK AT THE NUTRITION FACTS

How can you find out the glycemic index for a particular food? It is rare to find a GI number specifically listed on a package, but you can come up with an idea based on the nutrition facts on the food label. Like we discussed early in this section, look again for the "total carbohydrates" content that is usually broken down into several subcategories: sugar, sugar alcohol, and fiber.

Your body processes sugars relatively quickly, so foods with high sugar content will tend to have a high GI. Sugar alcohols are fermented sugars that digest slowly and contribute little to the GI value. Finally, fiber has a GI of zero. The human body does not digest insoluble fiber, so it does not contribute to any change in blood sugar.

If a high percentage of the total carbohydrates in a food are from sugars, realize that the food has a high GI and will spike your blood sugar quickly. If the food contains a high percentage of fiber or sugar alcohol, the food probably has a low GI and will cause blood glucose to go up more slowly. (Warning: consuming foods with large quantities of sugar alcohols may also cause gastrointestinal discomfort and possibly lots of visits to the bathroom, so consume in moderation.)

TIMING YOUR MEAL BOLUS BASED ON THE GLYCEMIC INDEX

FOODS WITH LOW GI (BELOW 55) tend to produce a slow, gradual blood sugar rise. The blood sugar peak is usually modest and may take several hours to appear. Examples include whole grain pasta, whole fat yogurt, beans, chocolate. The same slow, gradual rise in your blood sugar occurs when eating meals or snacks over an extended period of time (like a Thanksgiving dinner!), when you have very large portions (typically meals more than 60 grams of carb) or when meals are exceptionally high in fat (pizza, Alfredo sauce, etc.). In these instances, bolusing before the meal tends to cause a low blood sugar after the meal followed by a rise in your blood sugar a few hours later as the bolus wears off and food starts to take its effect. Try to use a combination or dual-wave bolus with 25 to 35 percent of the bolus delivered immediately and the rest delivered gradually over 2 hours.

FOODS WITH MODERATE GI (BETWEEN 56 AND 69) digest a bit faster than low GI foods, resulting in a more modest blood sugar rise about 60 to 90 minutes after eating. Examples include Quick oats, brown rice and popcorn. Bolusing too soon before eating these types of foods could lead to a low blood sugar soon after eating. Try to bolus about 15 minutes prior to moderate GI foods.

FOODS WITH HIGH GI (GREATER THAN 70) tend to raise your blood sugar fastest, with a significant rise occurring about 30 to 40 minutes after the meal. Examples include bread, pretzels, crackers, potatoes, breakfast cereal, white rice and sugary candy like jellybeans. For these types of foods, you should bolus 20 to 30 minutes before taking your first bite of food. Doing so will allow the insulin peak to coincide with the rising of your blood sugar. Bolusing for high GI foods just before, during or after eating is not ideal as the food will raise your blood sugar long before the insulin kicks in—this usually causes a significant after spike in your blood sugar right after eating followed by a marked drop a bit later.

Here's a chart to simplify things:

BOLUS TIMING IN RELATION TO MEAL	HIGH GI (>70)	MODERATE ON (56–69)	LOW GL (<55)
BG ABOVE TARGET (>160)	35–45 MINUTES PRIOR	20–25 MINUTES PRIOR	Correct the high BG 20 min before the meal and start the meal bonus at the time of the meal
BG WITHIN TARGET (80 – 160)	20–30 MINUTES PRIOR	10–15 MINUTES PRIOR	15 minutes after meal starts (or use dual wave bolus)
BG BELOW TARGET (<80)	0–15 MINUTES PRIOR	5–10 MINUTES PRIOR	20–30 minutes after meal starts (or use square wave bolus over 1 hour)

These recommendations provide a place to start and it can be helpful to establish a list of foods you prefer, where they fall in the glycemic index scale and then how your blood sugar responds to the food and the type of bolus you deliver. It's great if you have, and can use, a CGM to follow the post meal/bolus trend—it will provide good information to show exactly when the rise in your blood sugar started after the first bite of food and when the bolus was delivered. An insulin pump can be very helpful for bolusing appropriately and allowing a bit of extended delivery based on what you are eating. Using technology to your advantage with foods that are common in your meals can help you navigate better when you are eating foods out of the norm.

6 SIMPLE GUIDELINES TO ASSESS THE GI IN A MEAL

Besides reading the nutrition label, here are 6 simple guidelines that can help you estimate the GI of one food compared to another.

1. The GI of fruits and vegetables will increase as they ripen. This includes ripening during storage, so the GI of a banana will increase even as it sits in your house. They don't develop more sugar, but as the fruit ripens, the sugars will begin to break down and your body will digest them faster (the fruit might also be a bit sweeter).

2. Consider food preparation. Factors such as cooking time can influence GI. For instance, soft cooked pasta has a higher GI than al

dente pasta, mashed potato has a higher GI than whole baked potato, and juice has a higher GI than the whole fruit itself. Consider that the softer the food preparation, the easier it is for your body to break food apart and send it into your bloodstream as glucose.

3. Foods that are processed and stripped of their nutritive value, like white rice, and foods made with white flour, are considered very high glycemic index and are more likely to cause quick spikes. Many gluten free food choices are made with highly processed alternative carb sources—white rice flour, potato flour, tapioca flour, etc.

4. Remember that low GI foods still contain carbs and need to be counted and covered with insulin to prevent a rise in your blood sugar.

5. Understand that just because a food is Low GI doesn't mean it's always healthy. Consider a 1 oz portion of Peanut M&Ms has a GI of 33 (low because it's less than 55, right?). But, is this a healthy snack to replace something like fruit? A medium pear also has a GI of 33.

6. Try not to use the GI as a gauge of how 'good' or 'bad' a food is. Just because a food has a medium or high GI doesn't mean you can't ever eat it. Learn how foods affect your blood glucose by checking your glucose after a meal and make your own assessment.

OTHER BOLUS FACTORS TO CONSIDER

So here's the other reason ICRs aren't always so simple: it's not just carbohydrates that impact our blood sugar and insulin needs during a meal! To keep us on our toes—because type 1 diabetes isn't challenging enough already—it's important to know that certain meals can really throw your blood sugar for a loop. If you don't consider a few factors, you might be left thinking that the ICR you tested isn't working well, and you might think you need to make adjustments.

Here are two factors in your meals to keep in mind when determining your meal-bolus dose. *We will discuss more in-depth factors around the timing of "pre-bolusing" your meal insulin doses in Prep 5.

- **HIGH-PROTEIN MEALS:** Approximately half of the grams of a "complete protein" over 20 grams will convert into glucose, which should be counted in the total carbohydrates. As you will read in Chapter 5, a complete protein contains all 20 amino-acids and is usually derived from an animal product.

EXAMPLE: If a 5-ounce chicken breast has about 35 grams of protein, there are 15 grams over 20. Therefore, 50% of 15 grams is 7 grams of added glucose to the total carbohydrates of that meal.

EXAMPLE: If a 12-ounce filet mignon has about 84 grams of protein, there are 64 grams of protein over 20. Therefore, 50% of 64 grams is 32 grams of added glucose to the total carbohydrates of that meal.

That is a significant number of extra glucose to account for when you're calculating your insulin dose. You can see, then, how not taking that protein quantity into account would impact your blood sugar in the hours following that meal. Typically higher protein meals will cause a slow gradual rise in blood sugar after the meal and keep blood sugar higher hours after a meal if the protein isn't accounted for.

Bolusing for this "extra" glucose is another experiment. If you want to give it a try, a "starting time" for a protein/glucose bolus is at the end of the meal or about 1 hour post meal. For those on insulin pumps, an extended bolus can be delivered to cover 2 to 3 hours which is the typical time that protein will rear its head. For those using injections, taking a bolus of insulin about an hour after eating can give a similar effect to cover protein's conversion to glucose.

- **HIGH-FAT MEALS:** When you consume a meal with more than approximately 20 grams of fat, this can blunt your sensitivity to insulin. Determining how much more insulin you will need is less exact, but a good starting point is to give 0.5 or ½ a unit of additional insulin for every 10 grams of fat over 20 grams.

EXAMPLE: 1 cup of Ben & Jerry's Cherry Garcia ice cream contains 52 grams of carbohydrates and 28 grams of fat. That is about 10 grams over 20 grams, therefore I would add ½ or 0.5 units of insulin to my insulin dose after calculating the dose for the 52 grams of carbohydrates.

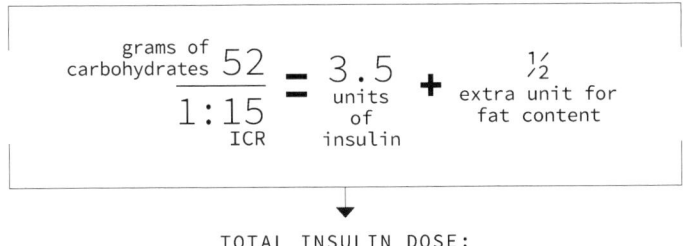

$$\frac{\substack{\text{grams of}\\\text{carbohydrates}}\; 52}{\underset{\text{ICR}}{1:15}} = \underset{\substack{\text{units}\\\text{of}\\\text{insulin}}}{3.5} + \underset{\substack{\text{extra unit for}\\\text{fat content}}}{^{1\!}/_{2}}$$

TOTAL INSULIN DOSE:
4.0 UNITS

The larger you are (height and weight), the older you are, and the more resistant you are to insulin will help you determine where to go from there. For instance, I know that I can add generally one full extra unit to any high-fat meal in order to help me prevent that high blood sugar spike two hours after my meal.

If I were less active, overweight, or older, I would probably need more than just one extra unit. If I were younger, active, and had a very lean body weight, I would probably need less than one unit.

The most important thing, though, whether you create an experiment around this or not, is to realize and remember that a high-fat meal can and probably will impact your blood sugar; therefore, if you want better control over your blood sugars, you can pay closer attention to this and adjust as needed.

As with protein, the bolus to cover fat is best taken after a meal since its impact is going to be about 2 to 3 hours after you finish the meal.

If you use an insulin pump, you can use the extended bolus feature which allows you to deliver that extra insulin over a 2 to 4 hour time frame. If you take injections, taking the extra bolus about 1 hour after you eat the meal can also be effective.

For very high fat meals—(think pizza, burger and fries or a thick cream sauce like Alfredo) an alternate strategy that is highly effective is to increase the basal rate for 6 to 8 hours. Basal insulin effect is decreased about 50% for the 8 to 10 hours following a very high fat meal. So if your basal is running at 0.50 normally, its effect will only be 0.25 if you've just had a high-fat meal. Increasing your basal by using the temp basal feature for several hours after the meal can offset the effect of fat and keep your blood sugar stable.

If you are on an insulin pump, try a 50% increase in basal by using your temp basal feature. Start this at the end of the meal and set it to run for 6 to 8 hours.

If you are using basal insulin via injection, you can adjust the basal dose of insulin if the meal is a dinner meal and your basal injection takes place at bedtime. Typically an increase of 2 to 3 units for high fat can cover the effect of fat, but because a basal insulin that is injected covers the 24 hours after injection, you might also find a bit lower blood sugar for the rest of that 24-hour time frame. This is not as effective as adjustment using an insulin pump.

NOTES

PREPARING FOR PREGNANCY
PART 3
STANDARDS FOR HIGH & LOW BLOOD SUGARS

There's been a longtime assumption that anyone with an A1C in the
5s or low 6s *must* be experiencing a tremendous number of low blood
sugars every day or every week, but the truth is that *that* is not an essential
ingredient to achieving an A1C at or *near* non-diabetic levels.

What it really comes down to is different goals, different standards for the
day, different ways of dosing insulin, of choosing what to eat, when to take
insulin and how much longer after that before eating...it's a variety of *habits*
that lead to an A1C in the 5s or low 6s. Those habits require a tremendous
amount of practice, discipline, and always being open to learning and
making adjustments.

If you are aiming for an A1C in the 5s and low 6s and you're constantly
experiencing low blood sugars then that is a sign that you're due for a little
help and fine-tuning on how you're approaching your diabetes management.
Frequent hypoglycemia is *not* an essential part of achieving a low A1C.

This entire book is designed to help you achieve a low A1C *without*
experiencing frequent hypoglycemia! It's all about blood sugar management,
fine-tuning your insulin doses, and learning as much as possible about
diabetes management during pregnancy and everyday regular life!

Okay, now that we've gotten that part out of the way, let's talk about the
A1C you're aiming for and the blood sugar goals you've set for yourself.

WHAT DO YOU CURRENTLY CONSIDER A "HIGH" BLOOD SUGAR?

```
  12% = 298 mg/dL (16.5 mmol/L)
11.5% = 283 mg/dL (15.7 mmol/L)
  11% = 269 mg/dL (14.9 mmol/L)
10.5% = 255 mg/dL (14.1 mmol/L)
  10% = 240 mg/dL (13.4 mmol/L)
 9.5% = 226 mg/dL (12.6 mmol/L)
   9% = 212 mg/dL (11.8 mmol/L)
 8.5% = 197 mg/dL (10.9 mmol/L)
   8% = 183 mg/dL (10.1 mmol/L)
 7.5% = 169 mg/dL (9.4 mmol/L)
   7% = 154 mg/dL (8.6 mmol/L)
 6.5% = 140 mg/dL (7.8 mmol/L
   6% = 126 mg/dL (7.0 mmol/L)
 5.5% = 111 mg/dL (6.1 mmol/L)
 5.0% = 97 mg/dL (5.3 mmol/L)
```

We're going to keep this straight-forward, cutting right to the chase: if you're trying to achieve an A1C of 6.0 but your blood sugar between meals and during most of the day is usually sitting around 150 mg/dL (8.3 mmol/L) or higher, you'll be as likely to reach an A1C of 6.0 as someone driving north when they're trying to get to Florida. It just doesn't make any sense. Your target blood sugar ranges and your A1C goals don't match.

What do you do when you see a blood sugar of 150 mg/dL (8.3 mmol/L) on your glucose meter two hours after eating? Do you take a correction dose of insulin or do you say, "Eh, that's fine"?

Take a look (again) at the following A1C translation chart from the American Diabetes Association explaining what the *average blood sugar level* and overall *range* is for each A1C result:

What is your A1C *right now?* If you're at 7.5 percent and you're extremely frustrated, ask yourself, "How often is my blood sugar sitting around 150 mg/dL (8.3 mmol/L)?"

Now, where do *you* want your A1C to be either prior to pregnancy or during?

Take a look at what your goal A1C translates to as an average blood sugar and blood sugar range.

For example, an A1C of 6.0 percent: That means your blood sugar is *rarely* over 150 mg/dL (8.3 mmol/L), and *very often* sitting around 120 mg/dL (6.6 mmol/L). That 30-point difference matters. If you've been telling yourself that a 150 mg/dL (8.3 mmol/L) isn't a big deal and isn't much different than a blood sugar of 120 mg/dL (6.6 mmol/L), then you now know exactly why your A1C hasn't budged from 7.5 percent.

Want to get your A1C in the 5s? That means you're aiming for non-diabetic blood sugar levels. It means you're spending the entire night near 90 mg/dL (5 mmol/L). You're waking up near 90 mg/dL (5 mmol/L). (Why consider the overnight? That 8 hour window of time that you are hanging out at a value, weights about 33% into what your A1C value is going to look like). An A1C in the 5s means you are pre-bolusing your insulin before meals so that your blood sugar does not rise too much past 130 to 140 mg/dL (7.2 to 7.7 mmol/L) for very long, or very often. It means when you correct a low blood sugar, you only consume enough carbs to bring yourself back up to 90 mg/dL (5 mmol/L) rather than 130 mg/dL (7.2 mmol/L). It means when you see a blood sugar level sitting steadily at 140 mg/dL (7.7 mmol/L), you take a tiny correction dose of insulin to bring it down to 90 mg/dL (5 mmol/L).

An A1C in the 5s means you're always *aiming* for non-diabetic blood sugar levels, *but* that doesn't necessarily mean that's where *you* should aim.

NON-DIABETIC BLOOD SUGARS?! *THAT'S CRAZY!*

We know, it sounds crazy! But here's the thing: you don't have to do it perfectly. (And frankly, you don't have to do it all—that's a personal decision that you're going to make for yourself. It can't be made for you!)

Instead of perfection, it's just the aim. The target.

Instead of telling yourself that it's impossible to manage your blood sugars that tightly, you're telling yourself that you *can* do the very best *that you can* do to achieve the tightest blood sugar levels that *you personally* can achieve for the sake of both your health and your baby.

You don't have to be perfect. You don't have to get your A1C in the 5s. It's okay if you never see your A1C in the 5s while you're pregnant—but the *intent* is what matters. The intent and the belief in your ability to do the best you can do is what's going to help you achieve blood sugar levels you've never thought you could achieve. Learning how to manage your diabetes is a non-stop, life-long learning process and if you believe in your ability to learn and improve, you could learn more about diabetes management during your pregnancy than you even realized there was to learn!

You just have to believe in your ability. Not the ability to be perfect, but the ability to improve, to achieve things you've possibly never achieved. That is all.

(And if you have a healthcare team that doesn't understand the aspect of "perfect blood sugars during pregnancy isn't possible" thing...you show them this chapter and you tell them what's up!)

And it's really about creating your own personal standards and goals.

YOUR PERSONAL GOALS

Above all else, you have to decide what is the right and safest goal for you. While we want to urge you to believe in your ability to manage your diabetes more tightly than you may have ever done prior to your pregnancy, it's also about finding your comfortable and *safe* zone.

WHAT IS THE RIGHT GOAL FOR YOU?

A target range of 70 to 130 mg/dL (3.8 to 7.2 mmol/L) for some who have lived with type 1 diabetes for 18 years and has been eagerly studying their diabetes in-depth for years may be a very different goal than for someone who was diagnosed with type 1 diabetes two years ago and is earlier in the lifelong learning process of diabetes management.

A target range of 70 to 130 mg/dL (3.8 to 7.2 mmol/L) for someone who has severe hypoglycemia *unawareness* (ie: doesn't feel the symptoms of low blood sugars) is not going to be as safe a target. This person may need to adjust their personal goals to 100 to 150 mg/dL (5.5 to 8.3 mmol/L). *That* decision may be what is safest and healthiest for both mom and baby. A fear of low blood sugars is a worthy fear. Low blood sugars are scary! Going to bed with a blood sugar at 80 mg/dL (4.4 mmol/L) can be nerve-wracking *if* you're not confident in your ability to wake up and treat your low, *and* if you're not confident that your overnight insulin doses are accurate. (And of course, nothing helps this situation more than having a CGM!)

We'll talk about high and low settings for your CGM technology in Prep 6, but we'd like to share how we personally decided on our own blood sugar goal ranges next.

GINGER & JENNY'S PERSONAL BLOOD SUGAR GOALS:

GINGER SAYS: "I set the high-alarm on my CGM to 140 mg/dL (7.7mmol/L) while I was preparing for pregnancy because I didn't want to burn out my energy on aiming for that 70 to 120 mg/dL (3.8 to 6.6 mmol/L) range before I'd even gotten pregnant!

Then, once pregnant, I set my high-alarm to 130 mg/dL (7.2 mmol/L) because even though I was aiming for 120 mg/dL (6.6 mmol/L) and below, I knew that I would over-correct with too much insulin if I was getting buzzed every time I was just sitting steadily at 122 mg/dL (6.6 mmol/L). Personally, I have a tendency to *over-correct* blood sugars and react too quickly when I cross over my high-alarm setting, taking more insulin before I know if I really need it. I know 120 mg/dL (6.6 mmol/L) is simply too much for me *mentally* to hear from my CGM that often! It leads me to making bad decisions rather than better decisions."

"As for lows," Ginger explains, "I have no problem going to bed with a blood sugar of 70 mg/dL (3.8 mmol/L) if I know I don't have a bunch of active insulin on board. Lows don't bother me. I've never had trouble treating a low or feeling a low, and I feel very safe going to bed at 70 or 80 (3.8 or 4.4 mmol/L), especially if I'm wearing my CGM."

JENNY SAYS: "I set my high-alarm on my CGM to 140 mg/dl (7.7mmol/L) while I was preparing for pregnancy. I also set a post meal bolus blood sugar reminder for 1 hour post bolus (on my pump) with the understanding that the 140 mg/dL (7.7 mmol/L) mark was where I wanted to be *below* at 1 hour post meal. CGM alarms are great, but if I tested my blood sugar at 1 hour after eating/bolusing it also gave me a good gauge for how well my CGM registered my post meal blood sugar rises."

"I also knew that once pregnant I might need to take some corrective action if my blood sugar was rising above that target goal. Testing at the 1 hour post meal mark also got me in the habit of testing earlier than I usually did after meals. Many OBs or High Risk Maternal Fetal Medicine doctors want to see the 1-hour (or sometimes 2-hour) post meal blood sugar as a marker for how much influence the blood sugar is having on fetal development. It was an early way for me to get ready."

"Once I was pregnant I set my high alert at 130 mg/dL (7.2 mmol/L)—again, a nice way for me to get an alert that my blood sugar was nearing that high mark—especially if it was around that 1 hour post meal mark and the trend on my CGM looked like it was still rising rather than flattening out."

"My low alert was set at 70 mg/dL (3.8 mmol/L) pre-pregnancy. I wanted to aim for maintaining my A1C without having blood sugars that were too low. Because I had my basal rates and my ratios tweaked pre-pregnancy I was comfortable going to bed with my blood sugar around 75 mg/dL (4.2 mmol/L) as long as I didn't have any IOB (insulin on-board) from a previous bolus and as long as I had accounted for heavier than normal exercise with a temp basal rate to prevent lows overnight. Once I was pregnant I set my low alert for 65 mg/dl (3.8 mmol/L). I sense low blood sugar well and since normal blood sugar in pregnancy is 60 to 120 mg/dL (3.3 to 6.7mmol/L) I wanted to continue to aim for that without getting low alerts while riding at 70 mg/dL (3.8 mmol/L) and sitting at my desk."

WHEN CONSIDERING YOUR OWN TARGETS BEFORE AND DURING PREGNANCY CONSIDER THE FOLLOWING:

- What do you think are going to be reasonable goals for you?
- What can you personally handle, both physically and emotionally?
- Prior to pregnancy?
- During pregnancy?

Remember: Don't just base your goals on what you've been able to achieve in the past. Nothing will inspire greater improvements in your diabetes management skills than a growing baby bump! You'll be surprised (and impressed) at what you're capable of achieving!

Meanwhile, be sure to anticipate a bit of frustration, too . . .

TALKING YOURSELF THROUGH THE FRUSTRATION

There will be many times during the next year that you're going to feel extremely fed-up, frustrated, and on the edge of throwing your glucose meter out the window. (Well, really, that's not all that different than a normal year with type 1 diabetes, eh?)

The frustration is going to happen. No matter how much you get frustrated when your blood sugars aren't cooperating during non-pregnant months, it's going to be twice as frustrating when you've got a bun in the oven. The emotional weight and pressure of trying to be the perfect diabetic so you can grow the perfect, healthy baby is immense. From start to finish. Even when your blood sugars *are* cooperating, you're going to feel that immense pressure and stress because we all know that they only cooperate for as long as you can get them to—and that whole "get them to" part is the result of a non-stop, remarkable effort on your part.

So, the point is: you've gotta learn how to talk yourself through the frustration when the number on the meter is not what you were hoping for—because giving up is *not* an option.

Here's the secret to surviving the frustration: reminding yourself *constantly* of a few very important facts.

FACTS TO FIGHT THE FRUSTRATION:

1. **YOU ARE NOT A FAILURE JUST BECAUSE YOUR BLOOD SUGAR IS TOO HIGH OR TOO LOW.**
   In fact, you're pretty amazing that you deal with this crazy, high-maintainance disease every day...especially during pregnancy!

2. **EVERY BLOOD SUGAR IS JUST INFORMATION.**
   That information is telling you that you got either too much insulin or not enough. A high after dinner? Not enough bolus insulin (perhaps the timing of the bolus with the food intake, etc.). A low after your walk? Too much insulin (or not enough carbs) prior to the exercise. A high that wouldn't correct itself after a whopping dose of insulin? Not enough basal insulin. A high an hour after eating? Not enough time between bolus insulin and eating. A low within an hour after eating after precisely taking your pre-bolus? Probably the frustrating case of a meal that is digesting really slowly due to high-fat content...too much time between meal and bolus insulin!

3. **THERE IS ALWAYS AN EXPLANATION— EVEN IF YOU HAVEN'T LEARNED IT YET.**
   As frustrating as diabetes is, it's not random. Our bodies are machines and every fluctuation is the result of another physiological process.

Some of those processes you may have already learned, but there are probably others you didn't even know existed! That's okay!

4. **YOU ARE ABSOLUTELY CAPABLE OF LEARNING THOSE EXPLANATIONS!**

Even if you don't know the scientific explanation for why your weight-lifting workout *raises* your blood sugar a hundred points, or why your spinning workout *doesn't* lower your blood sugar first thing in the morning on an empty stomach...you are still capable of pinpointing variables and creating your own understanding. The most freeing thing anyone can do as a person with diabetes wanting tighter blood sugar levels is embracing the idea that there is *always* more to learn about the physiology of our own bodies. With this mentality, you are never defeated. Instead, there are just challenges that you have to work your way through until you gain a deeper understanding on that particular issue!

5. **YOU ARE AMAZING!**

Every day throughout your pregnancy you are not only growing a human life inside you...you are working non-stop to "control" something that your body is supposed to be controlling perfectly on its own! It's *insane* to expect someone to do this perfectly day-in and day-out...and you are doing at the very same time as growing a human life in your body! The intensity and tremendous demand this is on one's energy, mentally and physically, can't be put into words. *Well, okay, it actually can be put into words:* **you're amazing!**

Deep breath. Pat yourself on the back (or go get a pedicure!). And keep going.

NOTES

PREPARING FOR PREGNANCY
PART 4

PREVENTING THE ROLLER COASTER RIDE

What's one of the worst rides at the diabetes park? The roller coaster. And during pregnancy it's crucial to avoid getting on that ride as much as possible. If roller coaster blood sugar levels are a regular occurrence for you in your non-pregnant life, that's definitely something you'll be thankful you addressed prior to pregnancy, or at least early in your pregnancy.

The over-treated low and the super-crazy highs are perhaps one of the most tedious, frustrating aspects of blood sugar management. Severe lows, followed by too much food, followed by super-highs, followed by too much insulin—it's just an exhausting mess. When you're working your tail off to manage your blood sugars tightly—for that cute little baby you haven't met yet—you don't want to needlessly increase your workload by accidentally putting yourself on a blood sugar roller coaster.

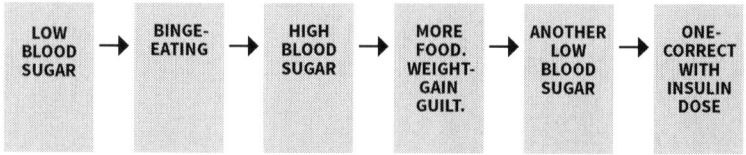

Those severe lows and super-highs aren't good for baby. They aren't good for you. The excessive consumption of calories every time you have a low blood sugar isn't ideal either. The whole ride is just *the opposite* of what we want when both our brains and our bodies are working so hard.

That's why it's *crucial* to establish good habits around how you treat and manage your low blood sugars *prior* to pregnancy, or at least, as soon as you learn that you're pregnant.

Can you prevent *all* the roller coaster rides? No—because on the days when your body is suddenly saying, "I need more insulin!" or "I need less insulin!" throughout your pregnancy, a roller coaster might be the exact indicator that it's time to make adjustments in your insulin doses. But there are *so many* things you can do to minimize those overwhelming days of swinging between super high and super low.

The very first step is simply acknowledging that *you* are in control and in charge of how you handle those highs and lows; to take a deep breath and remind yourself, "Okay, I really want to fix this low but I'm going to be thoughtful about it."

Let's dig into the details....

AH! FEED ME! MORE! MORE! EVERYTHING!

FACT: the human brain relies on a second-by-second delivery of glucose (sugar) in order to function properly, to think, to wonder, to know the difference between red and blue. This fact helps explain why, during a low blood sugar, we can feel as though no amount of food will ever possibly be enough.

Binge-eating during a low blood sugar is common—you're not the only one who's done it! It's easy to do because your brain keeps telling you: *"More. More. More. You might die if you don't eat more! More cake! More cereal! More candy!"* Until the symptoms or leftover icky feeling of low blood sugar is gone.

The low leads to overeating. Overeating leads to guilt and shame and frustration...and then a high blood sugar. The high blood sugar leads to more guilt, and then a massive over-bolus of insulin to help alleviate the guilt of over-treating the low. And then the glucose and excess calories from that high blood sugar will eventually be stored as body fat! Ugh.

Ay yi yi! It's brutal.

This is a roller coaster that *feels* impossible to avoid, but in the end, you do have a choice in how you treat your low blood sugars. Over-treating your lows is just a *habit* that you've given yourself permission to do over and over. It may feel like it's just your brain begging for food and you have no control over it, but somewhere in that process you're telling yourself, *"Go for it! Binge on everything and anything! You have permission!"*

You can change that habit. You can change the rules you've laid out for yourself. Before you become pregnant (ideally) it will be important to identify current habits that lead to over-treating the lows. You'll want to create simple guidelines for treating without overeating. Why? Because that roller coaster that doesn't feel good to you is even worse for your developing baby.

And like we mentioned earlier, this doesn't mean you'll never see a day of swinging highs and lows, but you control the simplest variable: how you treat your low blood sugars.

WHAT DOES THAT LOW BLOOD SUGAR BINGE COST YOU?

There's nothing like a good math presentation to really rub in the facts. Let's take a look at how many extra calories can be consumed from over-treating only one low blood sugar a week in these estimated examples:

AVERAGE LOW BLOOD SUGAR BINGE:

```
= 500 calories
```

ONE 500 CALORIE BINGE PER WEEK:

```
=  2,000 calories/month
= 24,000 calories/year
  24,000 divided by 3,500 calories it takes to lose or
         gain one pound
= 7 pound weight-gain per year from over-treating
    lows once a week
```

RECOMMENDED TREATMENT FOR LOWS

15 grams of carbohydrates = 60 calories. It's important to note that these are simple carbs *without* fat or protein. It's important to treat a low blood sugar with simple carbs to raise the level quickly (digestion is fast for simple carbs) and avoid excess calorie intake from other nutrients like fat and protein (which delay digestion and keep you feeling low longer).

Yes, you're going to gain weight during pregnancy, but if you find yourself continually binge-eating every time you have a low blood sugar, you're going to easily surpass the recommended 25 to 35-pound weight-gain parameters for pregnancy.

Why do you have to worry about your weight-gain during pregnancy? Why can't you just "enjoy the journey" and eat whatever your body craves? As people with diabetes, we need all the help we can get to keep our bodies as sensitive to insulin as possible.

The more weight you gain over that necessary 25 to 35-pound recommendation, the more complicated diabetes management will be, the more at risk your little bambino will be for other possible complications, the more at risk you will be for other complications, and the harder it will be to get back to your pre-baby weight after your baby is born. And *it's a lot easier to prevent excessive weight-gain during pregnancy than it is to lose that excessive weight-gain after the baby is born!*

CHOOSING TO TREAT LOWS DIFFERENTLY

You're probably not going to like this, but we're going to say it anyway because it's something we've both said to ourselves many, many times: you have control over what and how much you eat when you're low. Yes, your brain is begging for *everything* but your brain is also still thinking, "I really shouldn't eat *everything*..I just need a few grams of carbs."

For the past ___ years, you've been giving yourself permission to binge on food when you're low. You've decided it's okay. It's normal. It's allowed. It's reasonable. It's no big deal.

But that's just a habit. It's just something you're used to doing. Something you've decided is "okay" for the way you personally manage your diabetes. If you're sick and tired of riding the blood sugar roller coaster, then getting off that darn ride is as simple as deciding that binge-eating during a low blood sugar is *not* okay.

The truth is: unless you're so slow that you can't even say your own name out loud, you're not low enough to claim that you just have no control over what you eat.

Even when you're not pregnant, consider how the stress from your current habit of over-treating your low blood sugars truly impacts every different area of your life: relationships, career, energy, exercise, nutrition, etc.

It can ruin blood sugars for the next 24 hours if you really get stuck on that ride, and when you're pregnant, 24 hours of out-of-range blood sugars feels like 24 years.

The moment you decide to take responsibility for the amount of food you put in your mouth during a low is the same moment you decide to put these guidelines into action and take control of this part of your life. It is completely up to you. And the best part is that you'll actually *like* the results! You will *love* taking fewer rides on that horrible roller coaster!

ESTABLISHING GUIDELINES FOR TREATING LOWS

How would you *like* to behave during your low blood sugars? When sitting and thinking (with an in-range blood sugar), what do you envision as the best way for *you* to treat your lows?

HERE ARE A FEW OF GINGER AND JENNY'S PERSONAL GUIDELINES FOR TREATING LOWS:

1. LOWS ARE NOT OPPORTUNITIES TO EAT YUMMY TREATS.
Foods you love (like ice cream, donuts, etc.) will only be eaten when your blood sugar is in a safe range, when you can properly dose the accurate amount of insulin for the carbohydrates, and you can actually *enjoy* what you're eating. The foods you *love* will not be used to treat low blood sugars.

2. ALWAYS BE PREPARED FOR LOWS WITH THE FOODS MEANT FOR LOWS.
Whenever possible, try to keep sources of carbohydrates for low blood sugars nearby. These foods will be things you don't *mind* eating, but they will be foods that you don't necessarily love, either. If you have a low right before a meal, you will use these specific foods to treat your low rather than scarfing down your dinner, so you can enjoy your meal without overeating. If you need to *surround yourself with juice boxes* to feel more confident in your ability to treat your lows, go for it! Be as prepared as possible.

3. TAKE A DEEP BREATH, BE PATIENT.

Wait. Be patient and give your brain time to catch up with your blood sugar. A little mantra for you, while you wait, "I will not abuse my body with food during this low."

4. AIM FOR A NEW TARGET.

If your current goal after a low blood sugar is to get back up to 150 mg/dL (8.3 mmol/L), you'll find that during pregnancy your goal is to actually get back up to 100 mg/dL (5.6 mmol/L), so you're going to treat your lows with far fewer carbs than you have in the past. Once you start feeling more comfortable with your blood sugar hanging out around 85 mg/dL (4.7 mmol/L) all day, you'll find you only want to treat your lows with 5 to 8 grams of carbohydrates when you used to treat them with more than 20 grams.

5. IF YOU BINGE, ACCOUNT FOR IT.

Okay, sometimes overeating is *going* to happen. The best thing you can do if you know you're *going* to overeat is to take responsibility for it by paying attention to how many carbs you're eating beyond the necessary 15 gram mark, and cover those carbs with a carefully calculated insulin dose. That way you can at least *prevent* the super high that will follow that super-binge. Desperately need to eat a giant bowl of cereal, not even George Clooney could stop you? Okay. Fine. Just think about how much insulin you probably need to go along with that bowl of cereal so you can raise your blood sugar...but not raise it through the roof.

Nobody's perfect. Sometimes, over-treating lows happen...often because low blood sugars *feel awful* and the only thing we can do to help feel *safe* again is to eat carbs. Nobody's perfect. Think about what you can do to improve how you manage your low blood sugars and start there.

SUGGESTED FOODS FOR TREATING LOW BLOOD SUGARS

Did you know that *what* you choose to treat your low blood sugar can have a *huge* impact on just how long it takes for your blood sugar to come back up to a safe level?

Foods that are high in fat or protein are going to take *much longer* to be broken down and digested—which means they'll take much longer to raise your blood sugar! Not ideal when you're desperately trying to feel better so you don't binge on a bunch of other food.

Let's take a look at the best choices for treating lows.

- glucose gels
- glucose tabs
- smarties
- pixie sticks
- honey
- maple syrup

These sources are digested within 10 minutes because they contain dextrose or glucose—your body doesn't even have to break the glucose down into glucose...because it's already glucose! If you eat a piece of bread, your body has to first break that carbohydrate down into glucose before it can be absorbed into your bloodstream. Dextrose has a very similar "molecular structure" to glucose, so it's also very effective at raising your blood sugar quickly!

GOOD SOURCES OF CARBOHYDRATE:

- juice boxes
- soda
- dried apricots
- jelly beans
- gummy life savers

These sources can take at least 20 minutes to break down and get into your bloodstream. Jelly beans, for example, have a lot of additives and fillers, which your body has to break down first, so that will add to the time it takes for any glucose to get into your bloodstream.

LOUSY SOURCES OF CARBOHYDRATES:

- milk
- peanut butter sandwiches
- chocolate bars
- cookies
- ice cream
- spaghetti and meatballs

Loaded with fats and proteins, these sources of carbs are going to take well over 20 minutes to get into your bloodstream and help you feel better. They're also very high in calories that you don't need for the sake of raising your blood sugar.

BUT WHAT IF YOU CAN'T STAND GLUCOSE TABS OR PIXIE STICKS?

It's really okay if you don't use all the foods listed on the "best sources" for treating lows. At this point in your life with diabetes, even the mere thought of tasting another chalky glucose tab may make you nauseous.

But the point is to find sources of carbs that are at least "good" for treating lows (ie: low in fat and low in protein for fast absorption) and using those foods as though they are medicine, not a treat.

FINDING THE RIGHT CARB...FOR THE RIGHT SITUATION

Another tricky aspect of being prepared for lows is that some situations call for different types of food merely because of things like the *temperature of the space that food is kept in (summer or winter?),* the *size of the space that food is kept in (your purse or your desk?), and the quantity that food can be contained in (one fruit leather is only going to treat one low).*

HERE ARE A FEW IDEAS ABOUT WHAT AND WHERE YOU STORE YOUR FOODS FOR LOWS:

- Gummy Life Savers, for instance, are great for keeping in the car because they don't melt and they don't freeze! A bag of Gummy Life Savers can treat multiple lows, so you don't have to worry about restocking your supplies after each low. And 1 Life Saver is 3 grams of carbs, which means you can be very particular about how many grams you treat your low with. Sometimes 1 or 2 may be all you need to get back into your ideal range during pregnancy!

- Juice boxes in the car? Not such a good idea: because they will rot in hot weather and freeze in cold weather. They also aren't great for keeping in your purse because at some point someone is going to sit on your purse and that juice box is gonna be a big mess!

- Juice boxes are great for keeping next to the bed—but remember, if you're aiming for a blood sugar of 100 mg/dL (5.5 mmol/L), you may only need half of that juice box...which means you can save the other half for another low! So sip carefully!

- Bananas? Bananas are *impossible* to measure because they're all different sizes, and most lows do not need a whole banana so you're left with another half of a banana that requires severe willpower not to snarf down in one chomp. Not to mention that the ripeness of a banana actually changes how quickly the sugar in it is digested! Green bananas taste nasty because they aren't ripe enough to have quick digestible sugar, compared to an overly ripe banana which is super sweet.

- Pixie sticks are a good example of something that can be stuffed into a sports bra if you're walking and don't have pockets. Small. Discrete. And *fast.*

- Sliced mangoes? As delicious as these are, they come in a million different shapes and sizes, so it's very hard to know exactly how much carbs you're really consuming. You might find a way to ensure that you only consume one slice for a mild low, but if you're someone who wants a specific carb-measurement to help keep you in-line during a low, mango slices are probably not ideal.

- Raisins and dried cranberries can be useful, especially when you're treating a low on a full stomach after eating a meal! Merely 5 to 10 raisins or cranberries is all it takes, quick to chew. Done. Just beware of the serving size, because these compact sources of sugar can be easily over-consumed and thus over-treat your low.

Think about the foods you would like to think of as *medicine*, and what, where, and when you're going to use those for treating low blood sugars.

Now, while learning new habits for treating low blood sugars will *definitely* prevent many of those super-high blood sugars—and thus, the mega-dose of correction insulin—it's still worth taking a look at this other part of the coaster, too.

WHAT ABOUT HIGH BLOOD SUGARS?

Have you ever "rage-bolused"? This amusing term was created to describe when a person gets so mad that their blood sugar is super high that they take a huge amount of insulin to bring it down despite knowing that that's probably way too *much insulin*.

And of course, the rage-bolus can lead to any of the following:

1. You end up really low again, followed by binge-eating, and then *you're high again.* Rinse and repeat. Bleh.
2. As your blood sugar starts dropping, you start to think rationally: "I took way too much insulin!" so you eat, eat, eat in order to prevent going low again. Then you end up high. Rinse and repeat.
3. And of course, *occasionally*, it's possible your rage-bolus works perfectly because of other circumstantial factors affecting your sensitivity to insulin. During pregnancy it *might* happen especially during high-fat meals and during the last trimester when you are especially insulin resistant.

If you think you want that super-high blood sugar *down right now* when you're *not* pregnant, get ready, because that desperate, impatient, guilt-ridden feeling is only going to skyrocket when there's a bun in your oven!

The very first thing you can do to help prevent launching the roller coaster with a rage-bolus is by keeping your Correction Factor (which you read about in Prep 1) right in front of you at all times. If you need to write it on a sticky note and duct-tape that sticky note to your diabetes kit, go for it! (Although, keep in mind that it's going to change throughout your pregnancy, so...maybe don't use duct tape.)

While we will talk about pregnancy-related changes to your Correction Factor throughout the book, there are a few things to keep in mind when trying to correct a high blood sugar:

1. The number one most important thing to remember is that if you take a correction dose of insulin and nothing happens for 2

to 3 hours, and you're still high (and you didn't just eat a high-fat meal of pizza or nachos), then it's very possible you actually need another increase in your background insulin dose. Even 1 or 2 units added to your Total Basal Insulin or long-acting insulin dose can have a tremendous impact. Again, we'll talk about this in much more depth elsewhere in the book, but it's important to keep in mind when observing how your high blood sugars react (or don't react) to your correction doses of insulin.

2. What did you just eat? If your blood sugar is 230 mg/dL (12.8 mmol/L) and you just ate a meal that is high in both carbs and fat, it's going to take longer for that correction dose of insulin to take effect. *Additionally*, you may need more insulin than usual for that particular circumstance because of the food that your body is still digesting!

3. Lastly, if you are trying to dose your insulin for a *super-super-super high blood sugar* (generally anything above 250 mg/dL (13.8 mmol/L) could qualify but especially anything over 300 mg/dL (16.6 mmol/L)), you will likely need more insulin than usual. When your blood sugar is that high, your body simply needs more help getting back down because of additional variables like ketones and possible dehydration.

4. Speaking of dehydration, if you're high and you're frustrated and you want it down faster...drink some water! Plenty of water. The more dehydrated you are, the more concentrated the glucose in your blood becomes, and thus the higher it will be and the harder it will be to bring it down. Drink some water!

5. Take a deep breath. Be thoughtful. Be patient.

The blood sugar roller coaster is not a required experience in managing type 1 diabetes! It comes down to simply establishing good habits, personal rules, and personal goals for what you truly want your diabetes management to look like.

NOTES

PREPARING FOR PREGNANCY
PART 5
THE MAGICALLY AMAZING PRE-BOLUS

THE PRE-BOLUS. You've probably read about it in diabetes textbooks or lectures from your doctor when you were a teenager. Maybe your parents used to freak out about pre-bolusing your insulin when you were still under their watchful eye...but when was the last time you really did it?

(Okay, maybe you've been doing this for years, and you're ahead of the game when it comes to managing tighter blood sugar levels *after* eating and *during* pregnancy.)

If it's been a long time since you've even heard the term "pre-bolus," let's do a little review:

To pre-bolus your insulin means to take your insulin a certain amount of time *prior* to eating. Usually this timeframe is at least 15 minutes, because it takes about 15 to 20 minutes for most fast-acting insulins to begin working in your bloodstream, working on the carbs you eat and preventing a post-meal (postprandial) spike in your blood sugar.

Even if you follow a lower carb nutrition lifestyle, under 100 grams or 50 grams per day, pre-bolusing is still essential to staying in non-diabetic range after a meal.

If you eat a fairly medium-to-high carb-quantity most days, anything over 100 grams per day, then mastering the discipline required for pre-bolusing is an absolute must if you're striving to keep your A1C well below 6.5 percent.

LET'S PAINT A LITTLE PICTURE
FOR FURTHER UNDERSTANDING:

FIRST SCENARIO: Sarah sits down to a meal of steak, onions, and sweet potatoes. She calculates the insulin dose she will need for the 1 cup of sweet potatoes on her plate according to her insulin-to-carbohydrate ratio for her dinnertime meals. Then she immediately starts eating her meal.

After about 15 to 20 minutes, Sarah's blood sugar is going to rise. By the time her insulin starts to kick in, her meal is already *well on its way to raising her blood sugar.* By the time her insulin catches up with the carbs from her meal, it could be nearly an hour after eating. During that hour Sarah's blood sugar could easily have reached 200 mg/dL (11.1 mmol/L) or higher.

SECOND SCENARIO: Sarah thinks about what she's going to eat for dinner. She calculates her insulin dose for the carbs on her plate, *yada yada yada.* And then, 15 minutes later, she begins to eat that meal.

After 15 minutes of eating, Sarah's insulin dose has already been working in her bloodstream for 15 minutes. *Wait, what about going low before she even starts eating?* Fortunately, unless she started out *low*, it's very unlikely a dose of insulin would begin working *so quickly* that she'll actually see a measurable drop in her blood sugar after 15 minutes. *Instead*, what she'll see is that instead of spiking to 200 mg/dL (11.1 mmol/L) after eating, her blood sugar may only get up to 160 mg/dL (8.9 mmol/L) before coming back down into range (if your insulin dose was *accurate)* because of the pre-bolus! If you really master your pre-bolus technique, you can help your blood sugar stay under 130 or 120 mg/dL (6.7 mmol/L) after a meal—something your body, your baby, and your doctor will love!

(Now, there will be times during your pregnancy when you *won't* want to pre-bolus and times when you'll want to pre-bolus your insulin by nearly 45 minutes...but we'll talk about that in a few minutes!)

Someone may have once told you that a person with diabetes *can't possibly* keep their blood sugar under 160 mg/dL (8.9 mmol/L), and especially under 130 mg/dL (7.2 mmol/L), after eating a meal...but that person was severely mistaken. It is absolutely doable! Sure, it *does* take effort and thought, and there will be some situations where it's not ideal to pre-bolus (more on that in a moment), but for the majority of your normal meals, taking the time to pre-bolus is going to have a tremendous impact on your blood sugar goals!

The pre-bolus, we like to think, is kind of magical, because it has such a major impact on your blood sugars that it's going to quickly become one of the most important tools you have to keep your A1C and your overall blood sugars in your target range.

In other words: the pre-bolus is truly essential to diabetes management during pregnancy.

CREATING YOUR OWN PRE-BOLUS EXPERIMENT TO SEE THE RESULTS

To see the difference for yourself, let's do a little personal research. Next time you have a simple snack with an amount of carbohydrates you can clearly measure, create an experiment for yourself.

GINGER SHARES AN EXAMPLE: "I know I need 3 units of insulin for a Honey Crisp Apple with 2 tablespoons of peanut butter using *my current insulin-to-carbohydrate ratio*. If I take those 3 units and begin eating that apple with some peanut butter right away, my blood sugar is guaranteed to hit at least 180 mg/dL (10 mmol/L) within 45 minutes before it starts finally coming down after at least an hour since eating. The decline could take another 45 minutes so that's really almost 2 hours of hanging out *higher than my goal range* just because I didn't wait long enough between taking my insulin and eating the snack."

"However, if I wait 15 or even 20 minutes before beginning to eat, I can *easily* keep my blood sugar under 140 mg/dL (7.7 mmol/L)."

TRY YOUR PRE-BOLUS EXPERIMENT WITH A SIMPLE SNACK:

> **Note: these experiments will work best if you are starting with an "in-range" pre-meal blood sugar…such as a blood sugar at least below 140 mg/dL (7.7 mmol/L). But "in-range" can vary based on your individual goals. (Obviously, if you were low to begin with, waiting to eat is not a wise idea and you should try this experiment when your pre-meal blood sugar is in range!)*

EXPERIMENT #1: Eat your meal right after bolusing, check your blood sugar 45 to 60 minutes after eating. Likewise, if you have a CGM you can follow the rise and see more precisely when it started. Do not take a correction dose. Check your blood sugar again in *another* 60 minutes and see if you're still high. (If you are still high, chances are you might have needed a smidge more insulin with your meal!)

EXPERIMENT #2: The next day, choose that same simple snack at ideally the *same time of day.* Take your predetermined accurate amount of insulin. Wait 15 to 20 minutes before eating. Eat your snack. Check your blood sugar in 45 to 60 minutes after eating. Check your blood sugar again 2 hours after eating. Compare the results!

If you are *high or low* even after a proper pre-bolus, then you could consider one of these variables:

- **HIGH:** The meal was very low in fat and therefore digested *very quickly,* which means your body may need a longer duration of waiting after taking your injection.
- **LOW,** *THEN* **HIGH:** The meal was high enough in fat that it slowed down the rate of digestion and your insulin dose would be better administered right before eating and perhaps even a second bolus *after* eating. On insulin pumps this can be programmed as a "Square Bolus" or a "Dual Wave Bolus."
- **LOW,** *CONTINUED*: This is likely a combination of an inaccurate insulin-to-carb ratio and a meal that simply doesn't require much pre-bolus or delayed bolus, just a regular bolus when you begin to eat.
- **LOW,** *THEN* **HIGH**: Gastroparesis and pregnancy are both two conditions that can significantly slow down the rate of digestion and therefore complicate the timing of insulin dosing!

THE MORE PREGNANT YOU GET,
THE MORE PRE-BOLUS YOU'LL NEED

By the time you're in your third trimester, pregnancy hormones are so high and digestion is altered so much that you'll be much more resistant to insulin than normal, and your body will simply need more insulin to account for weight-gain, etc.

This means that the time between when you take your insulin and when you eat—if you're trying to keep your blood sugar in non-diabetic ranges—will need to be as long as 30, 45 and even 60 minutes depending on the meal.

A carb-loaded bowl of oatmeal in the third trimester will easily call for a 45 minute pre-bolus, even with two eggs added in. A grapefruit? Easily 60 minutes. A grapefruit with a handful of almonds eaten right before it... that could help *reduce* the amount of pre-bolus time you'll need during the third trimester. That's the magic of *dietary fat!* Sometimes you really *want* to slow down the digestion of those carbs in order to meet the abilities of your insulin and blood sugar goals. We'll talk about this in more detail during every trimester.

MEALS AND SITUATIONS WHEN
THE PRE-BOLUS *ISN'T* SO MAGICAL

Here are a few types of meals and situations for which pre-bolusing your insulin might not be a good idea. Keep in mind that we'll talk about this aspect of meal dosing throughout each trimester as well.

- **LOW BLOOD SUGARS:** It's definitely *not* necessary or safe to pre-bolus your insulin for a meal if your blood sugar is already below 60 mg/dL (3.3 mmol/L). If you are someone who is very uncomfortable even just sitting at 65 mg/dL (3.6 mmol/L), then maybe, for the sake of your sanity, anything below 70 mg/dL (3.8 mmol/L) is a good reason to not pre-bolus. Just keep in mind when you're eating that you just need to treat the low with 5 to 15 grams of carbs, depending on how low it is, and that you *will* need insulin for anything above that quantity. Starting a meal with a low blood sugar isn't an excuse to go nuts and throw caution to the wind with the rest of the carbs!

- **LOW-CARB MEALS:** A low-carb meal of steak and broccoli or bacon and eggs will likely still need a small dose of insulin (and more as you approach the third trimester), but pre-bolusing that insulin dose would be a very silly thing to do. Fat slows down the digestion of a meal, so while you may have 8 grams of carbs with your broccoli, the fat from the steak is going to significantly delay the impact of those carbs—especially when they are from vegetables!

Protein, like a steak, in large quantities (typically anything over about 20 grams) can be partially broken down into glucose, but not only is that process going to take much longer than breaking down a slice of bread into glucose, it's also simply not going to impact your blood sugar as significantly as true carbs.

If you currently don't take any insulin for meals like bacon and eggs, take a closer look at just how much your blood sugar rises after that meal. During your third trimester, a few slices of bacon can easily call for some amount of insulin in order to keep your blood sugar in non-diabetic range.

- **HIGH-FAT WITH HIGH-CARBS:** You know what makes things like lasagna or pizza or chinese food or cake with buttercream frosting so delicious? High fat content combined with high carb content = deeply soul satisfying food.

These kinds of meals call for a completely different approach to dosing insulin than practically everything else: If you are using injections you may need to dose a small portion of the bolus before the meal, with most of your insulin taken about an hour—if not *two* hours—*after* eating it. If you took your entire dose for the carbs in that pizza all at the same time, what will likely happen is your blood sugar will *plummet* an hour later, and then *four* hours after you ate that pizza, your blood sugar will rocket to the moon! This is because the fat content is severely slowing down the rate of digestion and absorption of the carbs in that pizza.

Instead, you may find you want a few units of your dose when you start eating, but the majority of your dose will really need to cover the carbs that are digested several hours *after* you finish your meal, because of the incredibly delayed digestive process due to the high fat content combined with the high carb content. How do you know what will work for you? Trial and error, check your blood sugar often, and take good notes so that you know how to manage your insulin around that type of food again.

For those using an insulin pump, this is the best time to learn how to use your extended bolus feature. Often called a *square, dual wave, combo* or *extended* bolus—each pump has its own term—but they all do the same thing. The extended bolus allows you to deliver the meal bolus with some insulin right away and then the rest in a drip-drip fashion over 1+ hours. This allows some of the insulin to get into your body now (like a normal bolus) and some over time to allow for the slower digestion and absorption of the food.

- **VEGETABLE-BASED MEALS:** A big bowl of veggie-packed soup that doesn't contain any real *starchy* vegetables will likely take a little longer for your body to break down because of all the fiber in the meal. This is a good thing! The reason a slice of bread breaks down so quickly is because it's so processed. When you're eating a bowl full of *real* food veggies, it's going to raise your blood sugar much more slowly because of the healthy fiber and wholeness of vegetables. Your body's gotta break all that down! This means that you'll likely be better-off taking your insulin at the same time you eat the meal.

- **EATING IN A RESTAURANT:** This is tricky, because certainly you need to pre-bolus for the carbs in your meal whether or not you're in a restaurant, but what if your meal ends up taking an hour to arrive because there was a big spill in the kitchen? What if you pre-bolus for a whole sweet potato you're expecting to arrive on your plate and it turns out that your sweet potato is one of the smallest sweet potatoes you've ever seen in your life? Now you've got too much insulin and not enough carbs. Overall, pre-bolusing for a meal in a restaurant should be done with a great deal of thought and caution—always better to underdose in a restaurant than overdose.

Even if the idea of a pre-bolus sounds tedious and annoying, and you choose to not bother with it during the first few months of your pregnancy, by the time you get to your third trimester you'll desperately want to pre-bolus because your blood sugars will feel completely unmanageable if you don't. Yes, it's annoying, but it will be one of the most important (maybe even *the* most important) thing you can do to reach your A1C goals and help ensure your baby is as healthy as possible.

> If you do nothing else to improve your blood sugars while pregnant, do your pre-bolus.

NOTES

_____

_____

PREPARING FOR PREGNANCY
PART 6

MOSTLY "CLEAN" & CONSISTENT NUTRITION

Regardless of diabetes, all of our bodies rely on good nutrition throughout each trimester for the sake of our own health, and the health of our growing baby. In fact, your nutrition is important even *before* that little baby has been conceived. First we're going to talk about your nutrition as a whole, and then we'll take a closer look at those essential vitamins and nutrients for pre-conception and fertility.

SO, WHAT DOES A *REAL-FOOD* DIET LOOK LIKE?

When was the last time you really observed your nutrition? Before we can improve our nutrition habits, we have to actually know where we're starting. Whether you use an app like *MyFitnessPal* or just a pad of paper and a pen, writing down what you eat for a few days, a week, or several months is a great way to really open your eyes to your current nutrition habits. Sometimes we might think we're only eating sugar or treats once a day when in reality it's really four times a day!

So, before you do anything else, we highly recommend tracking your nutrition for at least a few days and thinking honestly about where you're at and where you'd like to be. You don't have to obsess over calorie counts or carbohydrate goals, just write down the food you ate and the time of day you ate it at. Then take a step back and think about where you'd like to make improvements. Remember, you don't have to be perfect, you don't have to change everything at once (or ever). You're just looking for opportunities to improve your nutrition for the sake of improved blood sugars and improved health during pregnancy for everyone involved!

THE 80/20 OR 90/10 GUIDELINE FOR NUTRITION

We strongly believe the long-term secret to success in eating a healthier diet is the 80/20 or 90/10 guideline. This means that 80 to 90 percent of your nutrition comes from real, whole foods—preferably that you prepared yourself—and that leaves room for 10 or 20 percent of other less healthy foods.

For some people that 10 or 20 percent will come from bread and butter or fries or a slice of pizza. For others it might be from chocolate, ice cream, or candy. Or a little combination of both. The idea, though, is that you're aiming to *get the greater majority* of your day's nutrition from real, whole, healthy foods, but in order to sustain that disciplined nutrition, you're giving yourself room for imperfection, too.

Trying to eat *perfectly* for 30 days, let alone 9+ months, isn't usually a realistic goal for most of us. Will power does run out. Instead, focus on balance, not restriction. Focus on eating more whole foods, with a little room for a treat each day or maybe even every few days depending on what you personally need in order to prevent yourself from binge-eating junk foods or feeling obsessive about your nutrition.

What are *real*, whole foods? Here's a little list to give you an idea of what a 90/10 or 80/20 diet might contain:

- **VEGGIES (NON-STARCHY):** Bell peppers, broccoli, onions, Brussels sprouts, green beans, mushrooms, peas, carrots, etc.
- **BEANS:** Slow-cooked beans (cooked overnight in a slow-cooker on low with water), then used in soups, chili, salads, etc. You can get beans from cans, too, but remember those will be *loaded* with sodium, so cooking them yourself in a slow-cooker is more ideal...and *very easy!* If canned is your best option, go for the best quality you can buy (organic, etc.) because the price difference is usually pretty small. And be sure to rinse them thoroughly in a strainer to help reduce the sodium content.
- **NUTS:** Almonds, pecans, walnuts, cashews…oh my!
- **FRUIT:** Any of your favorite fruits...but of course eaten with awareness and moderation because they will spike your blood sugar, especially if you don't pre-bolus your insulin don't. HINT: adding *fats* to any snack of fruit will slow down the digestion and thus won't cause as severe of a spike in your blood sugar!
- **DAIRY:** Keep in mind when consuming dairy that products like milk and yogurt usually have a decent amount of added sugar. In addition to *real* butter and cheese, if you'd like to have a yogurt you'll be better off getting a *plain* Greek yogurt and adding your own berries for flavor. Great alternatives to cow's milk: unsweetened almond milk, flax milk, coconut milk.
- **ANIMAL PROTEIN:** Eggs, beef, chicken, breakfast sausage and most seafood. The higher quality animal protein you can buy (like cage-free organic eggs, grass-fed beef) the higher quality that animal protein will be for your body.
- **GRAINS:** There are so many great, healthy grains—oats, oat bran, quinoa, buckwheat, millet, brown rice...the list goes on and on. Something to keep in mind when it comes to eating grains is *how processed* is this grain? Instant oatmeal? Not a really a great source of a grain, highly processed, poor quality, added sugars, etc. Steel-cut

oats that you cooked on the stove or zapped in the microwave for a couple minutes? Much better. The more processed the grain, the faster it will digest and the less nutrition you're going to get from it.

- **BEVERAGES:** Water! Working towards a lifestyle where water is the primary beverage in your life will support your health goals in so many ways! You can add lemon or lime for a little added flavor, or flavored seltzers if you really need some more *pop* to your water. There's nothing wrong with drinking a cup or two of coffee, even while pregnant...but what are you adding to your coffee? A lot of creamer with artificial sweeteners? Black coffee on its own is basically a very whole food, but when we start adding lots of stuff to it—like cream and sugar and sweeteners and French vanilla flavored creams—it isn't quite so *whole* anymore. And protein smoothies? You bet...but beware of making your smoothie with too much fruit. 1 cup of frozen berries is only approximately 10–15 or so grams of carbs versus adding in a banana, an orange, etc. and stacking up over 50 grams of carbs in one smoothie! We'll talk about some great smoothie recipes later.

TREATS!

What can you have as a cheat or a treat in preparation for or *during* pregnancy?

The fact is that the more skilled you become in the "art of the pre-bolus," the more flexible you can be with treats. However, the other tricky part of blood sugar management when eating treats is that with foods high in both fat and sugar, like cake with buttercream frosting, the traditional pre-bolus won't help you. Instead, you may find you need to take some of your insulin dose with the cake and some after or even several hours *after* you eat the cake! Just like we mentioned earlier in Prep 5, those high-fat/high-carb meals, whether it's lasagna or cake, will require more creative bolusing techniques in order to keep your post-meal blood sugars in-range, or at least *near* your range.

But no one expects you to go 9 months without eating a darn cookie— be sure to remind your doctor that they probably couldn't go 9 months without dessert either. Instead, the most important thing you can remember when including treats in your day is to be thoughtful about those treats.

QUESTIONS TO ASK YOURSELF WHEN PREPARING TO EAT A TREAT:

- What is a reasonable serving size for this treat?
- How many carbs are in that treat?
- If you don't know how many carbs are in that treat, do everything you can to find out, such as putting the recipe into an online nutrition

panel tool (MyFitnessPal works great for this) or by creating a careful experiment with your insulin dose to determine how much insulin you need. For example: per cookie or per slice of cake, etc.

- Is there enough fat to cause a significant delay in when those carbs will raise my blood sugar? If so, how will I adjust my insulin dosing approach? If there's more than 20 grams of fat to go along with all that sugar...
- Have the majority of my other food choices today been from healthy, whole-food choices?
- Why am I eating this? Because it's delicious? Because I've been told it's "off-limits"? Because I'm pregnant and I can eat whatever I want? Because I'm craving it?

WHEN IT COMES TO TREATS, THINK ABOUT WHAT KIND OF PERSON YOU ARE: Does abstaining from something completely make you want it more and more and more? Do you end up binge-eating the thing you've tried to avoid? Are you better off when you know you can always have a few pieces of chocolate without going overboard? If you're that kind of person, then actually making sure you include regular treats in your nutrition plan is going to help you maintain a healthier relationship with food overall.

Or are you the kind of person who is all or nothing? Get the chocolate out of the house and you feel great, you don't need it if it's not there, and you don't end up binge-eating on bars and bars of it once you encounter it again?

Think carefully about which kind of person you are when plotting how to include treats in your daily nutrition.

FOODS TO LIMIT DURING PREGNANCY

- **SODIUM:** Sodium is found in abundance in most packaged/ processed foods, making it very easy to consume far beyond the recommended 1500 mg/day suggested limit. It's certainly not a nutrient that most people have to worry about consuming enough of unless your diet is truly entirely whole foods and only contains sodium that you add by sprinkling on your own salt—if that's *your diet*, make sure you're getting enough salt! For most, though, it's important to pay attention to your consumption because it can affect blood pressure levels. For women with diabetes, we're at a higher risk of developing pre-eclampsia, so eating a diet high in sodium from processed foods is only going to increase your risk.
- **FISH:** The primary concern with fish consumption is *mercury*. Mercury is found in most sources of seafood, but the fish sources with the *lowest mercury levels* are salmon, tilapia, shrimp, tuna, cod, and

catfish. Seafood consumption during pregnancy should be limited to 2 to 3 servings per week. *All raw seafood should be avoided completely.*

- **CAFFEINE:** A little caffeine each day is okay, but caffeinated beverages should be limited to a maximum consumption of 200 mg of caffeine (which is about 12 ounces of coffee or one very large cup of coffee).
- **UNPASTEURIZED CHEESES:** Unpasteurized cheeses, like brie, can contain the bacteria "listeria" that is very dangerous for a pregnant woman because listeriosis has been shown to cause miscarriage.
- **DELI—MEATS:** Like unpasteurized cheese, deli-meats can also cause listeriosis. If you do feel like making yourself a grilled ham and cheese sandwich during pregnancy, you need to actually *cook* your deli-meat by simply putting it in a pan and thoroughly cooking both sides of each slice of meat to the point that they are steaming hot.

A "DAY IN THE LIFE" EATING A MOSTLY-CLEAN DIET

Here are a few sample days of what a diet of *mostly clean, real food* looks like:

SAMPLE:

- **BREAKFAST:** protein smoothie of whey protein, blueberries, unsweetened almond milk, & peanut butter *(recipe in back of book)*
- **LUNCH:** big salad with chicken, spinach, kale, iceberg, bell pepper, cheese & ranch dressing
- **SNACK:** apple & peanut butter
- **DINNER:** steak, onions, broccoli
- **DESSERT:** homemade gluten-free chocolate chip cookies

SAMPLE:

- **BREAKFAST:** flaxseed muffin *(recipe in back of book)*
- **LUNCH:** tuna & veggie tortilla wrap (or lettuce leaves), potato chips & dark chocolate
- **SNACK:** protein bar
- **DINNER:** black-bean veggie burger with bun & strawberry/spinach salad
- **DESSERT:** frozen lemon Chobani yogurt cup

SAMPLE:

- **BREAKFAST:** two eggs & bowl of oat-bran/oatmeal
- **LUNCH:** gluten-free sandwich bread with chicken, cheddar, lettuce & mayo
- **SNACK:** plain greek yogurt with strawberries & blueberries

- **DINNER:** hamburgers with gluten-free buns & side-salad
- **DESSERT:** bowl of ice cream

SAMPLE:
- **BREAKFAST:** two eggs & two slices gluten-free toast
- **LUNCH:** chicken caesar salad
- **SNACK:** almonds & an orange
- **DINNER:** baked tofu & quinoa pasta
- **DESSERT:** 10 Hershey kisses

SAMPLE:
- **BREAKFAST:** gluten-free english muffin & two breakfast sausages
- **LUNCH:** taco salad in a bowl from Chipotle
- **SNACK:** carrots, celery, hummus & peanuts
- **DINNER:** gluten-free pizza
- **DESSERT:** microwave popcorn

ARTIFICIAL SWEETENERS DURING PREGNANCY

Is drinking a diet soda or a bowl full of sugar-free jello sweetened with aspartame the worst thing in the world for a pregnant woman? No, but it's not exactly something you want to be doing regularly either.

The research on sweeteners like aspartame (Equal and what's used in most diet sodas) and sucralose (Splenda) are really still quite inconclusive. When doing your own reading on sweetener studies, one thing to keep in mind is: who paid for this study? If the American Beverage Association paid for a study to determine how healthy or not healthy artificial sweeteners are, you can bet the results are going to be skewed in their favor considering how much money they make from selling diet sodas that use those sweeteners.

If you know you aren't willing to give up diet sodas and other products with these sweeteners…

First, remember there is the brand *Zevia*, which is diet soda sweetened with stevia (read below to learn about why this is a very safe artificial sweetener).

If *Zevia* isn't what you want…and you don't want to give up your favorite after-work beverage. That's your decision! At the very least, consider creating some kind of parameter around your consumption of artificial sweeteners or diet sodas.

For instance, you *love* your diet root-beer? Then consider limiting yourself to one glass of soda per night or three per week or one every weekend—you have to determine the right amount for you.

It's also important to remember the caffeine contents in some of these beverages. If you consume five or six Diet Cokes in one day, that's *a lot* of caffeine, let alone a lot of aspartame, and the caffeine limitations during pregnancy are clear: 200 mg per day. So this is something you'll want to work on reducing your consumption of prior to pregnancy or as soon as you become pregnant.

Remember, it's okay if you're not perfect when it comes to artificial sweeteners, but it's important to be aware of how much you're consuming and set reasonable limits for yourself.

THE SAFETY OF ALTERNATIVE SWEETENERS DURING PREGNANCY

- **STEVIA:** Stevia is a plant that happens to have a sweet taste. It does not contain any carbs but most of the stevia-sugar products out there are mixed with something else to add volume, because stevia itself is so sweet, just a tiny pinch could sweeten a whole batch of cookies. When buying stevia, look for brands that are mixed with sugar alcohol sweeteners like xylitol or erythritol rather than corn-based additives like maltodextrin. While stevia is safe to use during pregnancy, remember that even a good thing should be consumed in moderation—so don't go too crazy with your consumption, use it in small amounts. Chugging 8 cans of stevia-sweetened diet soda every day isn't "healthy" or "harmless" just because it's sweetened with stevia.

- **XYLITOL AND ERYTHRITOL:** These are sugar-alcohol sweeteners that will still show up in the total carbohydrate count on a nutrition panel (and will be identified as such) but they still raise blood sugar in some people so keep a close eye on your blood sugar after consuming foods or drinks with these sweeteners to determine how much they impact your blood sugar. Consuming these sweeteners in large quantities can also lead to a bit of digestive distress (aka: diarrhea) so...don't go crazy with this one either!

- **SUCRALOSE, ASPARTAME, SACCHARIN:** In general, these sweeteners are created out of chemicals and it's best to avoid them as much as possible during your pregnancy because the effects on the fetus are simply unknown. While it has been said that sucralose does not pass through to the fetus, there are plenty of studies to suggest it isn't harmless to mom. These are chemicals, simply put, and none of us benefit from consuming them regularly.

In the end, it's completely up to you how much artificial sweetener you consume during your pregnancy. When it comes to beverages, there's nothing your baby will appreciate more than a nice tall glass of water.

GETTING YOUR VITAMINS & NUTRIENTS

While there are certainly great pre-natal vitamins, your food matters, too, and a vitamin isn't going to make-up for a nutrient-poor diet. A healthy diet is one that provides a variety of nutrient-*rich* foods.

Eating a variety of foods will ensure you get a lot of these nutrients from a whole food source; however, taking a prenatal vitamin starting 3 to 4 months before you start trying to become pregnant will ensure your body is optimized for healthy fetal development from the get-go!

WHY ARE VITAMINS SO INCREDIBLY IMPORTANT PRIOR–TO AND DURING YOUR PREGNANCY?

Aside from the obvious reason—your baby needs vitamins for proper growth and development—it's almost crucial to understand that once you are pregnant, your body is going to send the nutrients from what you eat to the baby before sending any to your body! If your diet is lacking in nutrients, both you and the baby can suffer from vitamin deficiency.

But there are also certain vitamins and nutrients that are extra important for women with type 1 diabetes. Specifically: folate (folic acid) and vitamin D.

In addition to taking a great pre-natal vitamin (we'll suggest a few we're fond of in a moment), here are a few extra vitamins to be aware of as a woman with type 1 diabetes:

- **FOLATE (2000 MCG/DAY):** Non-diabetic women generally only need 400 to 800 mcg of folic acid, but very recent research has found that the need for folic acid is dramatically higher in the population of women with diabetes of any type. Fill up on this starting at least 4 months prior to when you try to conceive. This nutrient is very important for both fertility as well as early fetal development and prevention of neural tube defects.

- **VITAMIN D (400 IU/DAY):** It is especially important for those with diabetes to get a vitamin D level test prior to conception. Any result less than 30 means you should be taking a "therapeutic dose" of 4,000 to 5,000 IU/day in order to increase your body's vitamin D levels. Get your level re-tested 8 to 12 weeks later, and then, if your results are well above 30, continue a maintenance dose of about 2,000 to 3,000 IU/day. Vitamin D is especially important for diabetics—we are notoriously low in vitamin D levels, and research has pinpointed a connection between vitamin D levels and autoimmune dysfunction. Low levels of vitamin D in a pregnant woman can also set up her baby to have low levels, too.

- **CALCIUM (1000 MG/DAY):** If you think dairy is the only reliable source for your body's calcium needs: think again! Leafy green veggies (spinach, broccoli), almonds and almond milk all have plenty of calcium, too, and can actually be more easily absorbed by your body than dairy-sourced calcium.

Remember, the broader variety of *real, whole foods* you eat each day, the more easily you'll get adequate amounts of these nutrients. This can be harder once you're actually pregnant because some foods, even healthy things like vegetables, might be less appealing—so that's why a great whole-food based prenatal vitamin is as important as your nutrition.

There are so many vitamins on the market today, it's hard to know what's the best choice for you. It's also easy to get suckered into buy cheap vitamins online that may actually just be full of cornstarch and completely *counterfeit*—this is actually a significant problem in the supplement industry so don't be lured by cheap online prices!

Here are a few brands we personally recommend because they are high-quality.

RECOMMENDED VITAMINS & SUPPLEMENT BRANDS:

PRENATAL VITAMIN & FOLATE:

- **NEW CHAPTER / RAINBOW LITE /GARDEN OF LIFE:** These vitamins are derived from *whole food* sources rather than synthetic chemicals. They also contain a number of medicinal herbs, and probiotics, the good bacteria your gut needs!
  - They're not as inexpensive as many of the vitamins you're used to seeing on the shelves simply because they're much higher quality than a mainstream brand you'd see commercials for on TV, which are derived from *synthetic* sources (Vitamin C from car tires? Yuck.), not whole foods. These vitamins are worth every penny because you're getting the real deal and much more with added herbs and probiotics.
- You can also trust these brands for your additional folate (folic acid) supplement or B-vitamin complex, which will contain folate.

VITAMIN D:

- One of the easiest ways to get your extra vitamin D is in liquid form. It's actually very inexpensive to get 1 bottle of liquid D at any vitamin store such as GNC or Vitamin Shoppe or a health-food store. 1 drop is typically 400 to 1000 IUs.

OMEGA FATTY ACIDS:

- **NORDIC NATURALS / OCEAN'S MOM / NEW CHAPTER:** Omega fatty acid supplements can easily be counterfeited or contain a much smaller quantity of the acids than the bottle claims, so sticking with trusted, certified brands is crucial. Getting these healthy fatty acids are crucial for the "building blocks" of your baby's developing brain, and other parts of the body such as the retinas in their eyes!

It may sound *very overwhelming* if you've never taken vitamins before. If that's the case and you just want to stick with the basics, get yourself a great prenatal multivitamin and a great omegas vitamin and leave it at that. Do what you can personally manage and afford.

NUTRITION FOR FERTILITY

It can't be said enough that one of the *most* powerful ways to boost your fertility is through improving your blood sugar levels. The more stable your blood sugars are through diligent insulin dosing, checking your blood sugar regularly, and eating a diet of *mostly* whole foods, the less likely diabetes will get in the way of your ability to become pregnant.

But nutrition can help, too!

To optimize fertility once you and your partner have received the "green-light" from your doctor that your diabetes management and overall health are ready for conception, you can start to eat healthy foods that will also boost fertility.

THE BEST FOODS FOR FERTILITY ARE:

- **ARUGULA:** A good source of folate (about 30 mcg in a ¹/₂ cup), vitamin A and C.
- **ASPARAGUS:** A great source of folate (100 mcg in 5 spears) and vitamin C.
- **AVOCADO:** Women who ate more avocado were shown to have higher levels of fertility! Avocados are also *full* of healthy fats which are crucial to proper hormone levels for females.
- **BUCKWHEAT:** A gluten-free and low glycemic seed that can be found as flour or a toasted groat, is an excellent source of B vitamins (folate is one of these) and zinc. B vitamins can help with increasing fertility as well as increasing energy levels. Buckwheat is low glycemic and can help keep blood sugar levels better controlled. This provides an optimal environment for conception since high blood sugar levels increase risk of infertility.
- **ENDIVE:** A tasty type of salad green that is full of wonderful nutrients to help support fertility, folate in particular. Low folic acid levels is one of the many reasons that a miscarriage may occur, and as women with diabetes we want to do everything we can to optimize overall health for prevention. This wonderful stand-alone green is also packed with fat soluble vitamins (A, E and K—so eat with a bit

of oil or salad dressing to enhance absorption) as well as vitamin C, calcium and iron.

- **OLIVE OIL:** This nutrient-dense oil is wonderful from pre-conception all the way through pregnancy and the postpartum time. Olive oil is a plant-based fat – also called mono and polyunsaturated fats. Fat is important in the diet as it helps with absorption of our fat soluble vitamins A, D, E and K, which are important for many systems in our body. But remember there is always a limit, even with good things. Try to be aware and measure the amount of fat you eat because even though we need plenty of fats in our diet and fats are packed with essential nutrients, it's also very dense in calories and easy to overdo.

- **SPICES:** Food always tastes a bit better with some flavor or pizzazz added! Try a bit of cinnamon in your morning Oats or smoothie—research has shown benefit for improved blood sugar control. Another wonderful addition if you like a bit of spice is paprika. This bright red spice made from hot pepper is packed with iron, vitamin A and vitamin C.

THE WORST FOODS FOR FERTILITY ARE:

- **GLUTEN:** More and more research is connecting infertility and miscarriage to gluten. The reason is because in most people gluten causes at least some level of inflammation. The more sensitive you are to gluten (you can easily be unaware of this) the more affected by that inflammation you will be, especially when trying to conceive. It is not uncommon for women who are struggling to become or *stay* pregnant to overcome that struggle after removing gluten from their diet long enough for that inflammation to subside, which is generally 3 weeks to a month.

- **LOW–FAT DIETS:** As a female, eating adequate amounts of healthy fat is essential to your reproductive system. A severely low-fat diet will easily rob your body of the nutrients necessary to produce proper estrogen levels...and from there the whole show shuts down. This doesn't mean you should go hog-wild on butter and bacon, but it does mean you need to make sure you're feeding your body enough *real food* sources of fat from foods such as nuts, avocado, animal products, and seafood. (And if you don't like seafood, that's all the more reason to make sure you're getting an omega fatty acids supplement!

- **JUNK. JUNK. JUNK:** If your diet is full of junky, processed, packaged *stuff* rather than *real food*, your fertility is going to struggle just as much of the rest of your body is struggling to function on a diet that is lacking in real nutrients and vitamins. If you've never found the motivation to quit the fast-food lunches and create the time to make more healthy meals for yourself, let pregnancy be that motivation for you. Your blood sugars will thank you, too!

- **DIETING:** Simply put, consuming too few calories when you are trying to conceive will absolutely interfere with your body's ability to ovulate and nurture a fertilized egg. The same can be said with trying to maintain a level of body fat that is only attainable by consuming too few calories. Your body is *smart*—it knows that a mother whose body is in caloric deprivation isn't an ideal place to grow a baby. Growing a baby requires adequate calories and healthy levels of body fat, so getting *pregnant* with that baby is going to require adequate calories and healthy levels of body fat, too. Pre-pregnancy and pregnancy itself are not appropriate times for weight-loss efforts or calorie restriction.

IT'S NOT ABOUT PERFECTION

Remember in the end it's not about eating perfectly, it's about eating as healthfully as you personally can manage. The more *whole, real* foods there are in your diet that *you* prepared yourself...the healthier you'll be and the better you're feel throughout your pregnancy. Oh, and the healthier that adorable little bun in your oven will be, too!

NOTES

PREPARING FOR PREGNANCY
PART 7

EXERCISING WITH TYPE 1 DIABETES

Another one of the most useful tools you'll have to help you manage your blood sugars during pregnancy is exercise. Yes, yes, you've heard it before: *"Exercise is really important for diabetes management...blah blah blah."*

This isn't news, we realize.

But during pregnancy, when we say regular exercise is important...we *really, really* mean it.

For some of you, exercise is already a huge part of your life. You may not have to make any adjustments to your workout or you may completely change your workout to accommodate your physical needs while pregnant, but either way, you'll continue to be *active* during your pregnancy.

For others, exercise might be something you have yet to really make a regular part of your life. And that's okay. Starting to exercise shortly before you become pregnant or when you learn that you've become pregnant *isn't too late* to reap the many benefits of being *active* during your pregnancy.

3 REASONS TO BE ACTIVE DURING YOUR PREGNANCY

1. **POST-MEAL BLOOD SUGAR SPIKES:** Remember when we talked about how important keeping your post-meal blood sugar in-range will be for your A1C goals? In addition to pre-bolusing your insulin, simply going for a 10 or 15-minute walk after you eat will work wonders! Or standing in place and dancing during the commercial breaks after dinner, or doing a hundred reps with 3 lb. dumbbells while you're on a 30-minute phone-call for work.

2. **INSULIN RESISTANCE:** Throughout this book, you'll learn more and more about how your increasing levels of pregnancy hormones and natural weight-gain during pregnancy are going to lead to increasing levels of insulin resistance. Staying active can help lessen this part of pregnancy with type 1 diabetes. Not only will it help you maintain lower blood sugar levels and prevent excessive weight-gain, it will also help keep your total daily insulin needs lower as well. Exercising regularly throughout your pregnancy could be the difference between needing twice as much insulin by the end of your pregnancy versus needing three times as much insulin (or more) by the end of your pregnancy.

3. **ENERGY LEVELS:** When we're tired, it can be easy to think that the only solution is to be *less active* and conserve energy. While you certainly do need adequate amounts of rest during pregnancy (you'll feel this right from the start), staying active throughout your pregnancy is going to help you *feel* more energetic overall. Pregnancy shouldn't be an excuse to sit on the couch for 9 months—your body and baby will thank you in ways you can't even measure if you get moving every day.

THE SIMPLEST EXERCISE YOU CAN DO DURING PREGNANCY

Even if you were already incredibly passionate about a certain type of exercise prior to pregnancy, and your doctor has given you full permission to continue doing that exercise during pregnancy you may find that your body just doesn't feel right doing it now that you're pregnant. And that's okay—in fact, it's really, really normal, and it's something your body is telling you that should definitely listen to!

Some women can run half-marathons during their pregnancy and lift weights and play tennis. For others, it just might feel wrong. Your body and baby might be asking you to *not do that.*

That brings us to the simplest yet very worthwhile exercise almost everyone can do during pregnancy: walking.

Whether you walk on the road, on a treadmill, in a pool, in the woods, or up a mountain, you will be thankful you kept up with your walking by the time that baby is ready for its big debut, and long after you've met each other.

Whether you walk for 10 minutes after every meal, or 30 minutes in the afternoon, or an hour or more every day, it doesn't matter. Figure out what you can do and make it a priority.

MANAGING BLOOD SUGARS DURING EXERCISE

If you've been frustrated in the past because of low blood sugars and high blood sugars during or after you exercise, you're not alone! Balancing your blood sugar during *any* kind of exercise can feel incredibly confusing and overwhelming and impossible.

Even a 30-minute walk can send your blood sugar plummeting and 30 minutes of weight-lifting can leave you a hundred points higher than where you started!

You may have eased this frustration in the past by letting your blood sugar purposefully stay *high* during exercise. The problems with this are aplenty, but you can imagine that doing this while pregnant is *definitely* not an effective or safe method for your baby.

Whether or not you're pregnant, exercising with purposefully high blood sugars not only leads to gradual long-term complications you've been hearing about since you were diagnosed, but it's also going to get in the way of your body's ability to lose weight, perform properly during your workout, recover properly from your workout, and cause overall stress to your entire body. It's simply not a smart thing to do—and it isn't necessary either!

Successfully managing your blood sugars during exercise comes down to one thing: understanding the *simple physiology* behind the type of exercise you're doing and then...how to prepare properly for that physiology.

In this next section, we're going to give you the *need-to-know* details for balancing your blood sugar during basic types of exercise. What we aren't going to do in this section is talk about how to train for marathons, how to balance your blood sugar for a 100-mile bike ride or during your next CrossFit competition. Those levels of exercise are much more complex and simply not realistic for the average pregnant gal.

▌ *Now let's get to the good stuff.*

3 BIGGEST FACTORS THAT IMPACT YOUR BLOOD SUGAR DURING EXERCISE

Let's take a closer look at the three most important factors that will affect how your blood sugar responds to exercise and how easily you'll be able to stay in a safe and healthy range during exercise.

FACTOR #1: AEROBIC VS. ANAEROBIC EXERCISE

The primary way to predict how a form of exercise is going to impact your blood sugar comes down to understanding whether your chosen form of exercise is *aerobic* or *anaerobic.*

AEROBIC EXERCISE: Low to moderate level aerobic exercise burns glucose primarily for fuel and can lower blood sugar levels. Aerobic (or cardio) exercise uses glucose primarily for fuel because when your heart rate is persistently high, your body can't get oxygen to the fat cells quickly enough to use *fat* for fuel. Instead, it's forced to burn glucose. That's why when you go for a 30-minute jog and your heart rate is beating hard at 160 beats per minute, your blood sugar drops 100 mg/dL points. Types of aerobic exercise include: jogging, powerwalking, running, cycling, power-yoga, dancing, vacuuming, swimming laps, etc.

- **FOR EXAMPLE:** Ginger shares, "When I was teaching power-yoga, I knew that I needed approximately 15 grams of carbs *right* before teaching. If I ate the carbs too early, I'd end up high halfway thru the class, but if I ate *right* before teaching, my blood sugar stayed in-range. At the time, I used a small cup of yogurt or an apple with a small handful of nuts.

ANAEROBIC EXERCISE: Anaerobic exercise burns primarily fat for fuel and has no effect on or can raise blood sugar levels. You may be thinking the only type of anaerobic exercise is *strength*-training in the gym with weights, but that might still leave you wondering why your spinning class sometimes sends your blood sugar through the roof! Anaerobic exercise is defined by any type of exercise that you perform intensely for a small amount of time followed by a brief period of rest and then a period of intensity again. Types of this exercise would include weightlifting, sprinting, spinning and cycling (depending on how it's performed).

The reason anaerobic exercise generally does *not* raise blood sugar levels is because that constant rising and dropping of your heart rate allows your body to get oxygen to your fat cells (during the resting period) to use for fuel.

Some people will find they actually need a bolus of insulin prior, during or immediately after an anaerobic workout because of how it raises blood sugar. This is something you'll have to experiment with in your own body to determine the timing and insulin doses that work best for you.

- **FOR EXAMPLE:** if you're sprinting and your heart rate is only high for short periods of time, specifically 2 minutes or less, and then your heart rate decreases for a few minutes, and then you sprint again, this is actually *not* "cardio" or "aerobic" exercise, but instead it's really "anaerobic" because you're performing short bursts of really intense exercise. This will likely not lower your blood sugar, and it could even cause your blood sugar to rise!

- **FOR EXAMPLE:** Ginger shares, "When I do a weightlifting workout, even if it's just 30 minutes, my blood sugar starts to rise the moment I *finish* my workout. If I'm not going to eat right after my workout, then I usually need to take a really small bolus of insulin to prevent the post-workout spike. If I do eat right after my workout, I generally only need insulin to cover the food. This is because that post-workout spike is my body trying to cycle fuel to my muscles so they can start recovering. If I don't eat, my body has to make that glucose by releasing glycogen from my liver, and converting it to glucose."

FACTOR #2: THE TIME OF DAY & LAST INSULIN DOSE

This one's a biggie, and it's especially important because it's what helps you individualize your exercise and choose *when* you want to exercise based on your own schedule.

IN THE MORNING...BEFORE YOU EAT BREAKFAST: When you're not pregnant, exercising first thing in the morning on an empty stomach may sound like a *crazy* idea but it actually works really well for maintaining in-range blood sugars during aerobic exercise—as long as your background insulin doses are accurate. The reason it works is because if you don't eat breakfast (or even the few calories from cream in your coffee), your body remains in a fasted state; this means it continues to burn *fat* for fuel instead of glucose.

Sounds crazy? Don't be surprised if you've never heard this before, it actually comes from the bodybuilding world in which burning fat is a huge focus. Diabetic or not, exercising (particularly walking) first thing in the morning prior to eating will burn body fat primarily for fuel.

THE TWO CAVEATS TO THIS FOR THOSE OF US WITH FUNKY PANCREASES ARE:

1. You shouldn't do this if your blood sugar is *low*. Duh. Feed your blood sugar...*then* begin your workout. You benefit in the same way for the fat-burning sake, but you'll still benefit from simply exercising!

2. It won't be as effective if your blood sugar is *high* and thus you have to take a bolus of insulin to get your blood sugar down. You *can* still start the fasted workout and you *should* take that correction dose of insulin, but it simply isn't going to burn fat as efficiently... which is a great motivator to ensure you wake up with in-range blood sugars!

RIGHT AFTER A SNACK OR MEAL: Depending on the type of exercise you're going to do, the snack or meal you eat before exercise may need insulin to go with it, may need only half as much insulin as you'd normally take, or may need no insulin at all.

- **FOR EXAMPLE:** If you're about to go for a 10-mile jog, which is definitely going to primarily burn glucose for fuel, you'd likely want to consume a small amount of carbs prior to the jog and then likely another serving of carbs halfway through your jog depending on your blood sugar.

  But if you're going to go for a 3-mile jog, and you only need about 10 grams of carbs to keep your blood sugar steady during that exercise, you would probably need *some* insulin to go with your meal merely because the amount of carbs in your meal is greater than what you need for your blood sugar. This begins to get a little more complex in that exercise increases the efficacy of the insulin we take, so you may not need as much insulin for those excess carbs as you normally would.

2 HOURS AFTER A SNACK OR MEAL: If you ate a lunch or snack with the appropriate amount of insulin at 10 a.m., and you exercise at 12 p.m., that means that even though rapid-acting insulin stays in your body for up to 4 hours, it's past its peak efficacy. Preventing your blood sugar from dropping if you exercise after that 2-hour mark is going to be easier than exercising *right* after you ate and took insulin.

QUICKIE EXERCISE AFTER EATING: A 15-minute walk after a meal can also be tremendously helpful in curbing that post-meal blood sugar spike. It can be the difference between rising to 170 mg/dL (9.4 mmol/L) after eating and only rising to 130 mg/dL (7.2 mmol/L)—but the trick is to make sure there isn't a large gap of time between the meal and the exercise. If you wait too long to head out for that walk, your blood sugar could easily already have made its way up to 170 mg/dL (9.4 mmol/L). Use this simple little trick to your advantage!

FACTOR #3: HYDRATION, BABY! H2O!

Water. Even when you're not exercising dehydration can cause high blood sugars simply because the less water there is in your bloodstream the more concentrated the glucose in your bloodstream becomes.

When you're exercising and your water consumption is supporting *two* humans instead of one, get plenty of water. It's that simple.

SHOULD I REDUCE MY PUMP BASAL RATE DURING EXERCISE?

While your first instinct with an insulin pump might be to cut your basal insulin back by a certain percentage, this can actually cause more problems than solutions for your blood sugars.

The primary reason is because basal insulin stays in your body for *four hours*, and the insulin you get from your basal rate between 1 p.m. and 2 p.m. really doesn't impact your blood sugar until after 2 p.m. So, for example, if you're exercising at 1 p.m., and you set a reduced basal rate for your hour-long power-walk, you'll likely still go low *and* you're also likely to go *high* after your walk because your basal was reduced and it impacted a four-hour window of time after you set that reduction.

The only exception to this is for workouts that are well over 60 minutes, particularly aerobic workouts (anaerobic workouts over 60 minutes may likely need an increase in basal). But for the average 30 to 60-minute workout, a reduced basal rate isn't generally necessary and is likely going to cause more blood sugar trouble for you in the hours that follow.

KEEP MOVING!

Whatever works for you—weightlifting, walking or pole-dancing—try to stay motivated and *keep moving* as long as you feel comfortable and safe. By the end of the last trimester, you may find you're just doing a shimmy in front of your couch during the commercial breaks of your favorite show... but that's better than nothing at all!

NOTES

PREPARING FOR PREGNANCY

PART 8

SUPPORTING A PREGNANT WOMAN WITH TYPE 1 DIABETES

Being the husband, wife, boyfriend, or girlfriend to a person with type 1 diabetes comes with a variety of challenges and responsibilities...and those challenges are only magnified when your loved one with diabetes becomes pregnant.

This section is for both of you: the pregnant woman with type 1 diabetes and her devoted partner.

LET'S START WITH YOU, THE PREGNANT MAMA-TO-BE:

There's no denying that you'll be thinking about your blood sugars 24/7 when you're pregnant. If you thought diabetes flooded your brain on an average day, you'll find it never leaves your mind when there's a little fetus growing inside you! That much is obvious though, right? The reason this is extra important to consider when it comes to the support you'll be receiving from your partner is that we really do need to make sure we include them, give them a way to express their own concern and care, and give them helpful ways to support us throughout our pregnancy...because this is their baby, too! They care about *both* of you!

The reality is that we really can't tell our partner (who totally adores us) to keep out of our business, especially when it comes to blood sugars, during pregnancy. It's part of their role as "adoring partner" to be concerned about both mama and baby.

Trouble can start, though, if the kind of support your partner instinctively offers isn't actually the kind of support you want or the kind of support that actually feels...supportive!

So far, in your relationship prior to pregnancy, you've probably already established some sort of habit or pattern together in how your partner *is or isn't* involved in your diabetes care. And *now* is a great time to observe whether that habit or pattern has been positive or negative for your relationship. Take a look at whether it needs some attention *or* if it's already very effective and productive and benefits your relationship rather than adds more stress to it.

- When your partner asks you what your blood sugar is or how your blood sugars were today, do you feel as though they are invading your privacy and resent the intrusion...or do you feel as though they are expressing their love and concern for your well-being?
  - **FOR EXAMPLE:** An all too classic example of love and concern from a partner is concern that actually feels like nagging. "What were your blood sugars today? Were you high? How high? What'd you do!?" Yada yada yada. What your partner really wants to know is how you're doing and how they can help, but if we don't give them specific ways to support us it can easily come out like nagging. Instead, try, "How are you? How did everything go today?" and let the your pregnant partner divulge their blood sugars for the day at their own pace.

- When your partner reacts or comments to a blood sugar reading on your glucose meter, do you feel as though you're being judged and graded...or do you feel like they are part of your team, just observing the data together?
  - **FOR EXAMPLE:** If your partner currently says something like, "Wow, that's high. What the heck did you eat"? and that makes you feel horribly guilty, that is something you really want to express to them. The trick though, is expressing this in a way that teaches them what to say instead rather than just telling them to say nothing at all. There's a big difference between "Wow, what the heck did you eat?" and "Is there anything I can do to help you bring it down...like bring you a glass of water?"

- When you and your partner are eating meals together, do you feel as though the food you choose is impacted by the food they choose? Do you eat healthier or less healthy because of the way your partner chooses to eat?
  - **FOR EXAMPLE:** if you know your partner has a habit of bringing home fast-food when you're trying your darndest to eat healthier and cook more of your own meals, that would be a very good reason to have a clear conversation with your partner about not bringing home fast-food during pregnancy and at the very least, not bringing any home for you and eating that meal in the car before they get home. Or maybe you make an agreement together that you'll eat take-out once per week during your pregnancy as a treat and break from cooking, so it's clear and planned and gives

you a sense of control over your nutrition, rather than feeling like an impulsive decision.

- Do you and your partner make time for exercise together? Individually? Do you encourage each other to be more active or does one person tend to resent that the other chooses exercise over spending time together?
  - **FOR EXAMPLE:** If becoming more active has always been a struggle for you, would it motivate you to plan more exercise with your partner? Walking together for 30 minutes after dinner on Tuesdays, Wednesdays and Fridays? Joining a gym together? Meeting each other at the gym after work instead of at home on the couch?

- How well does your partner know your insulin doses? How to program your pump? How to support you during a severely high blood sugar or a severely low blood sugar? The little details of diabetes management that you know like the back of your hand…
  - **FOR EXAMPLE:** You certainly wouldn't expect your partner to know your insulin doses as well as you know them, but it might be helpful to just give them a little "insulin doses 101" lesson at the start of your pregnancy, writing down your current basal rates, insulin-to-carb ratios, correction dose ratio, and your total daily insulin. You could even keep the daily total on a note on the fridge, updating it each time you increase your doses just to keep your partner somewhat in the loop. You never know if you might have to go to the ER halfway through pregnancy from a bad stomach bug and your partner might need to communicate your diabetes management to the ER staff while you're under the weather and puking?

All of these questions and situations are simply to help you *think* about what areas of your diabetes management *and your relationship* you might want to change or improve, or at the very least just discuss with your partner. Do you and your partner need to score an A+ in every area of diabetes and health to be ready for pregnancy and parenthood?

Absolutely not!

But it might still be helpful to simply be *aware* of what areas aren't as solid merely for the sake of reducing as much risk as possible for stress or arguments or hurt feelings or frustration. You're a team, and as the one who actually has the baby in their belly and the type 1 diabetes along for the ride, you are the Team Captain.

HEY, BELOVED PARTNER: THIS SECTION IS FOR YOU!

Let's just get this one thing out of the way: while we won't specifically discuss foot rubs and pedicures...they are heavily encouraged!

Your partner's pregnancy with diabetes is going to be stressful in a different way for you, and perhaps even in a way that you wouldn't expect. You might be thinking, "Puhh-leeeze, I've never stuck my nose into my wife's diabetes management before. I've never stressed out about it. She's fine." But the moment she becomes pregnant you may suddenly find that you want to know what her blood sugars are while she was at work all day, while she was at dinner and desserts with friends, and especially while she's sleeping.

And that's okay—it's okay that you're concerned and that you care—but how you go about expressing your concern and care is going to either make things *more stressful* for you and your wife in your endeavor to manage diabetes during pregnancy or it'll make it less stressful.

Our goal is to help you create ways to express your concern without making your wife feel like she's being watched like a hawk, judged and scolded for "imperfect" blood sugars, or *nagged*.

The tricky part is this: **What feels like support to one person can feel like nagging to another.** What feels like plenty of privacy and space to one person can feel like *not enough* support to another. Together, you need to determine what that relationship looks like, and what you each need from that relationship.

CREATING YOUR DIABETES CONVERSATION GUIDELINES

Here are 5 conversations to have *together* to establish positive communication and the support you both need during pregnancy:

1. **"WHAT DOES POSITIVE DIABETES SUPPORT LOOK LIKE TO YOU?"**
Have you ever asked your partner what kind of diabetes support they'd like to receive during their pregnancy *or even prior to their pregnancy?* Maybe they have a hard time remembering to check their blood sugar before bed and they wouldn't mind having a reminder from you. Not only does this help them remember, it also takes one little task out of the *many* daily tasks of diabetes management off their shoulders.

Positive support doesn't just have to come in the form of you *doing* something for your partner, it can also simply be a conversation you have.

- Listening is absolutely the most valuable thing you can do for your partner. Not telling her what to do and giving her solutions, but letting her explain and talk out loud about the diabetes management challenges she's facing. By talking about them out loud, you're giving her a chance to think through what happened in a different light. By asking open-ended questions and continuing to listen, you may help her discover solutions to prevent or improve that diabetes situation in the future.

- Expressing major shock, disgust, or disapproval to a blood sugar reading that is *too high* or *too low* is only going to make your partner feel even more discouraged and guilty. Trust us when we say your partner feels enough guilt over blood sugars that are 5 mg/dL out of range as it is. Instead, offer support, a listening ear, ask them how you can help and if they would *like* help. And if you are truly, truly, truly concerned, calmly express that concern to your partner by encouraging them to seek help from their healthcare team or other resources rather than trying to beg or nag them to improve the habits that are negatively impacting their diabetes and pregnancy.

- Ask. Ask. Ask. Questions are always going to come off better than directions when you're both looking at a glucose meter with a less-than-ideal reading on it—but phrasing those questions is the tough part. Let's dig into this deeper...

FOR EXAMPLE, HERE IS A CONVERSATION WITH QUESTIONS THAT PROBABLY *DON'T* FEEL POSITIVE TO YOUR PREGNANT PARTNER:

"Hi honey! How was your day?"

"Stressful. My blood sugars were so f*%king annoying and stubborn today."

"Ugh. How bad were they? What'd you do? You've gotta stop doing that."

OR, A MORE POSITIVE VERSION:

"Hi honey! How was your day?"

"Stressful. My blood sugars were so f*%king annoying and stubborn today."

"Oh, I'm sorry. What can I do to help you?"

A SECOND EXAMPLE:

"Good morning, my love."

"Ugh, good morning. My blood sugar is 44 mg/dL."

"What! How did that happen? Why is it so low?"

(The snarky response would be: "Umm...because I have to measure out my own insulin because my pancreas doesn't work perfectly like yours! Roar!")

A MORE POSITIVE VERSION:

"Good morning, my love."

"Ugh, good morning. My blood sugar is 44 mg/dL."

"Oh, yuck. Can I get you a juice box?"

> **Remember:** Sometimes the most supportive, positive thing you can do is just ask an open-ended "How are you?" and listen. You don't need solutions. You don't need to do anything. Just listen.

The point at which you can get concerned and try to encourage your partner to think more deeply about the *cause* of that low is if they are happening frequently and becoming destructive to her day and she seems to have no control over preventing them. *But* it's important not to ask about those frequent lows or frequent highs when your partner is in the middle of managing one of those lows or highs! A human-being with a blood sugar of 40 mg/dL is not the kind of human-being you want to poke and prod with sensitive questions. And a human-being with a blood sugar of 250 mg/dL while pregnant feels enough guilt as it is in that moment. Let her numbers stabilize, let her feel better, then have that conversation.

In the end, diabetes management during pregnancy involves making constant little adjustments that are very hard to predict, so your partner *is* going to experience out-of-range blood sugars, but the frequency of those out-of-range numbers, and how destructive they are to her day, is what signals a red-flag.

2. **"HOW DOES YOUR DIABETES TECHNOLOGY WORK?"**
Preferably before she is pregnant, it would be wise to learn how all of her diabetes technology works *and* how to actually insert a new infusion site for her insulin pump or a new sensor for her continuous glucose monitor.

She might actually be very hesitant to let someone else step in on this part of her life—something she's been doing herself *to her own body* for years—but at a certain point in her pregnancy she may not be able to use the same areas of her body because of her growing belly. She may not be able to twist around enough to place a sensor in her upper glute or her thigh or her arm.

You may find yourself in the hospital during the last few weeks of pregnancy for induction or extra monitoring, etc. and she needs your help putting in a new infusion site. It's better to expect it and be prepared than encounter it and have no idea. (And, whether she likes it or not, it's always nice to find a part of diabetes management that you, the partner, can take on in an effort to lighten her burden.)

Tip: Use Youtube videos from the manufacturers of your technology to learn how to put it in properly for your partner!

3. **"WHAT ARE YOUR INSULIN DOSES?"**

While you shouldn't ever be in a position of managing all of your partner's insulin doses, you should know what they are (which will change constantly during pregnancy) so that you can help advocate for her when she is in the hospital ('cause believe me, you'll have to). Having two people adamantly saying *"Yes, I need two units of insulin for that banana!"* is going to come off much more firmly.

As her partner, you should also know her insulin doses in case there is a time when she can't speak for herself or is severely sick and needs to spend her energy breathing rather than explaining her diabetes management to an ER doctor.

Because these doses will change regularly, though, it will be helpful to have some kind of notepad where she makes her updates on dosage changes so that you always have access to those numbers. (Maybe there's an app for that?)

WORK TOGETHER: IT'S THE BEGINNING OF YOUR PARENTHOOD JOURNEY!

In the end, you and your partner are going to be "working" together on parenthood for the rest of your lives, and that parenthood journey really begins the moment you decide you want to even *try* to become pregnant. The moment that decision is made is that same moment that your diabetes becomes "everybody's diabetes" to a certain extent because those blood sugars are going to directly impact everyone involved: the mama, the baby and the partner!

Let the people who love you find a way to support you!

NOTES

MONTH 1
I THINK I AM...I THINK I AM...I THINK I AM!

Consider yourself normal if you are overwhelmed with frustration that you can't yet prove whether or not you're actually pregnant this month. A cruel, cruel waiting game that a woman could never understand until she's waiting on the confirmation of her own child's existence.

(For the record, that emotional waiting game counts if your own child is growing in the body of another woman, too! Or if you're waiting to hear your child was born from another woman, or if you're waiting for your child to arrive on an airplane to meet their new parents. However that child comes into your life, you know that one-of-a-kind waiting game.)

Try not to waste too many paychecks on bulk orders of pregnancy tests... in fact, if you just can't help yourself, at least save a little cash by using those cheap ones at Dollar Store. Sometimes the only way to relieve a little of that waiting game anxiety is to pee on a damn stick each morning.

MAMA'S MENTAL HEALTH

Below, you'll find a letter from Sarah, a.k.a. Sugabetic. Sarah is a type 1 and a mother of two. She's the go-to patient-resource for all things in diabetes technology (she's worn every pump that exists), and she's also just a regular gal like you and me. Sarah's letter is speaking to you the new mother-to-be even if you haven't gotten that positive pregnancy test yet, her words are worth hearing as early as possible in your pregnancy journey.

Dear New Type 1 Mama-to-Be,

So, you've found out that you're expecting a new little bundle of joy! Congratulations! I'm sure you're a bundle of nerves yourself.

It is completely normal for the nerves, worry, and panic of what a pregnancy for those living with diabetes can have in store—I know, I've experienced this twice myself—but I have to tell you, the biggest thing I learned between my first and second pregnancies is to be sure to take time to enjoy your pregnancy!

Sure, your pregnancy will be inundated with loads of appointments, tightened blood glucose requirements, and the carb-counting strategies of a carb-guessing ninja, but don't let all of this take over your experience of growing a tiny little miracle inside of you. Take a step back and be in awe of how pregnancy can teach you new things about your body, not just it's abilities to grow, but also to adapt to the stresses of such an awesome experience.

I didn't do this with my first pregnancy. From the day I found out until the day he arrived, my mind was overtaken with fear of the unknown. The fear of every high blood sugar, the fear of every missed carb-count, the fear of every little thing I was doing was going to hurt my baby. The fear that when he arrived, he would not be healthy, and the fear of knowing that I would have to live with that guilt took over me and I did not enjoy my pregnancy, and I regretted it later.

I still remember when he was born, and he had to be in the NICU because his sugar was too low for a day or so. I cried and cried. It was the worst low I had ever felt in all of my life with diabetes. It wasn't until the NICU's head physician came by and rested his hand on my shoulder to tell me that he was perfectly fine—no problems at all… and if he hadn't known it from his chart, he would have never known that my son was born to a mother with diabetes—it wasn't until this moment that I was able to let go of all of those emotions… and BOY did they let go! CUE the tissues!

I swore from that moment that if we decided to have another child, I would enjoy my pregnancy. Sure, I would still have to be vigilant, I would still have to be super careful about blood sugars and carb counts and all of the things that go along with being pregnant and being a person with diabetes, but I wouldn't let it completely envelop me and my emotions toward my growing child.

Four years later, I had that opportunity, and let me tell you, it was the best thing I could have ever done. Yes, it was still stressful, but I made sure to do things to help lessen the stress. I talked about it with more of my family and let them know the real emotions I had rather than keeping them to myself. I spoke more openly at my endocrinologist and OB-GYN checkups. If I became too stressed over the numbers, I didn't hesitate to let my endo know. I didn't try to handle so much of it myself. You're already a superwoman for carrying a tiny human, why try to prove it even more by handling the pregnancy own your own as well? Of course, part of it may have just been the difference between experiencing the first pregnancy versus the second one, and I knew more of what to expect.

Since I can't go back to my 26 year old pregnant self and tell her it will all be ok, I'm passing this little bit of comfort along to you. Take it. Hold on to it. Hug it. Take a deep breath, shed a few tears (ok, a lot), and scream at times if you must, but most of all, don't forget to enjoy this time.

It's short, and it goes by so quickly.

Sincerely,
Sarah
Sugabetic.me
DiabetesDaily.com

___

NUTRITION & FITNESS

Since fetal development starts before you can even confirm your pregnancy, you've taken some great steps up to this point to make sure you've given your baby a start in the right direction by taking a prenatal vitamin and getting lots of veggies into your diet.

In these first few weeks, the main features of your baby are being set up in the early weeks of pregnancy—the organs and spine are forming (folate/folic acid is a major player here!) and the limbs are budding. Iron and calcium are major players right now, too.

Thankfully, there are a lot of great nutrients that you can get from eating a good variety from vegetables, fruits, nut, dairy and protein/meat. However, if your cravings have already kicked in and your food aversions are present, too, green vegetables might actually be one of the last things you can bear to eat. That's okay—many women find vegetables an incredible turn-off during the first trimester. You can help compensate for this by taking that prenatal vitamin every day!

No matter what, remember your goal: mostly clean & consistent nutrition. It doesn't have to be perfect, but if at least 80 percent of what you eat are whole foods that you prepared yourself, your body and baby will thank you.

As women with type 1 diabetes, this means that we should try to be creative when attempting to satisfy those early cravings. If your body is desperately craving salt, that doesn't mean your only option is greasy potato chips! Consider healthier foods that contain salt such as nuts, salted cucumber, or even a gluten-free cracker like sea salt rice crackers! Even a processed cracker is going to leave you better off than a bag of potato chips.

- banana or apple with peanut butter
- 1 fruit with a handful of nuts
- rice crackers and nut butter
- 5 thin slices swiss cheese and fruit
- 1 scoop protein powder with unsweetened almond milk & peanut butter
- 2 eggs and a choice of fruit
- 1 avocado with salt…and a spoon!
- 2 rice cakes with avocado spread on top (and hot sauce!)
- 3 frozen breakfast sausage, microwaved/sauteed
- plain greek yogurt mixed with fruit
- plain greek yogurt with fresh berries/stevia
- plain greek yogurt with nuts/seeds
- small bag of nuts and a string cheese
- nuts and small scoop of chocolate chips
- veggies and hummus
- veggies and salad dressing to dip

WEIGHT–GAIN & CALORIE RECOMMENDATIONS

Yes, you're eating for two, but the newest human in this duo doesn't need much more than you're already consuming. Instead of trying to eat more during the first few months of pregnancy, it can often to be helpful to actually think about just consuming a normal amount and focus on getting those calories from good quality sources.

It's very easy to overeat during pregnancy, largely because of your gradually increasing appetite, sure, but also because we've all been taught by society that pregnant women should eat a lot! When you have type 1 diabetes, and insulin resistance is already inevitably challenging during the second half of pregnancy, being thoughtful and wise about your increased calorie consumption and weight-gain is especially helpful!

Most women who start a pregnancy at a healthy bodyweight need about 250 to 300 extra calories per day to ensure adequate baby growth and supply enough energy for mother's health. This increase will account for a total 25 to 35 pound (11.3 – 15.9kg) weight-gain over the course of the entire pregnancy.

For a woman who begins her pregnancy overweight, the weight-gain recommendation is a bit less at a total 10 to 20 pounds (6.8 – 11.3kg) by the end of pregnancy.

For a woman who begins her pregnancy underweight, weight-gain recommendations can vary as much as 30 to 40 pounds by the end of pregnancy.

In the end, it's about being thoughtful with your choices around food. You don't have to be perfect! If you want to eat a slice of cake, there's nothing wrong with that...but at least be thoughtful about eating that slice of cake by trying to count the carbs, take the appropriate amount of insulin, keep your serving-size in-check, and check your blood sugar frequently after eating it. And take notes so you're even better prepared to dose your insulin for that slice of cake if you choose to eat it again: how many units did you take, how long did you take your insulin before eating, and what was your blood sugar
an hour and two hours after eating?

FATIGUE VS. EXERCISE

Whether you were a Crossfit enthusiast, a runner, an average gym-goer or someone who just loves going for walks, finding the right type and amount of exercise for you during each stage of your pregnancy is important.

As women with type 1 diabetes, zero exercise isn't a wise idea, of course. On the other hand, don't be too hard on yourself if one of your friends was able to run half-marathons throughout her entire pregnancy, and you're struggling to stay motivated for daily walks. Everyone is different— but the most important that is that you keep moving somehow, each day. (Dancing to Justin Bieber in your kitchen counts, too! We won't tell!)

Well, if the fatigue of pregnancy has hit you already, you might start to realize just how tired your friend really felt! Now, we're not saying everybody is going to stop doing their favorite workouts, but don't be surprised if you need to make adjustments.

Yes, you want to push through the fatigue to a certain extent, because sitting on the couch all day for the next 9 months is definitely not going to benefit you in anyway, but, on the other hand, you need to listen to your body, too.

Your body is telling you, loud and clear: "I need more rest than I used to need!"

Things to consider when you adjust your workout routine:

- If you used to exercise for two hours a day, you may need to cut down to one hour a day.
- If you used to do hill-sprints and HIIT workouts, you may need to do go for a light jog and do your HIIT exercises but without the time-constraining intensity of a normal HIIT workout.

- If you used to lift heavy weights for an hour a day, 5 days a week, you may need to cut down to light/medium weights for 45 minutes a day, 3 days a week. And then add in walking on the days in between.
- You may just need to walk. Walk. Walk. Walk.

Listen to your body. The fatigue is there for a reason: your body is doing an amazing thing right now! It's creating life. It's creating eyes, a head, a liver, a pancreas, bones, feet with adorable little toes! The list goes on! It's an amazing thing. So give your body rest with a balance of physical activity that doesn't leave you in a heap of tears because you're so exhausted by the end of the day. If all else fails, go for a walk.

INSULIN MANAGEMENT

This month's changes in insulin needs are fairly simple: within a few days of becoming pregnant (but long before you can prove it with an at-home test) you'll likely see your blood sugars rise and sit stubbornly 100 to 200 mg/dLs above your normal range. This is because of the sudden change in hormone production your body is now experiencing.

EXPECTED INSULIN ADJUSTMENTS

BASAL/BACKGROUND INSULIN DOSES: For most, a slight increase in your background insulin doses will do the trick. Remember, when making adjustments in your background insulin doses, always start with an increase no greater than 1 to 2 units, then wait a day or two to increase again if necessary.

On average, you will notice they need about a 20% increase in their total background insulin dose. To calculate your 20% increase, you would take your current total daily dose (example: 30 units) and multiply it by .20 (example: 30 units x .20 = 6 units). This means that you can anticipate an increase in your background insulin dose by about 6 units. Again, this is an average.

TDD x .20 = the number of units that equals a 20% increase

Jenny, for example, had an average increase in insulin needs in the first trimester of her first pregnancy, but she also experienced significant insulin resistance and much higher increased insulin needs during the beginning of her second pregnancy.

Ginger had a very average increase in her insulin needs during her first pregnancy, and a little lower than average for her second pregnancy. You have to watch the fine details and adjust based on the evidence of your blood sugar, taking the dose you personally need to attain healthy blood sugar levels for you and baby.

OTHER DOSES: Most likely, your other doses such as insulin-to-carbohydrate ratios and correction factors won't need any adjustments if your basal background dose is accurate.

Over the course of the next few weeks, now that the pressure is really on, you're going to become acutely aware of whether or not your blood sugars are where you'd like them to be. This means that you're also going to become acutely aware of whether or not you're getting enough insulin. This brings us to the on-going, non-stop chore of assessing your insulin needs.

Remember: During pregnancy, you want to make a change in your doses after seeing a trend of higher or lower blood sugar levels over the course of two days rather than three or more days when not pregnant. It's also important to never make increases of more than 1 to 2 units in one day. Make an adjustment of up to 2 units, assess its efficacy over the next day or two, and adjust again as needed. Within each trimester, you will likely see a total increase in your basal/background insulin needs of anywhere between 3 to 7 units. Those with higher levels of insulin resistance and weight-gain will see the greatest increases in their insulin needs.

Let's take a closer look at 7 helpful things to keep in mind for the entire rest of your pregnancy (and your entire future as a person with type 1 diabetes!) that will help you determine if it's time for an adjustment in your background insulin needs.

7 THINGS TO REMEMBER WHEN ADJUSTING YOUR BACKGROUND INSULIN

Throughout most of your pregnancy, your background insulin is only going to increase (we talk about when it will likely decrease in Month 2). You will be increasing your background insulin often: sometimes once in a week, sometimes twice in one week, and some weeks not at all. Learning when and by how much to change your background insulin comes with a few guidelines:

1. Having a lot of low blood sugars can actually imply that you need more background insulin. If your blood sugar is constantly high after meals, and you're constantly trying to correct it with small correction boluses, you can wind up having a tremendous amount of lows because of stacking meal boluses on top of correction boluses. Be aware of this quirky issue throughout your entire pregnancy: ask yourself, am I having all these low blood sugars because I keep trying to correct highs? Probably time to increase my background insulin doses!

2. Never increase your total background insulin dose by more than 1 to 2 units in one day. This means that even if you're on a pump,

you want to look at the total basal insulin before making any adjustments, and then make sure that you're adjustments didn't add up to more than a 1 to 2 unit increase. If, over the next day or two, you're still seeing your numbers settling higher than your target range, you can make an additional increase by 1 or 2 units.

3. Don't be afraid to make changes. One unit up or down isn't going to ruin your blood sugars entirely, but a simple 1-unit increase could actually solve the issue of blood sugars running generally higher than you'd like.

4. If you're on an insulin pump, keep in mind that the insulin you get between the hours of 8 a.m. and 11 a.m. (for example) don't just impact your blood sugar between 8 a.m. and 11 a.m. Rapid-acting insulin stays in your system for up to 4 hours as a bolus. For basal, any change to the rate (for those on a pump) will have impact at least an hour to 2 hours after that rate change. This means that the insulin you got in your basal rate at 10 a.m. is going to impact your blood sugar all the way until 11 a.m. or 12 p.m. Therefore, when making adjustments, remember to look at the bigger picture of how your insulin is impacting you and at what times of day.

5. If you're on injections, keep in mind that some long-acting insulins are inconsistent. For example: 20 units of Lantus insulin might be what you need to keep your blood sugar from rising in the morning and evening, but it might be causing you to experience lows at lunch-time. This is a fairly normal issue merely because your dose can't be fine-tuned by the hour like basal rates in a pump, so some times of day will pay the price. What you can do though is decide if you'd rather take more insulin with your breakfast to combat the highs before lunch or reduce your background insulin dose which will leave you running a little higher at 8 a.m. which means you might have to take an extra little bolus of rapid insulin to prevent that high when you wake up at 6 a.m.

6. Just because you increased your background doses two days ago doesn't mean you won't need to increase them again two or three days later—especially during your third trimester. Don't get frustrated. Try to keep your mind open to the fact that everything is going to change constantly, and you're doing the best that you can.

7. Measure twice, cut once? Well, you know what we mean: double-check your doses before hitting "confirm" on your insulin pump. It's also a good idea, especially if you feel overwhelmed by how many different rates and times of day you have programmed, to write them down on paper so you can look at all of them together clearly before confirming those changes.

Now that you've got a fertilized egg on-board, you may find you're ready to commit to tighter blood sugar ranges in your CGM settings. Think carefully about what you personally can sustain and achieve without completely losing your mind and without sending yourself on a blood sugar roller-coaster ride every single day.

Ideally, we'd all be superstars and have our range set from 70 to 120 mg/dL. But if you don't feel your lows and hypoglycemia is a generally nerve-wracking issue for you, then your "low alarm" might be more appropriate at 80 or 90 mg/dL.

If staying under 120 mg/dL after eating a meal feels utterly stressful and impossible to you, think about changing your "high alarm" to anything between 130 mg/dL to 150 mg/dL. You might find after a couple weeks of aiming to stay under/near 150 mg/dL that you actually feel comfortable with lowering that high alarm to 140 mg/dL. And so on.

Yes, tight blood sugar control is ideal for your baby's development, but tight blood sugar control at the expense of mom's sanity and safety is not ideal for anyone.

THINK ABOUT WHAT IS RIGHT FOR YOU AT THIS STAGE OF YOUR PREGNANCY.

And remember: the number on your CGM isn't always accurate! Before taking correction doses of insulin for high numbers or eating for low numbers, confirm that number with your glucose meter.

AT THE DOCTOR'S OFFICE

Depending on your personal health background and the medical team you're working with, you may be asked to schedule an appointment to come in as soon as you become pregnant. This would usually happen if you are working with a high-risk maternal fetal medicine department.

The general standard for all pregnant women when you're working with a regular OB-GYN team is that you'll call after that first positive pregnancy test and schedule an appointment for when you're 8 to 10 weeks along in your pregnancy.

Of course, if you suspect any types of issues or problems, you should request to visit your doctor right away. Listen to your gut and get the support you need.

Very recent research has recommended that most women start taking 81 mg of asprin (1 baby asprin) once per day either prior-to or at the start of pregnancy to significantly reduce your risk of pre-eclampsia and other conditions. Ask your healthcare team if this is a good idea for you.

Otherwise, you've just gotta wait for that first exciting appointment!

GINGER'S PREGNANCY DIARY

PLEASE READ: This next section, titled "Ginger's Pregnancy Diary," is a section you will find at the end of every month chapter in the book. The goal with this diary was to share real-life diabetes management effort and obstacles and problem-solving. It's important to remember that these notes are about my pregnancy, not yours. While the science of all our bodies is ideally the same, our insulin needs and how we react to different foods, exercises, and phases of pregnancy are very different. My pregnancy diary is not medical advice, but I do hope it inspires you to do your own problem-solving when your blood sugars aren't cooperating. Don't get mad....get clever with you how you adjust and dose your insulin!

MONTH 1

WEEK 1-4: I have no idea when I ovulated. Despite using both an ovulation kit and basal body temperature testing, it appeared to me as though I hadn't ovulated at all...and so I assumed it was totally unlikely that I'd actually manage to get pregnant at the end of May. I was so sure it wasn't possible that I stopped thinking about it, and was bummed that I'd have to wait until my next expected ovulation date in June.

It turns out that I actually ovulated far past when my period app told me I would, which is why the ovulation test wasn't very useful!

Sure enough, a few days after when I now realize I ovulated, I kept spiking up over 200 mg/dL, sometimes as high as 250 mg/dL for no apparent reason. By this point I had already spent a great deal of time testing my basal rates and making sure everything was where it needed to be to maintain an A1C at or below 6.0 percent. But these insane spikes that persisted three days in a row—especially in the middle of the night when I hadn't eaten in several hours—had me puzzled...and incredibly irritated.

At first I blamed myself. I had eaten ice cream two nights ago...maybe it had a delayed impact on my blood sugar...even though I'm not exactly new to the task of balancing my blood sugar around Haggen Daz' Strawberry Ice Cream, and I'd never had this kind of trouble with it before.

But last night, I ate a very clean, low-carb, and wholesome dinner around 7 p.m. My blood sugar was around 110 mg/dL when I went to bed. Then by midnight, my blood sugar was up over 250 mg/dL. And these highs would hardly budge in response to any specifically calculated correction doses of insulin. I had to take twice the normal amount of insulin I'd usually need.

AND THEN IT DAWNED ON ME: OH! I MIGHT BE PREGNANT!

When I took a step back and really looked at when the highs were happening, it was whenever I went longer than 3 hours between taking fast-acting insulin injections for meals, which tells me that my background insulin dose wasn't doing its job.

This of course was before I had hired Jenny as my pregnancy coach, so I did a little searching and found a wonderfully specific article that explained how women with type 1 diabetes generally need a 20% increase in background insulin due to the rising level of progesterone and hcg hormones that the body starts producing during the first month of pregnancy.

I raised my Lantus insulin dose from 17 units to 20 units and voila! My blood sugars came back to hanging out between 70 to 120 mg/dL between meals. (Just to be clear, I definitely still saw my blood sugars go up between 140 to 170 mg/dL right after meals, this first month, if they were a carb-quantity I couldn't count or if I didn't take my insulin soon enough before eating, but with a small correction dose I was able to get them easily back into my ideal pregnancy range.)

Considering most women don't notice much or any symptoms during the first month of pregnancy—and it's too early to show up on an at-home pregnancy test—this consistent rise in blood sugar and increased need in background insulin is one of the benefits to being a type 1 diabetic mama-to-be.

HERE ARE THE FIRST SYMPTOMS I PERSONALLY NOTICED:

FATIGUE

The other symptom I noticed was fatigue. Now, because of my fibromyalgia, feeling totally exhausted isn't a rarity for me, but with fibromyalgia fatigue I can take an hour-long nap and usually feel significantly better. Fibromyalgia fatigue also tends to carry a dose of depression and dysfunction with it, but this fatigue was very different. With this fatigue, I found I could sleep for 3 hours in the middle of the day if I let myself, and I'd wake up feeling just as tired as I did before the nap. Emotionally, I felt perfectly content. I simply wanted to sleep.

The solution? I never found one. I did find that not every day felt like this. More like every other day. I continued exercising and tried to schedule time for a 45 minute or hour-long nap on the days I felt truly wiped out. I had already cut caffeine out of my diet 6 months or so before trying to get pregnant (for both the sake of fibromyalgia and pregnancy), so turning to coffee was not an option.

CRAVINGS

And then...the craving. I've made a very purposeful effort to eliminate all artificial sweeteners from my diet for several years now. When I had last tasted an artificial sweetener it tasted like absolute chemicals to me instead of the flavor I used to love and drink quite often in my teens and early 20s. Today, normally, you couldn't pay me to have a sip of a drink flavored with aspartame or sucralose.

But all of a sudden, I wanted a Diet Coke. What? Where is this coming from? I haven't had a diet soda in several years! Why on earth would I want this? There's no nutritional benefit. Nothing my body is seeking in a diet soda that would actually benefit my body in any way...but the craving wouldn't stop. I went three days ignoring it, and then I drove to the store and bought one. I was hoping I'd take one sip and think, "Bleh! My body was lying to me! I don't want this!" but instead, I guzzled it down quickly and loved every sip.

And that was the last one. I still crave it daily but I refuse to put that in my body. I don't know why my body thinks it wants this, and frankly, I have to not care, because logically, I know the ingredients in that product are absolutely not something I want in my body, let alone my growing baby's body.

On another note, I also started eating romaine lettuce like crazy. One day I ate 2 huge salads in a row (seriously, in a bowl the size of my head) with a homemade dressing and I would've eaten another one if I hadn't run out of lettuce. Fortunately, that's a craving I'm happy to indulge.

HUNGRY

In addition to that silly diet soda craving, I simply noticed that most days I am truly hungry. One morning I even woke up at 5:30 a.m. (90 minutes earlier than my normal schedule demands), because I was so hungry I desperately wanted to make myself breakfast. Even my husband noticed that one!

Normally, I can easily put off eating breakfast until 9 or 10 a.m. (Not ideal, but my body is rarely hungry in the morning these days, possibly a result of fibromyalgia). And it would usually be a small low-carb breakfast of either eggs or all natural pork sausage.

But this hunger wanted every macronutrient: fats, carbs, and protein. I found myself eating 2 eggs on gluten-free raisin bread with a slice of melted Swiss cheese almost every morning for two weeks straight. Fortunately, the hunger wasn't an overeating kind of hunger, instead it was just an obvious voice in my head saying, "You cannot go too long without eating! And you better not forget breakfast, missy!"

HELLO, LITTLE EMBRYO?
ARE YOU REALLY THERE?

Congratulations! So you've confirmed your pregnancy with an at-home-test and your partner can't help but smile every time they look at you—with an extra little twinkle in their eye. Things are getting exciting!

You may find it's sort of hard to believe you're really pregnant—even if you're experiencing a variety of classic symptoms. The hardest part, particularly for those of us with type 1 diabetes, is that the reality of the positive pregnancy test means we've really gotta get down to business in our blood sugar management.

Now, get ready for another mini-pep-talk. (Pep-talks, by the way, are something you should feel free to give yourself regularly throughout the next year, whenever you need to!)

In addition to the overwhelming excitement and joy (and possible nausea) that most pregnant women feel in this early stage of pregnancy, we know this news also comes with an overwhelming responsibility.

As we prepared and practiced for pregnancy, we could slack off a little here or there because it was just practice. But now it's real. Now our blood sugars no longer impact only our body but also the body of that growing little embryo. If the pressure to be the impossible "perfect diabetic" was heavy enough in ordinary life with diabetes, that pressure can feel much heavier now.

Simply the sight of the positive test may be all the motivation you need to apply as much discipline and routine to your diabetes management as possible, but you might also find that getting your "head in the game" so to speak might require a little pep-talk, a "start-day," or the support of someone else.

Regardless, remember that even though there's no better time in your life to be obsessive about your blood sugars than while you're pregnant, you don't have to be perfect in order to be doing a great job and in order to experience a safe and healthy pregnancy.

MAMA'S MENTAL HEALTH
THE PRESSURE TO BE PERFECT DURING PREGNANCY

As if the pressure to be "perfect" in life with type 1 diabetes isn't intense enough, adding pregnancy to the recipe can really push your diabetes-management-stress-levels over the edge.

In our non-pregnant diabetic life, a blood sugar of 200 mg/dL is obviously "higher than ideal" and can be tedious to see on your glucose meter, but in pregnancy it's easy to see 200 mg/dL on the screen and feel like the worst mother in the world. And the baby's not even born yet!

First, you should know that it's totally and completely normal to experience both a) frustrating blood sugars during pregnancy and b) frustrating feelings of momentary failure during pregnancy.

It's hard to imagine that you could possibly achieve your pregnancy A1C goals if your blood sugars aren't constantly near 100 mg/dL, but it's important to remember that even though high blood sugars will happen— because even the most obsessive, diligent diabetic can't predict hormonal fluctuations, slowed digestion, and weekly changes in your insulin needs— as long as your blood sugar isn't high all day long and you're quick to take corrective action (insulin or exercise) for the highs you do experience, the majority of your blood sugar levels throughout the day can still be within target range!

So...how can you tackle that guilt and frustration?

Early in your pregnancy, try to create a habit of how you talk yourself through those moments:

1. Take a deep breath! Every time you see a high blood sugar on your meter, take a deep breath. Or three. Whatever it takes to help prevent you from overreacting to the number and get you back into a thoughtful state of mind. (Yes, this is a lot harder than it sounds!)

2. Take your corrective insulin dose (based on a logical calculation and not an emotionally driven calculation!) and set a timer for 90 minutes. As much as we'd like to get that blood sugar down right now, it's important to give the insulin enough time to do its job before reacting again.

3. Repeat to yourself: "I don't have to be perfect in order to experience a healthy pregnancy!"

4. Contact somebody awesome and vent. Literally, think of someone in your life who "gets" diabetes whether they live with it themselves or not, and just vent a little. It might be a simple text message: "Arg! Today is so frustrating and my blood sugar is being a little %*&$#%!"

5. Ask for help. Are your latest blood sugar frustrations something that's happening day after day, or was it the result of a miscalculated carbohydrate count or another variable you're aware of? If the blood sugars on your screen are consistently out of target range for three days in a row, it's probably time for a few adjustments in your insulin doses. Even the smallest adjustment can have a tremendous impact! Contact your healthcare team!

6. Keep good records when you're having trouble. In order to make sense of the fluctuations in your blood sugar as the months roll by, it helps to log food, blood sugars, insulin doses and activity—especially around the times of day you're having the most difficulty staying in range. With these records, you'll be able to evaluate what is or isn't working well. One of the most important things to log, especially if you haven't ever before, is your food intake. Sometimes in pregnancy food will affect blood sugars differently because of slowed digestion. If you can establish a pattern around those specific types of foods, it will help take the guesswork out of how much insulin you need and help prevent any unwanted fluctuations.

NUTRITION & FITNESS

Food has probably been on your mind a lot since you became pregnant—perhaps even before you realized you were pregnant! Even though your body doesn't actually need more calories at this stage of pregnancy, your body is definitely going to be loud and clear about the calories it does need. Skipping meals or pushing dinner back a few hours is going to leave both your stomach and your growing little embryo desperately begging for food!

In your preparation for pregnancy, you may have been focused on improving your nutrition habits and choices or you may have been struggling and still find yourself trying to make improvements.

As we mentioned earlier in Month 1 and Preparing for Pregnancy, cravings are going to come and go, and everyone's cravings are different, but for those of us with type 1 diabetes, we really need to put as much thoughtful consideration into every bite we take because indulging in the wrong thing can leave us spending hours—if not the whole remainder of the day—trying to get blood sugar back into a safe and healthy range for the baby's development. Every bite counts.

In some ways, this make us more fortunate than our non-diabetic friends because we have an extra incentive to make healthier choices throughout pregnancy and it can help us resist that urge to eat every calorie-laden junk food item that crosses our path. You may find it's hard to resist at first but after a handful of experiences simply trying to get your blood sugar back in range, you'll hopefully find it easier and easier to say no to the cupcakes and opt for something healthier.

That being said, no one expects you to make perfect decisions throughout your pregnancy, but even when choosing to indulge in something delicious, being extra thoughtful about how you dose your insulin for that food and how much of that food you choose to eat can make all the difference in your overall blood sugars.

This is a topic we'll tackle in every single chapter because the way we feed our bodies has a tremendous impact on our blood sugars every single day.

MANAGING NAUSEA

On average, that nausea you've seen in just about every movie with a pregnant woman can strike around your 6th week of pregnancy. For some women, it can start barely a week after implantation, others may not experience nausea until week 8, and some of you lucky lady ducks may not experience nausea at all!

For a woman with type 1 diabetes, we have several extra concerns when it comes to nausea and vomiting.

Since the day of our diagnosis, we've been encouraged to take our insulin at least 10 to 15 minutes before eating for the sake of preventing that post-meal spike, but if that tedious nausea strikes and we lose our meal, that insulin has nothing to soak up, leaving us at risk for severe hypoglycemia. So severe, in fact, that may need more than just a juice box or two to bring our blood sugar back to up to a safe level.

Additionally, excessive vomiting can quickly throw the body into a state of diabetic ketoacidosis (DKA) because of dehydration combined with "starvation ketones," which on their own aren't necessarily an emergency but when combined with DKA from high blood sugar and dehydration, certainly don't help the matter!

Therefore, being extra prepared to handle any nausea or vomiting you may experience is key.

HERE ARE 5 WAYS TO PREPARE FOR AND DEAL WITH NAUSEA:

1. Frequent meals: First and foremost, eat more often! Smaller meals, more often, have shown to help prevent and alleviate nausea in pregnancy. Your body needs fuel to help that little embryo become a fetus, but because your digestion slows down early in pregnancy due to pregnancy hormones (which help your body extract all the necessary nutrients for you and your growing baby), you'll want to avoid eating big meals, as you'll just feel very full and uncomfortable for longer than your non-pregnant days (plus, there's not as much room in there with your uterus getting bigger each week!). Small meals and snacks, every 3 to 4 hours can help keep mild nausea at bay.

2. For mild levels of nausea, keeping ginger-based items such as ginger-lemon tea for brewing, ginger hard candies and ginger chews can settle a rumbling stomach. Other sources of glucose that are known for being gentle on the stomach include pedialyte, apple juice, and glucose tabs. Glucose tabs in particular can start to get absorbed when you chew them, so the glucose can get into your bloodstream more easily.

3. For moderate levels of nausea that include vomiting (and therefore the scary risk of severe hypoglycemia from active insulin on board that has no food to soak up, or on the other end, ketones because the body isn't getting any fuel from food) but, still allows you to keep at least some food and drink down, both glucose tabs and honey are gentle on the stomach, making them a smart way to soak up any insulin or any mild low blood sugars.

4. For severe nausea and the risk of severe low blood sugars, especially when you're unable to keep anything down, using a glucagon kit can be vital. The full dose in traditional glucagon kits are designed to treat severe low blood sugar in people up to 250 lbs. If you've ever used one in the past, then you probably know that a glucagon injection is likely going to leave your blood sugar sky high for hours and hours after its been administered—definitely not ideal in pregnancy! So, for severe low blood sugars during pregnancy, using only ¼ or a ⅓ of the solution in the glucagon kit depending on your body-weight can be a safe way to treat severe hypoglycemia during pregnancy, especially when you can't eat.

5. For extreme cases of persistent vomiting, Call your doctor to discuss options. There are several prescription medications that can be

taken. You can also ask your doctor about taking Unisom, a mild over-the-counter sleep-aid that happens to help with nausea, too.

6. A Drive to the ER: Last but definitely not least, having a friend or family member drive you to the ER to receive evaluation and possible use of IV with fluids and/or glucose. This is a wise and logical decision for a pregnant woman with type 1 diabetes! Refer to "Month 5" for tips on managing your type 1 diabetes at the ER and communicating your needs to the ER staff.

WHEN THERE'S NO SUCH THING AS "JUST A LITTLE BITE"

When you're trying to keep your blood sugar between 70 and 120 mg/dL for as much of the day as humanly possible, having "just a little bite" of anything will cause more trouble than it's worth.

During your non-pregnant days, it was no big deal to take a spoonful of that leftover apple pie on your way out the door to work. It was no big deal to grab a couple hershey kisses from the candy bowl on your co-worker's desk, or to munch on a small handful of cherries from the fridge while making dinner.

But when you're pregnant, those extra 8 grams of carbohydrate aren't so little anymore. Merely 8 grams of carbohydrate could raise your blood sugar 30 or 40 or 50 points! Merely 8 grams of carbohydrate could take you from that "perfect" stable 85 mg/dL blood sugar and leave you sitting at 139 mg/dL. Sure, 139 is a pretty awesome number in life with type 1 diabetes, but for a woman with type 1 diabetes whose body is working hard to make a baby, a blood sugar of 139 is considered high, and that 85 mg/dL will be desperately missed.

So there's no such thing as a just little bite. There isn't such thing as grazing or munching or a nibble here and there.

While pregnant women on T.V. are celebrated for impulsive eating decisions, we, as women with type 1 diabetes, have to think ahead. We need to have clear intentions: what are we going to eat, how much are we going to eat, and when are we going to eat it?

It's not easy. It might sound easy to an onlooker—"Oh, so you just have to know what you're gonna eat and take your insulin 10 minutes beforehand"—but in reality, in our culture, we eat in a rush. Even a pre-packed lunch for work doesn't come with the extra 10 to 15 minutes we need to take our insulin and then twiddle our thumbs until our body is ready for food. Instead, we work, work, work until the clock strikes the lunch hour and then eat, eat, eat quickly so we can get back to work.

NOT AN IDEAL SETTING FOR A PREGNANT GAL WITH TYPE 1

As tedious as it may be, the more you can establish control over what you're going to eat, how much, and when, the more success you'll have with your post-meal blood sugars. And learning this art sooner in your pregnancy is helpful because around month 5 and 6 your body is going to start needing more insulin, more time between when you take your insulin and when you take your first bite, and more thoughtful intentions when it comes to what you eat.

OVERWHELMING? Sure, but what if we take a step back and think of it as simply what it is: intentions. You don't have to do it perfectly all the time. You don't have to control every situation around food. You don't have to have everything planned out...but you can have the intention. With that intention, you'll hit the target more often. When life gets in the way and the target feels impossible to hit, you'll do the best you can afterwards to compensate, and then next time, you'll try that much harder to get back on track with your clear intentions.

Perfection isn't the goal...but effort and thoughtful intentions will go a long way.

A MUCH-NEEDED TIP FOR YOUR CRANKY DIGESTION SYSTEM
FEELING A LITTLE BOUND-UP?

The increased production of progesterone early in pregnancy is telling your digestion system to slow down. This helps to ensure that plenty of nutrients have time to be absorbed and make their way through the placenta before your body gets rid of all the waste. (More on how this affects your blood sugar later.)

One of the unfortunate side-effects of this natural pregnancy symptom, though, is constipation (and possibly hemorrhoids down the road). Sure, it's important to get plenty of fruits and vegetables in during pregnancy, but not only can that be hard based on any food aversions, it's also probably not going to be enough to conquer true constipation.

And the last thing we want to put in our bodies are a bunch of chemical-based laxatives.

And if you're thinking, "Maybe I can chow down on more vegetables to get things moving…" keep in mind that it isn't uncommon for pregnant women in the 1st Trimester to steer clear of vegetables. One possible theory for this veggie-aversion may be that fresh and raw vegetables are a natural source of bacteria and therefore unappealing to the pregnant body. (This is also why taking a prenatal vitamin is crucial, to ensure you're getting plenty of vitamins and minerals in a possibly bland diet.)

Instead, here are two simple things you can do to improve your digestion and find some relief:

1. Drink plenty of water consistently throughout the day. (This will be easy for many of you because pregnancy naturally increases your thirst—by the third trimester, you may feel constantly dehydrated even though you're chugging water all day long! Just make sure your thirst is leading you to good things, like water or tea, rather than juice or diet sodas.)

2. Get yourself a bottle of psyllium husk capsules. Psyllium husk is the natural fiber found in corn. They sell giant bottles of these capsules at wholesale stores like CostCo or BJs and are often labeled in big letters as "FIBER SUPPLEMENT." Be sure to look at the small-print and the ingredients, because you're looking for a capsule that is 100% psyllium husk and nothing else. Start gradually, taking 1 capsule in the morning and 1 capsule at night, until you increase the dosage to an amount you find helps you have at least one healthy bowel movement a day. By the third trimester, when hormones are even higher, you may find you need to up your fiber intake to keep things comfortable.

Note: the capsules do not work instantaneously. They can help move things along about 6-8 hours after being taken, which is why it's helpful to spread the dose 8 hours apart. If you find your natural bowel movement has turned into more of a diarrhea event, that means you're taking too much!

3. Iron can be another reason for constipation in pregnancy. Look for a prenatal vitamin without Iron. Despite an increase in need for iron, more often that is needed more in the 1st Trimester. If you have low iron stores, or just want to continue having iron as supplemental form look for one that is a liquid form which isn't constipating - such as Floradix.

INSULIN MANAGEMENT

This month is the first full and "true" month of pregnancy because the egg is implanted and your body is fully aware that its pregnant now. (And you're fully aware thanks to the exhaustion and the nausea you might be relishing at this point!)

By now, you may have increased your insulin doses a little bit, or you may have not needed much of an increase at all. You may be eating less food because of nausea and that balanced out the slight increase you might've needed in your background dose due to increasing hormones! Everyone is a little different.

The general rule of thumb, however, is that you'll see a small increase in your background insulin doses during these first 6 weeks.

And then, the next few weeks to come will get a bit more complicated.

EXPECTED INSULIN DOSE ADJUSTMENTS

While this section will be simpler to explain in future chapters, we're going to really dig into all the details of the upcoming weeks and how they're going to impact your insulin needs.

> * *Remember: During pregnancy, you want to make a change in your doses after seeing a trend of higher or lower blood sugar levels over the course of two days rather than three or more days when not pregnant. It's also important to never make increases of more than 1 to 2 units in one day. Make an adjustment of up to 2 units, assess its efficacy over the next day or two, and adjust again as needed. Within each trimester, you will likely see a total increase in your insulin needs of anywhere between 3 to 7 units. Those with higher levels of insulin resistance and weight-gain will see the greatest increases in their insulin needs.*

OH MY GOODNESS, I'M PRODUCING....INSULIN!

Starting at any point between 6 to 10 weeks, it is likely your body is going to start producing some of its own insulin again. Yup! You read that right! Go ahead and read it again just to make sure it really sunk into your beautiful diabetic noggin'.

You are going to start producing some of your own insulin.

THERE ARE TWO REASONS THIS HAPPENS:

THE FIRST REASON is that as soon as you become pregnant, your body begins producing more progesterone, which is what causes that initial rise in your blood sugars due to insulin resistance in the first few weeks of your pregnancy that we've mentioned in Month 1. Progesterone is initially produced by the corpus luteum—a component of the ovaries. However, around weeks 7 through 9, this progesterone production suddenly drops as the placenta takes over production of the progesterone, and thus your insulin resistance decreases as well. Some women experience a decrease in insulin needs that lasts for about 4 weeks, and others may experience this decrease for a shorter amount of time, or the decrease may be more subtle rather than dramatic.

THE SECOND REASON for low blood sugars in the coming weeks is that during your first trimester of pregnancy, the immune system actually starts to "back off" in order to protect your growing embryo. As lovely ladies with type 1 diabetes, our immune systems are usually constantly attacking and destroying the beta cells residing in our pancreas that are responsible for the production of insulin. Constantly. That means that as soon as the immune system backs off, there isn't as much of an attack on those remaining beta cells, and they can actually start producing bit of insulin which will bring injected or pumped insulin needs down.

AND POOF: We become semi-insulin-producing type 1 diabetics.

It's an amazing, awesome thing. (Now if only they could bottle it up and use it as a cure...wonder how our fellow male type 1 diabetics would feel about that one!)

Unfortunately, we don't start producing enough insulin to totally cover our body's needs, which means you still have to monitor your diabetes just as rigorously and be just as mindful of what you eat and the doses you take, but your pancreas is may actually (for once) be helping you out instead of totally abandoning you.

The challenging part of this awesome little miracle is that it will mean you can easily experience very low blood sugars that come on quickly until you and your healthcare team reduce your insulin doses accordingly to help prevent those recurrent lows. While it's a very cool thing, it can also be tricky and stressful because you'll be taking the insulin you normally need for your lunch and unbeknownst to you your pancreas is going to release a little insulin for that lunch, too. As women with type 1, we're not really used to insulin coming from anywhere besides our own syringes, pens, or pumps!

HOW MUCH INSULIN WILL I PRODUCE?

This is a tricky question because the answer is different for everyone. The possible production of insulin from your pancreas is going to start gradually, and the amount of carbohydrates you may be able to consume without taking a dose of insulin is going to vary from woman to woman. Factors that can affect just how much insulin your produce include body weight and overall sensitivity to insulin prior to pregnancy.

But even if your weight is healthy and your insulin sensitivity is high, you may experience very little of this insulin-producing phenomenon simply because your body may not have as many viable beta cells remaining. This could be due to the length of time you've had diabetes or just another one of the mysteries of type 1 diabetes, but regardless, don't panic or be too concerned if you aren't producing much.

Regardless of the changes in progesterone effect and how much insulin you miraculously begin to produce, you'll notice the amazing decrease in insulin needs through one or several of these symptoms:

- treat a low blood sugar (mild or severe), watch it rise to a nearly "perfect" level between 70 and 100 mg/dL (3.3 to 5.5 mmol/L), and then within an hour or so later, watch it start to drop again
- between meals, when no insulin doses for food are on-board, your blood sugar will suddenly begin to plummet—this can happen several times within one night or day until doses are reduced
- take your normal insulin dose for a meal, watch your blood sugar "flat-line" at/near non-diabetic levels on your CGM or glucose meter, then watch it plummet about an hour after eating

Some women will find they produce enough insulin that it is tremendously noticeable and the lows they experience are overwhelmingly low. Their newfound insulin production enables them to eat 10, 15, even 20 grams of carbohydrate without taking a bolus of insulin while seeing a very flat line in their blood sugars. Pretty nifty.

For others, the amount of insulin produced can be very subtle. The inexplicable lows will happen but once the background dose of insulin is reduced, these women may find they still need the same amount of insulin at meals and they can still experience high blood sugars just as easily if their dosage doesn't match the carb-count consumed.

The extra frustrating part of all of this is that there is no one-size-fits-all approach to adjusting your current insulin doses for the sake of this change in hormones and possible newfound natural insulin production. And it gets even more fun when that insulin production increases very gradually over the course of a week or even two weeks, rather than all in one day or two. Everyone is different!

There is no predicting how each of our bodies will respond to pregnancy.

HOW DO I ADJUST MY INSULIN DOSES FOR HORMONE CHANGES & NEW INSULIN PRODUCTION?

Of course, like all things in diabetes, insulin doses are very personal and specific from one person to the next, but there is a step-by-step process you can follow for determining your own insulin needs when you suspect your insulin needs have dropped in this time period. It is easiest to recognize due to recurring low blood sugars:

- FIRST, reduce your background insulin dose by no more than a total of 1 unit per day until you're able to prevent the recurrent lows. If you are on a pump, pay particular attention to the time of day when the lows are more prevalent.

- SECOND, if lows are more noticeable in the aftermath of a meal and bolus, increase your insulin-to-carbohydrate ratio by 1 to 2 grams ratio. For example: if you were using a 1:10 ICR (1 unit for every 10 grams of carb) you would reduce the amount of insulin being given at meals by increasing the number of carbohydrates in your ratio, making your new ICR 1:12 instead of 1:10. This means that you would be eating more carbohydrates with less insulin per each gram.

- THIRD, if lows still persist severely especially after meals, you may find you can skip your insulin dose entirely for 5, 10, 15 or even 20 grams of carbohydrate. Be sure to test this theory carefully with extra blood sugar monitoring until you're certain. You may also notice that lows occur around only one or two meals of the day rather than all of them. If this is the case, you can adjust your insulin-to-carb ratio around these meals instead of all your meals.

Unfortunately, as cool as this entire phenomenon sounds, it can be really frustrating because you're so used to managing your diabetes based entirely on the insulin you actually dose that it can be pretty aggravating and even scary to manage your diabetes when your pump or syringe or pen is not the only source of insulin.

But don't give up: if the lows persist this simply means you need to reduce your insulin doses further until you can sit steadily between meals and overnight between 70 to 120 mg/dL. One tiny adjustment of merely 1 unit of insulin less per day in your background insulin can make all the difference!

Some of you may find it's an easy adjustment because of how your body is responding to pregnancy and how it's begun producing insulin, and some of you may find yourselves desperately wishing you could fast-forward several weeks to when this freaky phase is less intrusive and more like a wonderfully temporary "vacation" from the usual demands of blood sugar management!

SO...HOW LONG WILL THIS AWESOME INSULIN-PRODUCING PHASE LAST?

Unfortunately, not all miracles are forever. You may also notice that lows occur around only one or two meals of the day rather than all of them. If this is the case, you can adjust your insulin-to-carb ratio around these meals instead of all your meals.

Starting at week 16, your insulin needs may start to increase, likely a little bit each week, throughout the remainder of your pregnancy. By the last couple of months of your pregnancy you could be taking anywhere from 1.5 to 3 times the amount of insulin you needed prior to being pregnant. And then, once that little baby arrives, your insulin needs will quickly decrease back to your original doses or even a bit less. This of course also depends on how much weight was gained during pregnancy and how quickly some of that weight comes off—just like normal weight-gain when you're not pregnant, pregnancy weight-gain that lingers postpartum will increase your insulin needs due to increased insulin resistance from increased body fat.

But we'll talk more about all of these details when we get there.

Meanwhile, enjoy getting an amazing kind of "help" that no one else could have possibly provided except for your own pancreas (and thankfully, your very reluctant immune system).

AT THE DOCTOR'S OFFICE

Most gals aren't invited into the doctor's office until 8 to 10 weeks, so depending on the protocol of your OB-GYN team, you'll either have a very exciting doctor's appointment this month to confirm your pregnancy or no appointment at all. But we do want to talk about another reason you may find yourself in your OB-GYN office earlier than 8 to 10 weeks: miscarriage.

MISCARRIAGE:
THE HEARTBREAKING EVENT THAT IS ACTUALLY VERY COMMON

You probably have friends who have experienced miscarriages, and you inherently understand how heartbreaking it can be, but experiencing it firsthand is an altogether different feeling. Sadness. Heartbreaking sadness is really the only words that really convey the pain of miscarriage.

As a woman with type 1 diabetes, it can be really easy to think that somehow you caused the miscarriage with an imperfect blood sugar, but the reality is that miscarriages can happen to anyone. More often than not, it has nothing to do with your diabetes.

The American Pregnancy Association (APA) says that most women have a 15 to 20 percent chance of experiencing miscarriage. 20 percent. That's a pretty significant percentage. In other words: miscarriages are actually quite common and are simply a natural part of the journey for many women. For women age 35 to 45, the risk is as high as 35%, and women over 45 years old have a 50% chance of experiencing a miscarriage.

Could your diabetes cause miscarriage? Yes, but likely only if your blood sugars are persistently high. DKA, blood sugars over 300 mg/dL (16.6 mmol/L) for days on end will put your pregnancy (and you) at risk.

But the average high blood sugar here and there? No, that's very unlikely related to a miscarriage you experienced. Instead, miscarriages are the body's way of saying, This isn't a viable pregnancy." Period. Typically early genetic reasons that the body can identify is the reason the pregnancy will not continue – there's nothing you have done to cause this.

When is it a concern? As with all women, if you experience 3 or more miscarriages in a row, the APA recommends talking to your OB-GYN team to identify any clear problems interfering with your ability to become and stay pregnant.

Don't lose hope. Many, many women experience miscarriage and go on to conceive and deliver healthy, beautiful babies!

MONTH 2
GINGER'S PREGNANCY DIARY

WEEK 5

Dear ridiculous body with 3 autoimmune conditions,

I just wanted to thank you, dear body of mine. Despite your issues, you've surprised me before, but this surprise is perhaps the best of all surprises: I'm pregnant. I can't make insulin. I can't digest gluten. I have weird, illogical pain in my joints and my bones and my muscles that stir up a slew of other weird symptoms...but I can do this: I can create life.

Thank you, body. You're full of surprises, and this is my favorite surprise by far.

With love and gratitude,
Ginger

WEEK 6

When your daily goal (and obsession) is to keep your blood sugar under 140 mg/dL at all times, the difference between waiting 4 minutes to eat after taking your insulin and waiting 15 minutes to eat is actually painfully significant. Halfway through week 5, my family came to visit, and nothing takes the control and consistency out of your schedule like hosting out-of-town company.

Not only was I juggling more things during the day as a host, I was eating foods I don't eat regularly—not necessarily junky or high-sugar foods, just foods I simply don't eat regularly, like watermelon. Turns out watermelon spikes my blood sugar like whoa, which I wasn't expecting—and will add to the "eat with caution" food list—but it definitely requires a good 15 minutes between insulin dose and actual consumption. The rest of my "eat with caution" list is simply grapes and cherries. Both delicious, and both fruits that spike my blood sugar faster than cotton candy! (Jenny refers to grapes as "sugar bombs." Based on how my blood sugar reacts to grapes, they might as well be Sour Patch Kids or Skittles!)

But these tiny little food details, I believe, are worth observing closely. Knowing which foods are easy to manage my blood sugar around and which foods require much more work and attention means I can choose more wisely when I need things to be simple, and I can choose the trickier foods when I know I have the time and patience to be ultra attentive, and when I don't have the ability to take my insulin 15 minutes ahead of eating. In some situations, that's harder to do than it sounds.

For instance, if you're eating in a restaurant, it can be very hard to know when the food is actually going to arrive at the table. Some restaurants are predictable while others are not, and the last thing I need is 6 units of insulin in my bloodstream when the food is still 20 minutes away from being served because the kitchen is backed up and the new busboy just dropped five dozen plates.

And of course, just to keep things interesting, there's also the rare issue of taking your insulin and waiting 15 minutes when it actually would've been better off taking my insulin immediately before eating because of the specific type of food and how quickly (or not quickly) it reaches the bloodstream!

THIS MONTH, I STARTED NOTICING TWO ISSUES WITH TAKING MY INSULIN TOO EARLY.

The first is when I eat the simple meal of two eggs and two slices of gluten-free toast—a meal I started craving and eating for breakfast the moment I conceived, perhaps because it's a good combination of fat, carbs, and protein. During the first few weeks of pregnancy, I had no trouble taking 3 units of insulin 15 minutes ahead of time for this meal and keeping my blood sugar in range. But around week 5 or 6, I noticed my blood sugar began plummeting 10 minutes within finishing the meal! And then of course, over an hour later, my blood sugar started spiking wildly up to 200 mg/dL.

What was causing the mess? Pregnancy was naturally slowing down my digestion system (as it does in all women, diabetic or not) and causing a very delayed breakdown and release of the glucose into my bloodstream because of the equal combination of both fat and carbohydrates. Fat naturally slows down digestion even when we aren't pregnant, and when you add that to the slow digestion of a pregnant woman, you can easily find yourself on an expected rollercoaster when you know you've taken exactly how much insulin you need for that meal.

This post-breakfast plummet followed by the spike an hour later occurred several days in a row —enough so that I knew there was a pattern and I could ask Jenny for help.

Jenny suggested I try taking 1 unit 10 to 15 minutes before eating, and the remaining 2 units about 10 minutes after eating. And presto, problem solved. (Jenny is brilliant.)

The other time this can happen is with a meal that is high in carbohydrates from vegetables.

Jenny explained that this is because the extra fiber in the vegetables (especially beans) can mean it takes longer for the meal to breakdown. So, when consuming vegetable-based meals—that aren't also high in starchy carbohydrates like rice or white potato—I can take my insulin dose closer to the time when I'm actually going to start eating rather than 15 minutes beforehand.

As far as cravings go, I'd say nothing major really hit in the start of this month except for the little voice begging for Diet Coke...which I must continue to ignore. The early morning hunger and the hunger between meals is getting stronger. I'm eating breakfast within 30 minutes of waking up and have definitely found that the low-level of nausea I've started feeling goes away as soon as I get two slices of toast with butter and two eggs into my belly.

But mostly, I'm just tired. Tired like...I don't want to get out of bed, and after my morning 45 minute walk with the dogs, I think about how much I'd love to get back into bed. But usually I resist the urge and try to do some low-key activity or work instead. Usually...well, okay, maybe like half the time. A nap can be so wonderful, you know.

WEEK 7

Who ate all the fruit? Oh, that was probably me. Peaches don't stand a chance in my home right now. I don't need all of them at once, but at least two peaches a day is what my body is begging for. Perhaps for the vitamin C, suggests Jenny (who is now referring to the baby as Peach).

I also must share that I've never wanted water so much in entire life. I've always been a devoted water drinker but now I keep a water-bottle-like container with me at all times and fill it up at least 5 times a day. Yes, I have to pee even more desperately, but my body wants that H20!

But I have to tell you, I'm really frustrated that I still haven't started producing insulin! It's week 7 for crying out loud! Hello, pancreas? Beta-cells? Please? Is it too late for my body? Am I past the point of no return? I know women who've lived with diabetes longer than I have and yet...they still produced insulin during their pregnancy. On the other hand, I haven't been puking so perhaps that's my trade-off? Did I trade "no puking" for "producing insulin"? I guess I should thank my lucky stars but I really did want to experience that insulin-producing phenomenon.

WEEK 8

A lot of things started changing this week. For instance, I hold my breath each time I open the garbage can. Then, as soon as I close it, I dash at least 5 feet away from it to prevent that post-trash-can smell that seems to linger even after it's closed from reaching my nostrils! Bleh.

My breakfast changed, too. For the past 7 weeks I've been eating toast and eggs every morning, but this week I don't want that anymore. I'm not sure if it's that I don't want that or I just desperately want to eat another peach, but I can't seem to go 5 minutes from the moment I open my eyes in the morning before I start thinking about how delicious my next peach or nectarine is going to taste. (Update: By the end of week 8, I have grown sick of peaches and have set my sights on oranges instead.)

And I'm learning repeatedly, it seems, that I cannot just "push back lunch an hour or two" just because I want to get a bunch of things done and can't be bothered to stop and eat. Merely pushing lunch back by 90 minutes consistently leads me to feeling as though my stomach is boiling and my throat is contracting, as though it's preparing itself for an upcoming hurl.

I've been prepping meats ahead of time by grilling 4 days' worth of steak or chicken, for example, and putting them in 4 small tupperware. Veggies are easy to prep by slicing up a lot of bell peppers on Sunday so I can easily grab them for lunch when I don't have time to cook other veggies like broccoli.

> **NOTE TO SELF:** you must must get food in every 3 hours! 4 hours is too long! 5 hours is unimaginable. Eat. Small meals. Often. You'll feel better! And p.s. I'm still not producing any insulin! Roar!

GINGER'S 2ND PREGNANCY

Note: This is the only entry of my 2nd pregnancy simply because I found out I was pregnant two weeks before the completion of this book! Read more about Ginger's 2nd pregnancy at DiabetesDaily.com by searching "Pregnancy with Type 1 Diabetes."

WEEK 5

We had been trying since early Spring of 2016 to get pregnant with our second bundle. And we tried all summer without any success. My period had become very irregular, some months 28 day cycles and other months were 31 or 33 or even 35 day cycles. I was frustrated and growing increasingly stressed with each month's arrival of my next period. I was telling myself to get ready for IVF or other fertility treatments, because surely, something was wrong.

So we decided that September to stop trying—to actually even make sure (mostly) that we didn't get pregnant—and instead wait until January so we could regroup, get our heads back into the right state of mind of feeling excited but relaxed.

I also decided to try switching from Lantus insulin to the newer Tresiba insulin once I knew I wasn't going to try to get pregnant. The switch was easy and definitely worth it. My dose was essentially the same, and I didn't have to deal with the acidic burning of Lantus anymore, or the 5-hour post-injection peak that often left me low at 3 a.m. However, several weeks into my pregnancy, I realized that my dose being the "same" may have actually been that many people need a 20% decrease in their Tresiba dose compared to their Lantus dose….and most pregnant women need a 20% increase in their basal dose shortly after implantation of an egg! So they could have cancelled each other out, and that's why I didn't notice a significant rise in my blood sugars shortly after conception.

Also in September, I decided to increase the "clean" part of my diet from 80 percent to 100 percent. I cut out all sugar, all dairy, and was preparing my meals, eating 5 to 6 times a day, and hoping the result would be that I could drop at least 5 to 10 pounds of the "squishy" that was on my belly. Despite being the exact same weight as I was before my first pregnancy, my midsection was squishier than I'd like. (In other words: I stopped eating dessert, and I started planning my meals ahead of time...and eating way more vegetables!)

Well by the end of September, I'd attributed my increased hunger between meals to the fact that I was eating so clean...but the scale hadn't budged. I was eating vegetables three meals a day, high-quality protein 3 times a day, and homemade bone broth from grass-fed beef. After breakfast of eggs, vegetables sauteed in broth-fat, and a cup of bone-broth, I was getting hungrier more and more as I waited for the arrival of my 2nd daily meal: a perfect honeycrisp apple combined with a handful of salted nuts.

When I woke up on October 1st feeling bloated like I was 6 months pregnant, and it was day 35 of my cycle with no period in sight, I decided to pee on one of those cheap little pregnancy strips.

Two lines. Pregnant. Holy...smokes.

Needless to say, the moral of my story is simply this: There's something to be said for letting go, relaxing, and letting life do its thing. Certainly, many women will face a heart-wrenching struggle during the pursuit of pregnancy—my heart goes out to you!—but if you're still in that first year of trying, take a deep breath, close that damn pregnancy app that keeps telling you when you ought to be shagging your partner, and just live life. At least for us, it worked much better that way!

HERE ARE 5 THINGS I PLAN TO DO DIFFERENTLY THIS TIME:

1. I'm not going to force myself to eat carbs (like gluten-free pasta) unless I truly want it. This time I'll make sure to eat at least 50 grams of carbs per day, but I won't make myself eat 100 like I did last time. As long as I'm eating lots of really healthy, whole foods and plenty of nutritious calories, baby will be happy! I'm sure I'll naturally eat closer to 100 grams per day than 50 grams, but I'm going to let my body decide that rather than the guidance of traditional OB-GYN textbooks.

2. I will ask for help with insomnia sooner! I struggled with insomnia big-time in my third trimester, and now in my first with baby #2 I'm already experiencing wicked insomnia. I didn't know last time that there are prescription-strength sleep-aids that are safe to take during pregnancy. Now I have a prescription for when my sleep is really out of whack or I've gone too many nights in a row with 4 or less hours of sleep.

3. I will speak-up sooner about who has the final say on insulin doses during delivery and postpartum. You'll read in the last entries of my pregnancy diary that I had to be a real b-....force...when it came to getting the insulin doses I knew I needed. This time I'm going to start this conversation during month 7 and really explain how many times I had to sneak extra insulin last time in order to keep my blood sugar in a healthy range. I also learned that I could've called the Patient Advocate Hotline and someone would've come to help me advocate for my insulin needs as an in-patient.

4. I turned off the alert on the my CGM that tells me if I'm increasing at a certain rate or decreasing at a certain rate. For me, those arrows just cause me to overreact and over-treat the blood sugar. Instead, I'll just use good old-fashioned blood sugar logic: when I'm low, treat with 5 to 8 grams, then another 5 to 8 if it's a severe low. Wait 15 minutes, treat again if necessary. With highs, take extra insulin if I'm rising only if I know I pre-bolused properly and I possibly ate something that contained a lot of processed carbs and thus could spike my blood sugar more than I expected.

5. Lastly, I'm not going to buy one of those damn Diaper Genies. They're tedious and fill-up too quickly. A good old fashioned trash can is not only sufficient, it's better! ☺

I'm still getting back into the groove of pre-bolusing for my meals. It is not my favorite part of this little adventure, especially with a nearly 2–year old to chase around. I can keep my A1C around 6.0 without much pre-bolusing effort—at least when I'm not pregnant because I don't eat many carbs—but if I plan to maintain an A1C in the mid-to-high 5s while eating more carbs, then I need to get back in this routine.

▎Okay, here we go again! Yahoo!

WEEK 6

Well, I took my CGM off last night. After 3 days in a row of crazy roller coaster blood sugars from 250 mg/dL down to 45 mg/dL and back up again, I needed to take that thing off. I've never had this problem quite so severely with CGM data, but man, this time I cannot handle it. And my blood sugars have been nearly perfect before I put it back on (I was off it for a couple months prior to learning I was pregnant) and now that I'm off it again, nearly perfect blood sugars resume.

I THINK IT'S A COMBINATION OF A FEW THINGS:

1. I have Lucy to care for now, so the sight of my blood sugar dropping makes me more anxious that it used to. I've never had concern with my ability to manage and treat a low, but I do have concern over managing and treating a low while I'm chasing my daughter down the driveway on her tricycle. And on the flipside, when I see it rising, I think in the back of my head I'm afraid it'll keep rising and I won't have time to notice and correct before it's too high—and I hate high blood sugars—and then it'll take all day to come down. So I'm over-treating the lows that were the direct result of taking too much insulin because I thought my blood sugar was spiking after a meal when it was really going to hit 145 mg/dL and come back within range. I mean, for the past 3 days, I was impulsively grabbing extra carbs I would've never needed because I was afraid my blood sugar was dropping.

2. I feel really confident in my ability to manage my blood sugars more tightly now because of my last pregnancy and everything I learned about managing my diabetes "super tightly" compared

to "average tightly." When I just use good old fashioned logic, thoughtful food choices, and intelligent insulin management, I have no problem seeing that my blood sugar is 75 mg/dL after a meal because I know that I took the amount of insulin I need for that meal. Why I'm getting so screwed up just because there's a screen with some delayed arrows on it, I don't know, but I don't think I need that screen nor the data right now.

I will likely put my CGM back on in a month or two—we'll see. But every time I checked my blood sugar today, before and after meals, I was between 70 to 100 mg/dL. I mean every time, and that's how my previous weeks were before I put my CGM back on, even more so after switching to Tresiba. So I'm just going to keep things simple until I see a clear reason to get more data by wearing my CGM again.

Why wear it if right now my blood sugars are exactly within my goals? I'm so relieved to take it off, honestly. I wouldn't have said that during my first pregnancy, but this one, I just don't need it the same way I did back then. Before getting pregnant with Lucy, I got my A1C down to 6.4 without a CGM, but getting a CGM is really what helped me getting to the 5s. After giving birth to Lucy, I've maintained an A1C around 6.0 with and without a CGM (I've taken several 3-month long breaks from it) because of what I learned about managing tight blood sugars during pregnancy. I just don't need it the way I used to.

Until the end of this week, I haven't had cravings as intensely as I did with my first pregnancy. I'm definitely not craving fruit like before, and even though I wake-up feeling hungry in the morning, I don't want to eat food like before either. But the cravings that have struck are for my homemade soup which is very boring: chicken broth, onions, carrots, celery, beans, and a variety of spices and herbs. I am starting to crave gluten-free pasta a little bit but I'm not actually making it for myself, only my kiddo, so far. Otherwise, I just want nutrient-dense, clean calories like my apple with freshly ground peanut butter, or two eggs with a giant bowl the deliciously boring soup...and steak. Oh, stead. (I also made tacos tonight and it was like whoa. So good. But that might have been because I barely had time to eat all afternoon besides a bowl of soup—which is pretty light—and an apple. I was chasing Lucy non-stop! This pregnancy will be very different for that reason alone!)

I'm feeling very queasy this week, especially when blood sugar starts dropping too quickly or cross the threshold to "low." And boy, when 4 p.m. hits, that's it. My brain is like, "Okay, I'm going to start shutting down now...but I'll stay halfway on so you can cook your family dinner, take your plethora of vitamins, and finish writing this book."

By the end of week 6, I'm happy to report that not wearing my CGM is continuing to work really well for me: staying within my target ranges without obsessing or stressing out, checking my blood sugar with my meter about every 2 hours, and using good old fashioned logic for eating and dosing. My husband was a little unnerved when I told him I'd take my CGM off but I assured him I'd put it back on as soon as I started needing more dramatic pre-boluses or if my blood sugars started being unpredictable and rollercoastering for several days in a row—a sign that I needed more data on a daily basis. And I'll definitely wear it in the last trimester. But right now, not wearing is working well for my sanity and my blood sugar goals.

WEEK 7

Ugh, I went nearly 4 or 5 days this week without eating vegetables because just looking at the raw broccoli in my fridge made my stomach churn. But I finally sauteed some frozen veggies (I recommend the higher quality choices from Costco!) and they were delicious.

I ate them up before I even at my steak. So I think that's the simple trick there this time for getting enough veggies in.

And I really want to just eat gluten-free bread from the moment I wake up, but I'm trying to resist the urge.

Nothing wild to report in terms of insulin doses changing. They've only gone up a few units since the beginning.

I think when I do finally put my CGM back on, I will turn it to "silent" so it isn't beeping at me. Instead, I'll just check it when I need to and that'll hopefully help prevent me from reacting too quickly to arrows or alert screens.

Next week is the ultrasound! On my 31st birthday!

NOTES

MONTH 3

OVERWHELMING BLOOD SUGAR OBSESSION

If you haven't already experienced at least a few days during which trying to achieve near-normal blood sugars felt not only impossible but also painfully agonizing...then you are not alone. If only we could all hire Jenny to just come live with us and manage our blood sugars for 9 months! Oh, that would be nice.

Alas, day-in and day-out it's up to us. Sure, husbands and wives and moms and friends can support us, encourage us, and help us...sort of. But in the end, we are the ones in charge. We are the ones who choose what and when we eat. It's up to us to be thoughtful about everything we eat and time every insulin dose as carefully as we can. It's up to us to treat low blood sugars mindfully, with just the right amount of carbohydrates to prevent a rebounding high. It's up to us to get at least a little exercise every day and keep our blood sugar in a healthy, safe range during that exercise. It's up to us to make good choices around food in the evenings to help ensure our blood sugars run smoothly and in-range all night long.

IN OTHER WORDS: there are a lot of little details that are entirely up to us.

But you need to know: rough days can happen. Rollercoaster days can happen. And just as you start getting used to the flux in hormones and some possible newfound insulin production and finally get your insulin doses adjusted to prevent all the lows...you'll start the next phase of pregnancy in which your insulin needs start increasing! We can't settle into any insulin routine for long because it's bound to change, at least slightly, each week.

And while we will each inevitably focus most heavily on the numbers we don't like, remember that you can still meet your A1C goals despite those frustrating hours, agonizing 2 a.m. highs, and rollercoaster days that all feel as though they're going to sabotage your big plans. We can work to make sure the highs aren't high for too long, and the lows aren't too low for too long.

The goal isn't 100% perfection, but instead working hard to help ensure that the greater majority of your blood sugars fall into your goal range and that you make adjustments with your healthcare team when you notice patterns in any low or high blood sugars. Don't forget to give yourself a little credit for all those in-range blood sugars!

MAMA'S MENTAL HEALTH

TEACHING YOUR PARTNER: HOW TO BEST SUPPORT YOU & YOUR DIABETES DURING PREGNANCY

If you and your partner already have a great tango when it comes to your life with diabetes and how they support you, that's awesome, and will probably continue to be awesome during pregnancy.

However if diabetes discussions or diabetes in general has never been an easy topic between the two of you, or perhaps there are certain aspects of diabetes that come between you, there's no better time to iron those out and try a new approach than during pregnancy. Sure, the real responsibilities day-in and day-out come down on your shoulders, but letting your partner support you and finding ways they can support can be helpful for both of you.

HERE ARE A FEW IDEAS AND ISSUES TO THINK ABOUT:

SHARING (AND TRAINING) IN DIABETES TASKS

Used to do everything yourself when it comes to diabetes? Even something you can do on your own, like placing a new CGM sensor, can help make the demands of diabetes during pregnancy feel more like a team-effort rather than a solo performance. Particularly in the third trimester, when you can't use your belly for infusion sites or cgm sensors, having your partner well-trained in placing these things can be imperative because you may find you just can't twist and turn like you used to! Making sure they know now how to apply those infusion sites and sensors, when you are fully able to teach and demonstrate, is going to give them plenty of time to practice before you really need their help.

CARB-COUNTING & OTHER FOOD DUTIES

Does your partner do a lot of the cooking in your household? Teaching them how to determine carbohydrate counts for the meals they're serving you could provide such a simple yet valuable reprieve from the carb-counting you do all day long.

Also in the realm of food, you may find that in addition to the foods you simply can't stand the sight of due to first trimester nausea, there may also be certain foods you just can't control yourself around that drive your blood sugars wild. Consider asking your partner to specifically not bring certain foods in the house because they're too tempting for you and cause too much trouble in your blood sugar goals.

HOW TO REACT TO BLOOD SUGAR READINGS & CGM SCREENS

It's their baby, too, right? So they do have every right to be concerned about high blood sugars and low blood sugars, but we need to provide them with ways they can express that concern that don't leave us feeling judged or embarrassed or guilty. (We're doing the best we can and we ain't perfect!)

3 THINGS TO HELP YOUR PARTNER REMEMBER:

- Panicking over a quickly rising blood sugar helps nobody. A high blood sugar here and there—even a high blood sugar for a few hours every day—isn't going to harm baby unless it's so high that you're both in need of hospitalization. High blood sugars are going to happen during pregnancy. It's impossible to prevent them all.
- The question "What did you eat?" or "What did you do?" or "Are you sure you should really eat more carbs for that low?" aren't going to feel supportive to mama. Guilt-tripping and shaming isn't going to help. Instead, you're almost always safe in asking this: "Honey, are you alright? Is there anything I can do to help?"
- Mama has a lot of stress on her shoulders right now—more than she can possibly convey and more than you can see through finger pricks and insulin doses. All day long she feels like she's taking a non-stop test, and her score on that test can affect someone else's well-being instead of just her own.

You're in this together! Let your partner know when their version of support doesn't fit the type of support you need. Try to keep your cool when explaining this to them and be sure to let them support you in other ways.

So by now, you're well aware of just how all-consuming managing your blood sugar during pregnancy can feel. Even for those who were super diligent about their diabetes prior to pregnancy will likely feel an extra added pressure or stress now because a) hormones make everything more complicated and b) you know your blood sugars are affecting more than just you now.

Now is actually good time to really think about how you can simplify your schedule and your life in general during the coming months, especially starting around month 6 or 7 when insulin resistance starts amping up and your energy isn't so ample.

Sure, maybe right now you feel totally capable of handling your normal workload, house-chores, social activities, volunteer work, etc. And the energy you'll have during the second trimester can be deceiving; remember: the third trimester is different! You will be tired—not because you're diabetic, but because you're pregnant! And the energy you will have in the last few months is going to be consumed by taking good care of your blood sugars, your nutrition, and your overall health. Nothing else will be as important.

Start thinking now about where in your life you can cut back later in your pregnancy, and begin having those discussions where (and with whomever) necessary. (If you're pregnant with twins, feel free to add several exclamation marks to every sentence in the following paragraphs!)

HERE ARE A FEW AREAS TO CONSIDER:

WORK: Certainly the biggest priority in our day is how we earn our paychecks. Many women work right up until the day they deliver—which is incredibly awesome and impressive—but you may want to consider leaving work a bit sooner merely because your blood sugars in that last month will be so imperative to your baby's well-being and your overall delivery. Can you afford to leave work a few weeks earlier than your due-date? Can you cut back to part-time? If your job currently involves standing on your feet all day, is there a way your role in your company can be adjusted so you can be sitting for some of the day instead?

HOUSE–CLEANING: By month 6 or 7, the idea of vacuuming and mopping your whole house might feel like a monumental chore—especially when simply carrying a basket of dirty clothes to the laundry machine can leave you huffing and puffing. Fortunately, it is one you can hand-off pretty easily to someone else, at least for a few months and a few bucks. Hiring a house-cleaner now rather than after the baby is born can be really helpful, both physically for you but also because it'll be nice to have that all straightened-out once you desperately need a little help postpartum.

OTHER CHILDREN: If this isn't your first kiddo, then you already know fully well just how tired you're going to be towards the end. If there are friends or relatives you can talk to about helping you out with a little extra childcare, introduce the idea sooner than later. Even if it's just for month 8 or 9, getting a little more help in this area will mean you can get a little more rest and keep your battery charged to manage your blood sugars for the baby in your belly just as much as you already do for the kiddo on your lap!

SOCIAL ACTIVITIES: Do you volunteer every week or host a book club? Whatever your usual social activities are, you might want to take a look at which ones you can cut back on in the upcoming months when you find yourself desperately wishing you could crawl into bed just minutes after you get home from work every day. No matter how fit or active you may be, simply resting, even if it's just sitting wide-awake on the couch, is going to be a pretty big priority by month 6 or 7. (And yes, your friends might be a little miffed that you're bailing on everything lately, but you've got your priorities! They will have to get used to that!)

PET-CARE: Depending on how many pets you have and how they normally get their daily exercise, having a dog-walker come by to help ensure they get the attention they need could be helpful both in the last few months of pregnancy and of course, for the month or two following your pregnancy depending on how quickly you're back on your feet.

COOKING: Oh, this is a big one, because ordering take-out every night especially during the third trimester when blood sugars are stubborn and insulin needs are high, is not ideal for a gal with diabetes. (Trust us: nothing will make life more frustrating during pregnancy with diabetes like a constant consumption of fatty, carb-loaded, greasy, fast-foods! Your blood sugars will fight you for hours!) If cooking is already something you find to be tedious and exhausting, then let's make sure you have a plan in mind for the third trimester. First and foremost: learning to make meals simpler (which we definitely hope the nutrition sections in this book will help you do!). If your partner is used to luxuriously home-cooked meals every night of the week, you may want to warn him or her that in the third trimester, things are gonna get simpler. Do you have a friend who seems to rock at cooking simple whole-food meals? Call them and ask for suggestions, guidance, even a lesson in the kitchen. Are there one or two restaurants in particular that serve fresh, healthy meals to go that you can budget for during the third trimester? Nutrition is a huge part of a life with diabetes, and it will only get bigger as the months progress. Think about your current life around cooking and how you can ensure that things are manageable and healthy when energy isn't as ample.

NUTRITION & FITNESS

Have those cravings hit full speed yet? We're going to say this because we're probably the only ones who can say it to a pregnant woman without being slapped across the fact: easy does it, girlfriend!

Yes, you're hungry, and yes, you want ice cream and French-fries. But trust us when we say you'll be thankful later on in your pregnancy (and after) if you don't indulge every time those cravings hit.

Now is a good month to really start thinking about how to manage those cravings in way that is both reasonably satisfying and as healthfully as possible.

THE ONCE A WEEK METHOD:

Desperate for a huge plate of _____? Okay, but what if you chose a special day each week to indulge in that less-than-healthy plate of _____? Let's take pizza for example. Pizza is pretty satisfying, especially to a hungry pregnant woman. Carbs and fat and protein and… cheese…oh my!

Okay, so enjoying some pizza with some extra tedious insulin dosing around it is no big deal, but enjoying pizza several nights per week could become a big deal. Instead of giving in altogether or avoiding it altogether, think about choosing one night each week that will be your treat night for whatever food you're most desperate for that isn't very healthy and isn't very easy to manage blood sugars around.

CREATE YOUR HEALTHY VERSION METHOD:

Dying for a chocolate milkshake? The average milkshake you'd get from a restaurant will pack in anywhere from 60 to 100 grams of carbs, at least 30 grams of fat, and will ruin the rest of your day as you struggle to get your blood sugars to cooperate.

Make your own healthy milkshake in a blender at home by mixing 1 scoop of chocolate whey protein powder (preferably sweetened with stevia rather than sucralose), 3–4 ice cubes, 2 scoops Breyer's vanilla ice cream (or other naturally lighter ice cream) and fill to the brim with unsweetened vanilla almond milk. This version of a chocolate milkshake will have barely 30 grams of carbohydrate, lots of protein, and less than 10 grams of fat.

THE 10% METHOD:

Okay, so you want chocolate. All day long. All. Day. Long. You. Want. Chocolate. But of course, while chocolate has its benefits, chocolate ain't exactly a "health-food." Fine—no big deal.

Instead, do your best to eat your healthier choices throughout the day and save room in your day's nutrition for a reasonable serving of chocolate at night—or whatever that 10% treat is that you're desperately craving.

THE POINT IS: identify what's going on and what you're craving and then, create a plan around that craving so you don't go insane trying to resist it and you don't go overboard trying to satisfy it. Think carefully about what you can do to satisfy the craving while still being thoughtful about your needs as a woman with diabetes.

INSULIN MANAGEMENT

This month you will likely see continued insulin sensitivity as hormones fluctuate and your body continues to produce a bit of its own insulin as described in Month 2. For many, you might not even notice the insulin sensitivity until this month when it really starts to ramp up.

Just because there is a bit of extra insulin now shouldn't mean you're constantly experiencing devastating low blood sugars every day. Those lows are a sign that you are getting too much insulin in either or both your background insulin doses and your meal doses and that something needs adjustment.

EXPECTED INSULIN ADJUSTMENTS

The tricky part about producing your own insulin is trying to figure out where you need to cut back on your insulin doses...which can actually be far more confusing and frustrating than trying to figure out where you need to increase your insulin during the later months of pregnancy.

What makes this part of pregnancy particularly complicated is that everyone's "newfound" insulin production varies greatly from one person to the next, so one woman may reduce her insulin needs by 40% during this part of pregnancy while another woman may only see a 10% reduction in her insulin needs.

Here are a few things to keep in mind when assessing your insulin doses.

- "Am I going low 1 to 2 hours after eating a meal?" Too much insulin with your meals: start by adjusting your insulin to carb (I:C) ratio up by 1 to 3g. This will give less insulin at the meal and you can reassess if this worked, or if further adjustment is needed.
- "Am I going low in between meals, when I haven't eaten for 3 to 4 hours?" Too much background insulin: start with a reduction in basal insulin of 10 to 25% OR if on a pump, reduce the basal in that specific time period of the day.
- "Am I going low because I'm constantly correcting high blood sugars 1 to 2 hours after eating?" Not enough insulin with your meals:

decrease the I:C ratio for that meal to give more insulin coverage. For example: instead of 1 unit of insulin for every 15 grams of carbs, trying 1 unit of insulin for every 12 grams of carbs.

- "Am I going low because I'm constantly correcting high blood sugars when I haven't eaten for 3 to 4 hours?" Not enough background insulin: start with an increase in basal insulin of 10-25% OR if on a pump, increase the basal in that specific time period of the days.

This is just a balancing act. It's frustrating and exhausting, but you've just got to fine-tune and adjust...and keep adjusting as needed!

* *Remember: During pregnancy, you want to make a change in your doses after seeing a trend of higher or lower blood sugar levels over the course of two days rather than three or more days when not pregnant. It's also important to never make increases of more than 1 to 2 units in one day. Make an adjustment of up to 2 units, assess its efficacy over the next day or two, and adjust again as needed. Within each trimester, you will likely see a total increase in your insulin needs of anywhere between 3 to 7 units. Those with higher levels of insulin resistance and weight-gain will see the greatest increases in their insulin needs.*

AT THE DOCTOR'S OFFICE

By now, don't be surprised if a medical professional has unintentionally tried to shame you or guilt-trip you into being the perfect diabetic. Maybe it's a nurse or doctor who knows a lot about gestational diabetes...but not type 1 diabetes. Or maybe it's a nurse or doctor who knows nothing about diabetes except what they learned in their courses in school but haven't had to use that information in everyday practice with patients.

Take a deep breath. And then try to express to them as clearly as possible why that type of conversation isn't going to help you become the perfect pregnant diabetic.

HERE'S ONE LONG YET STRAIGHT-FORWARD EXAMPLE OF COMMUNICATING THIS VERY IMPORTANT POINT TO YOUR MEDICAL TEAM

"Doctor, I completely understand your concern for my blood sugars and the baby. But I have type 1 diabetes...I produce pretty much zero insulin. Keeping my blood sugars in non-diabetic range isn't just about eating healthy and taking insulin a few times a day. I'm constantly counting carbs to determine my insulin dose, assessing the fat and protein content in that meal to determine how far in advance I should take that insulin dose so the timing of the insulin matches exactly with the timing of the food hitting my bloodstream!

That's not an easy thing to do, and I'm trying to do it all day long. And that's just one tiny aspect of what goes into managing blood sugars in a body that produces no insulin. I'd really appreciate if the conversations we have around my blood sugars never involve trying to shame me or guilt-trip me for having imperfect blood sugars. I have type 1 diabetes, I'm doing the very best I can, and it's challenging every single day."

Or, use the above statement to inspire your own way of communicating with your medical team. Regardless of how you do it, the point is that you speak up for yourself.

ADDITIONAL TESTING FOR HIGH-RISK AND ADVANCED MATERNAL AGE:

For pregnant women who qualify as high-risk or are over the age of 35 years old, additionally blood-tests can be done around this time to detect early signs of potential birth defects.

The Mayo Clinic explains additional testing options for high-risk pregnancies as the following:

- **SPECIALIZED OR TARGETED ULTRASOUND:** "This type of fetal ultrasound—an imaging technique that uses high-frequency sound waves to produce images of a baby in the uterus—targets a suspected problem, such as abnormal development."

- **AMNIOCENTESIS:** "During this procedure, a sample of the fluid that surrounds and protects a baby during pregnancy (amniotic fluid) is withdrawn from the uterus. Typically done after week 15 of pregnancy, amniocentesis can identify certain genetic conditions, as well as neural tube defects—serious abnormalities of the brain or spinal cord."

- **CHORIONIC VILLUS SAMPLING (CVS):** "During this procedure, a sample of cells is removed from the placenta. Typically done between weeks 10 and 12 of pregnancy, CVS can identify certain genetic conditions."

- **CORDOCENTESIS:** "This test, also known as percutaneous umbilical blood sampling, is a highly specialized prenatal test in which a fetal blood sample is removed from the umbilical cord. Typically done after week 18 of pregnancy, the test can identify chromosomal conditions, blood disorders and infections."

- **CERVICAL LENGTH MEASUREMENT:** "Your health care provider might use an ultrasound to measure the length of your cervix at prenatal appointments to determine if you're at risk of preterm labor."

- **LAB TESTS:** "Your healthcare provider might take a swab of your vaginal secretions to check for fetal fibronectin—a substance that acts like a glue between the fetal sac and the lining of the uterus. The presence of fetal fibronectin might be a sign of preterm labor."

- **BIOPHYSICAL PROFILE:** "This prenatal test is used to check on a baby's well-being. The test combines fetal heart rate monitoring (non-stress test) and fetal ultrasound."

Some of these tests, such as the CVS or amniocentesis, do carry a small risk of actually causing miscarriage. Many women don't have any of these additional tests done. They are not required or even necessarily recommended for women with type 1 diabetes—they are simply an option. The constant mention of high-risk during pregnancy with type 1 diabetes can feel suffocating. It's important to remember that it's far more likely that you will give birth to a happy, healthy, perfect little baby.

This is simply about an increased risk based on statistics from pregnancies across the country. The things you can do to drastically reduce that increased risk include taking good care of yourself during pregnancy by managing your blood sugar, eating mostly healthy foods, exercising, and avoiding things like cigarettes, alcohol and other drugs.

Don't let all this high-risk talk fill you with fear. Instead, let you fill you with motivation to take good care of yourself and your baby.

ESSENTIAL PAPERWORK PREPARATION: PUMPS & CGMS DURING LABOR

While we'll talk in great detail about how to create your own "birth plan" later in this book, there are a few details that you'll want to get started on now: the paperwork that will ensure you can wear your diabetes technology during labor.

For both insulin pumps and continuous glucose monitors, your OB-GYN will want to discuss the use of this technology with nurse manager of the labor and delivery ward of your hospital. There may be forms to fill out, or you may even be the first patient they've ever had with that type of technology!

Depending on the hospital's experience with that type of technology, this process may be very easy or a bit tedious, and that's why it's important to start the conversation early on so that everything is settled and clear by the time you're 7 or 8 months pregnant.

GINGER'S PREGNANCY DIARY

WEEK 9

I have to remind myself that most of the time I'm doing an awesome job with my blood sugar control...but when things are not so great, it can be really hard to remember that most of the time it's usually much better.

ALLOW ME TO PAINT YA'LL A PICTURE OF THE OPPOSITE OF THE PERFECT PREGNANT DIABETIC:

Earlier today, my blood was 73 mg/dL and dropping very slowly. Right as the "below 70 mg/dL" alarm chimed on my DexCom, I took a bite of a peach. I had taken an insulin injection just moments before that bite figuring that since my blood sugar was already dropping, waiting 10 to 15 minutes before eating the peach might simply add to the low blood sugar. I finished the first peach within 15 minutes, before that first dose of insulin even had time to get going. Then I ate a second peach and took more insulin—now I'm just being impulsive, not thoughtful, and certainly not The Perfect Pregnant Diabetic.

Sure enough, 20 minutes later there are two up-arrows on my screen and my blood sugar eventually makes its way up to 200 mg/dL. Lovely. So, instead of being patient for my not-early-enough bolus of insulin for the peaches to kick into action...I take one more unit of insulin, just to help... you know...get things rolling in the right direction. And yup, sure enough an hour or so later I'm down at 50 mg/dL.

It's frustrating, because while an outsider might look at the situation and say, "Well, geez, just freaking wait before you eat those darn peaches! You could've easily prevented that 200 mg/dL blood sugar!"...it's simply not that simple.

How often do you see a 200 mg/dL on your meter and feel like a horrible mother of a baby you haven't even met yet?

How often in your non-pregnant life do you think about eating 15 to 20 minutes before you're actually going to eat? Sure, you might know what you're going to eat sometimes, perhaps because it's packed in your bag, but in our day-to-day life we often just stop and eat. We don't stop 20 minutes beforehand and think, "Okay, in 20 minutes, I'm going to eat."

Making this a habit every single day during pregnancy isn't easy. It's the every-day part that is hardest because while we can put all our intentions into make this happen during a specific day—especially a day when we don't have a lot going on and the day is free—it's much harder due to the simplest little variables like: eating at a friend's house while lying by the pool or eating on the road while you drive four hours to your brother's house or celebrating July 4th at the parade, then the fair, then your family's enormous celebratory barbeque.

These are all just real life events that make that whole "take your insulin at least 10 minutes before you eat" (and hope that it's a type of food that actually digests quickly enough to make 10 minutes the appropriate amount of time!) really, really challenging.

I think, as I step into my third month of pregnancy, this inconsistency in when I should take my insulin is proving to be the most challenging aspect of striving to be that Perfect Pregnant Diabetic.

WEEK 10

My first A1C test since becoming pregnant came back at 5.7 percent, down from months ago at 5.9—which was the lowest I'd ever gotten it in my 15 years with type 1. I'd never had an A1C below 6.0 until this year, when I knew I wanted to get pregnant. Before this year, my A1C was usually somewhere between 6.4 to 7.3 percent.

As I think about the 5.7, despite that I know I've put every ounce of my energy into getting it there, I find it painfully amusing that all I can really remember are all the "awful" blood sugars I've accidentally caused.

I can remember the 250 mg/dL after the first (and last) time I ate Ben & Jerry's Ice Cream during pregnancy and learned how well that slowed digestion system can wreak havoc on my blood sugar after a high-fat/high-sugar dessert. (Since then, I've sworn to indulge occasional ice cream cravings with nothing other than Breyer's ice cream, which is naturally lower in fat and sugar and therefore much easier to manage within my blood sugar!)

I can remember that one day a few weeks ago when I went up and down from 50 to 250 mg/dL at least 3 times through the afternoon, stuck on the rollercoaster, trying my damndest to get off, but clearly struggling! (I've learned to be a little more patient and less anxiety-driven when dealing with high blood sugars during pregnancy...letting my corrective insulin doses do their job before reacting again.)

I can remember the midnight 270 mg/dL after eating gluten-free pizza for the first time during pregnancy...again learning the lessons in slowed digestion with the high-fat/high-carb meal. (I don't even really care much for pizza so it won't be hard to skip this darn food for the next 9 months.)

I can remember just last week when I ate two oranges with two chunks of cheddar cheese and I suspected I was starting to make insulin because I'd kept dropping to 60 mg/dL all morning, so I cut back on my insulin dose for the oranges out of fear of yet another low blood sugar. Sure enough, I cut back wayyyyyy to much and my blood sugar quickly skyrocketed to 250 mg/dL within an hour. My CGM, sadly, said 100 mg/dL at the time and was running way behind…just to add more frustration to the afternoon. (This taught me that, duh, I need to be super thoughtful when eating fruit every day and be sure my insulin is timed well because fruit is digested so quickly!)

So what I'm trying to say is: I can remember all the mistakes. The goofs. The high blood sugars that I feel like I should've been able to prevent had I only thought that much more carefully (or if I could become psychic) about what I was eating and how my body was going to receive it. What I'm remembering most are the less-than-healthy food items when in reality I know that the majority of my diet has been very clean and healthy foods. Fortunately, observing those frustrating blood sugars from the junk food choices provides easy inspiration to avoid them!

So when I saw that 5.7 percent A1C I was reminded that not every day is filled with mistakes. That the most of each individual day is filled with plenty of in-range blood sugars. I'm reminded that the mistakes don't make up the entirety of the past few weeks even if they do feel as though they weigh the most on my shoulders and my mind.

There are more in-range blood sugars in there than high blood sugars—I must remember that.

That I'm doing a great job, doing the best I can.

FINALLY! I'M PRODUCING INSULIN

Just when I thought my pancreas' beta cells had been totally wiped clean, my body started producing a little insulin during week 10. A little late to the party, if you ask me, but better late than never I suppose.

Unfortunately, I have to say I'm far less impressed by this phenomenon than I was expecting to be. First, I was really kind of hoping the production of insulin would announce itself with rainbows, glitter, and frolicking unicorns…you know, so it would be really clear that it was happening. Instead, it arrives with recurrent low blood sugars throughout the night (like, every 2 hours my blood sugar suddenly started to plummet. I'd treat it with 10 or so grams of carbs, and then it'd plummet again), followed by multiple lows during the day reaching 40 mg/dL or simply "LOW" on my CGM which implies below 40 mg/dL. Not my idea of a good time.

And the most obnoxious part was that after a day or two of new lows, I reduced my background insulin by 1, then 2 units, experienced a much steadier diabetic existence for a day or two, and then the recurrent lows started to happen again. In other words: my insulin production was coming on very slowly, and increased every couple of days over the course of almost two weeks. By the start of this two weeks I was taking 16 units of background insulin, and by week 12 I was down to 10 units of background insulin which is keeping me sitting steadily, for the most part, around 90 mg/dL.

Despite the tedious hypoglycemia (which I found can easily lead to hyperglycemia at first because I was so terrified I just wouldn't stop dropping if I didn't treat with 30 grams or more of carbs at certain points), I'm definitely not experiencing the "flat line" I've heard several women talk about before. I can still just as easily reach 200 mg/dL if I don't get exactly the right amount of insulin.

Twice during the recurrent hypoglycemia phase, I tried eating an apple or an orange without any insulin and sure enough, I went plenty high just like I would when not pregnant...so despite seeing a tremendous reduction in my background insulin, the reduction in the amount of insulin I need for meals has been fairly subtle. Seems like there ought to be a friendly middle-ground where both are decreased but that hasn't been my personal experience. Perhaps it's different because I'm taking a long-acting insulin rather than getting my basal insulin from a pump? Who knows! (I later asked Jenny about this and she confirmed that my insulin-reduction experience will definitely be different compared to a person on a pump who is getting that constant dose of fast-acting insulin.)

Needless to say, I was actually starting to miss the days where the only insulin I received was from my own syringe because after 15 years of managing my blood sugars myself, this whole "partial participation" thing from my pancreas is actually really obnoxious. Until, that is, I finally found things settle down when I got down to 10 units of long-acting insulin.

Meanwhile, I've noticed that the first thing I do when I wake up in the morning—and for the following 5 minutes as I get out of bed and putz around—is put my hand on my lower abdomen. It's such a unconscious little act, but it's one of the first most obvious things, so far, that reminds me I'm becoming a mother. As Jenny says, "You will never be a non-mommy ever again." (Except of course to my small herd of canines.)

Becoming a mother. I don't feel like I'm really a mother yet, but I do feel as though each day is a gradually deeper step into motherhood.

WEEK 11

To date, my cravings haven't included anything too crazy. But mostly, it seems pretty normal: any fruit packed with vitamin C and folate doesn't stand a chance when I'm around. I feel an irresistible desire to now eat two oranges a day instead of nectarines or peaches.

And carbohydrates in general draw my attention more than fats or proteins, but I'm trying to ensure the majority of my carbohydrate consumption is coming from good sources like brown or wild rice, sweet or white potatoes (sometimes the sweet variety turn me off, so white potatoes are more doable), fruit, and during a recent sore throat I indulged in a bit of yogurt which I'm really on the fence about because most yogurt contains so much unnecessary added sugar. I try to cut the sugar by mixing a plain yogurt with a strawberry yogurt...and always ensure it's a high-quality brand that isn't full of corn syrup.

However, I am truly thankful I've spent a great deal of energy in the past several years on establishing what I will and won't consider putting into my body when it comes to things like fast-food and other restaurant garbage, because driving down one of the main shopping strips that is lined with fast-food joints is a different experience in this pregnant body.

Usually, when I get a whiff of fast-food burger grease or french fries, I find myself saying, "Ugh! Bleh! Gross!" But now, as I drive down the road passing each restaurant, I can envision something I'd like to eat in each and every building—buildings I haven't stepped into for 10 years. The burger there. The fries there. A milkshake there. Chicken nuggets there. Anything. All of it. I don't crave these things when I'm at home and they're out of sight, but when they're right in front of me (and mealtime is approaching) I am grateful that my other inner voice (the one not controlled by my tastebuds) says, "Whoa, that's not the kind of stuff you'd normally put into your body because you know it's not good quality, clean, real, whole food. Keep driving!"

Just because I'm craving it, doesn't necessarily mean I need that version of that food. A craving for a fast-food burger is not my body's way of saying, "Mmm, that fast-food is actually filled with valuable nutrients! Honest!" Instead, it can simply mean I'm hungry and need to get home and make myself a nutritious and satisfying lunch of grilled meat, some veggies, and maybe a handful of pecans.

WEEK 12

So despite the major reduction in my background insulin dose (down from 16 to 10 units per day), I do need more insulin at breakfast now that I'm getting less background insulin at that time of the day—whatever, diabetes!

If you were wondering if it's near impossible to experience really high blood sugars when your body is producing insulin, I can assure you: it's totally possible.

This week, I experienced the highest blood sugar I've had in probably a year, back when I was trying out a different long-acting insulin that seemed to impact my blood sugar levels as strongly as pure water might. And naturally, this super-high came after several days in a row of staying "perfectly" between the target lines of my CGM!

At 1:45 a.m. I woke up to my CGM alarm letting me know that my blood sugar was 400 mg/dL or "HIGH" as the neon light seemed to enjoy flashing at me.

Earlier that night, around 8:30 p.m., I had eaten about 6 oz. of steak, a good pile of sauteed green beans, and a bowl of coconut rice. Well this was the first time I'd ever made and eaten coconut rice, and I should've known better because it involves cooking a can of coconut milk (naturally high in fat) with the rice.

Well that fat must've really slowed things down in my gut because I was low by 9:30 p.m.

I treated the low with 15 grams of carbs. When I went to bed at 10 p.m. my blood sugar was sitting steadily at 145 mg/dL, so I took a small correction dose of insulin to get back near 100 mg/dL and quickly fell asleep. Because I was already above my high-alarm setting of 130 mg/dL, the CGM didn't buzz again as my blood sugar kept rising for another 60 minutes. I must've ignored that in my sleep or pressed the button in my sleep so it wouldn't buzz again for another 60 minutes!

It took all night to get it back down again because it was enough that my normal correction dose wasn't enough. By 3:30 a.m., it took a second correction dose of much more insulin than I'd normally need to correct an average high blood sugar. (The higher the blood sugar, often the more resistant to insulin we can become!)

By 7 a.m. I was down at 100 mg/dL...which was a nice way to end the very frustrating sense of feeling like a pregnant diabetic failure. No matter how much I know I can't do this perfectly for 9 months, seeing a 400 mg/dL on the screen feels like failure. The best I can do—both for my growing baby and my sanity—is do everything I can to get back in range by morning. Being "there" by morning helps ensure the next day starts off on a positive note.

The next morning, Roger, who was well-aware that I was waking up repeatedly through the night to deal with my raging blood sugar, had a very important question that I hadn't yet explained the answer to:

"When your blood sugar is 400...do I need to worry about the baby? What does that mean for the baby?"

I explained that of course being at 400 mg/dL regularly would be very unkind to the baby because it would mean the baby is getting far more sugar than it would be getting from a non-diabetic mother's body. And no baby wants to work on creating healthy organs in an environment with 300 more milligrams of sugar than necessary. Fortunately, my blood sugar is definitely not regularly that high so we don't need to be concerned about this one event beyond doing everything possible to get my blood sugar down quickly (insulin dose + water + waiting). I also explained to Roger that the baby makes its own insulin, so even when my blood sugar is high, the baby's blood sugar is never actually high. Instead, again, it just means the baby is getting more glucose and thus having to produce more insulin and thus storing more glucose as body fat compared to what it would be getting and doing if I wasn't diabetic.

I'm glad Roger asked this question because it's important that he understands the specific science of how blood sugars affect or don't affect a growing baby.

WAIT, WHO IS GONNA MANAGE MY BLOOD SUGARS DURING LABOR?

Meanwhile, for some reason, I've started thinking more about the actual birth and getting a little anxious. You're probably thinking I must be anxious about the whole concept of pushing a watermelon out something the size of an orange, but that reality hasn't sunk in yet. Instead, I'm worrying about who is going to be managing my insulin doses and my blood sugars during the whole hospitalization.

Maybe it's just me, but I am the only person I really like to have making decisions about my diabetes. Jenny is one of the few CDEs I've ever found who I would also actually trust to take over my insulin dosing for a day or a week. And the only other person besides Jenny is our CDE friend Mara, who also lives with type 1.

So when I give birth, my blood sugars are going to be managed by…who? A group of nurses I've never met? A group of nurses who may or may not have much experience in blood sugar regulation beyond textbook protocol they're taught to follow? Can't I be in charge? I know somebody else has to know what's going on in case for some reason I can't take care of myself, but honestly, the idea of anyone, even a medical professional, making decisions about my insulin doses and my blood sugar readings terrifies me.

And my fears aren't exactly unwarranted! The two other times I've spent at least a night or two in the hospital, the staff on duty were beyond reckless with my diabetes. The first experience was when I was in DKA as a teenager after not receiving any insulin all night long through a malfunctioned pump site cannula. Two med-students decided they were going to give me 10 units of insulin per hour for the next several hours. I begged them not to because I knew that was way too much insulin for my tiny teenage body. They went ahead anyway and within one hour they were giving me an I.V. of glucose.

The other, a few years later, was after I woke up from reconstructive jaw surgery. My head was the size of a basketball due to the swelling. My jaw was wired shut. And I was puking up blood all over myself. But I still remembered that I needed my long-acting insulin dose. I managed to tell the nurse, "I need my Lantus. It's right there in my bag."

She said it wasn't on my list of medications so she would have to consult the surgeon first. The surgeon said, "I've never heard of that before—don't let her take it."

Ugh. You can imagine the fit I threw—despite my physical condition—and sure enough, the surgeon (without apology) relented and let me take my damn insulin.

So...the point is....I really don't trust other people, even most medical professionals (except for Jenny and Mara) to manage my diabetes. The idea terrifies me.

Fortunately, I expressed this anxiety to Jenny and she assured me that she and I were going to write-up a thorough "Birthing Plan" that we would get my doctor to sign-off on. And part of that plan would dictate who and how my diabetes would be managed during pregnancy.

And then, Jenny reminded me to simply enjoy this part of pregnancy and the gradual evolution of becoming a mother. Deep breath.

NOTES

MONTH 4

A LABOR OF LOVE... IT'S ALL FOR THE BUMP!

At this point, you've probably forgotten what it's like to go more than 30 minutes without thinking about your blood sugar and desperately needing to know exactly where it's at. The intensity that comes with managing your blood sugars during pregnancy is constant.

You are working so hard all day long—all day long—to keep your blood sugars in the best range for your growing baby. After 3 months of that intensity, that level of daily stress may have become your new "normal." Not to say that it feels easy—definitely not—but perhaps you've really forgotten what it's like to not obsess about your blood sugar all day long...or on the other hand, maybe you're feeling really frustrated. Struggling. Exhausted.

You're definitely not alone if you've found yourself thinking: "Oh my gosh, obsessing about my blood sugar every second for another 6 months? Can I make it?"...but you're also probably getting even more attached to that tiny little bump that may or may not be starting to appear.

Fortunately, just as the stress of obsessive-pregnancy-blood-sugar-maintenance really starts to build up, it's immediately slapped back into reality by the love you're already feeling for that little human you've never even met. A nice little game of ying and yang that helps keep us focused on why we're working so insanely hard every day.

Every thoughtful decision you make around nutrition, exercise, and insulin is an act of love and concern for your baby. If reminding yourself of that helps keep you motivated, use it! Focus on that. Write it on a stickie note and put it somewhere you'll see it every day.

It's all worth it. You're working this hard for the well-being of someone else and for the well-being of that someone's mother! YOU!

MAMA'S MENTAL HEALTH

The best thing about this month of pregnancy is that you should start to get some of your energy back—physically and mentally. That overwhelming fatigue of the first three months can feel like you've been walking up a hill all day—when does the hill end? Here, this is where that hill starts to flatten out. Sure, you won't necessarily be skipping down the side-walk or jogging 10 miles, but you'll feel a bit more like you.

Of course, to keep you on your toes, diabetes management will start to be more challenging this month, too, thanks to increasing hormone production and consequential insulin resistance...but we'll talk about that in a bit!

Mostly, just remind yourself that you're about halfway there.

NUTRITION & FITNESS

Thank goodness: you know that queasy stomach thing that's been pestering you since before you even confirmed your pregnancy? Around weeks 12 to 13, that should really fade dramatically or disappear entirely.

HELLO, APPETITE!

What comes instead is an increased appetite. And the joys of being a type 1 mama-to-be is that an increased appetite means an increase in the daily challenge of eating mostly what will support your blood sugar goals.

HERE ARE A FEW THINGS TO CONSIDER IN YOUR NUTRITION HABITS THIS MONTH:

Re-introducing some veggies: One of the biggest benefits of the aforementioned decrease in your first-trimester nausea is that you can make different choices around food. It's not uncommon for vegetables be a stomach-churning object in those early months, but starting in Month 4 you might want to give them another chance.

If cooking veggies on a daily basis isn't something you're especially comfortable with or experienced in, here are a few simple ways to eat delicious veggies:

- **2-MINUTE SALAD:** Buy a head of iceberg lettuce and a small box of "spring mix" salad greens, and mix several handfuls of each in a big bowl. Choose your favorite salad dressing—yup, you read that right, real salad dressing—and remember that less is more when it comes to salad dressing. (Tip: instead of buying low-fat, get the regular kind. There's more sugar in low-fat salad dressings, they don't taste as good, and they aren't nearly as satisfying. If you need salad dressing in order to eat a bowl full of salad greens, then that's better than no salad at all!) If you want, buy a cucumber, too. Every time you make a salad, slice 10 chunks of cucumber into it, too.

- **10-MINUTE STEAMED & SAUTEED BROCCOLI:** Buy one head of broccoli and chop it up, place it in a frying pan, and add a ⅓ cup of water. Cover with a lid and steam the broccoli on medium-to-low heat for about 5 minutes—until it's vibrant green and the water is essentially gone. Next, so it tastes good, drizzle a bit of oil on it (coconut, olive, avocado, butter or sesame, etc.) and turn the heat up to medium. Saute for 5 minutes until it starts looking a bit crispy. Once it's ready, you can add a little salt or your favorite herbs and seasonings, dip it in a little mustard—whatever floats your boat! (Tip: You can apply this simple approach to any variety of vegetables, not just broccoli! Green-beans sauteed with a sweet onion is Ginger's personal favorite! Jenny ate broccoli with mustard almost every day while pregnant!)

- **PRE-CHOPPED VEGGIES:** One way to reduce the work of getting more veggies in your diet is to buy them already pre-chopped. Costco, BJ's and most grocery stores sell pre-chopped broccoli, bell peppers, carrots, cauliflower and celery! Yes, it will cost more money, but if that approach fits in your budget and puts more veggies on your plate, then go for it.

- **2-MINUTE MICROWAVED VEGGIES:** Don't want to deal with preparing and cooking all those fresh veggies? Grabbing some frozen veggies at the store and microwaving them is far better than no veggies at all! If this sounds like the best option for you, peruse the frozen veggie aisle and choose the ones that ideally don't have a layer of manufactured cheese on them. You can always buy plain frozen veggies and then add your own butter and salt!

- **O – MINUTE VEGGIES & HUMMUS:** If cooking veggies just isn't going to happen, there's no reason why you can get your veggies in raw. Carrots, bell-peppers, celery, tomatoes—whatever raw veggies you love—all taste great with the right flavor of hummus for your tastebuds! Hummus is made primarily of chickpeas (garbanzo beans), so you'll be getting a lot of great fiber with the carbs in those beans, and far more nutritious calories than a traditional dip. Either way, a veggie is a veggie—even if you're dressing it up in hummus! (Tip: If you're not sure if you actually like hummus, one of the most popular flavors of hummus is Roasted Red Pepper flavor.)

THE POINT IS THIS: there are times during your pregnancy where particular healthy foods are simply not going to make it onto your plate. Month 4 is a great time to give those foods another chance for the sake of a healthy 80/20 or 90/10 approach to your nutrition choices.

BLOOD SUGARS DURING EXERCISE GET EASIER...

Now that your own magical insulin production is "tapering off or gone, and hormones continue to increase insulin resistance,, you'll notice over the course of the next few weeks that you don't need to worry quite as much about low blood sugars during exercise.

In fact, eventually, some of you might find that the balance between your insulin resistance and your exercise that normally burns glucose ends up being the perfect combination for not having to do anything for your blood sugar before and during exercise!

For now, during this month, just keep in mind that you definitely won't need to consume as many carbohydrates specifically for keeping your blood sugar up during exercise or cut back on your insulin doses as much as you have in the previous two months.

WALKING IS STARTING TO SOUND MORE APPEALING, YES?

If you are someone who has been keeping up with her usual jogging or CrossFit routine, you may find that this month is when that starts to feel less comfortable. All that bouncing and intensity might either feel physically uncomfortable in a supremely obvious way or just instinctively uncomfortable, as if your body is saying, "Um...why are you doing this? You really don't need to be doing this to me (or us) right now. Just, like... go for a walk!"

Or you might be one of those people doing cartwheels when they're 9 months pregnant...to which we say: Yowza! Rock on!" But most of us aren't one of those people—and that's really okay!

Walking is your friend. Go for a walk, sweet mama. Just go for a walk.

INSULIN MANAGEMENT

As we mentioned in the previous section, this month is where that funky insulin-producing phenomenon begins to wane when faced with the placenta's increasing production of ultra-powerful hormones that leads to gradually impressive insulin resistance.

You've spent the past few weeks being able to eat a reasonable portion of carbohydrates without having to work too hard to keep your post-meal blood sugar in-range because your pancreas has been helping. Next, however, is when things really start turning in the other direction: in other words, everything you eat is going to require an increasingly great deal more planning and thought around when you take your insulin and how much you take.

EXPECTED INSULIN ADJUSTMENTS

Here are a few things to keep in mind when assessing your insulin doses this month:

- **BACKGROUND INSULIN DOSES:** The variety of hormones your body is producing right now are going to impact your overall insulin needs in addition to impacting how you dose for your meals. This means that you'll want to pay very close attention to when your body is saying, "I need more basal insulin, please!" You'll likely find you need an increase at least once or twice.

- **SIGNS OF NEEDING MORE BASAL INSULIN INCLUDE:** correction doses for high blood sugars that seem to have no impact after two hours, blood sugar levels rising slightly when you haven't taken insulin for food in more than two hours, and recurring hypoglycemia because you're taking a lot of correction doses of insulin to correct stubborn highs that won't budge.

- **PRE-BOLUS IT, BABY!** If you haven't been making time for that 15-minute pre-bolus between taking your insulin and when you begin eating, around week 14 or 15 is a good time to make that a serious priority. In fact, at this point it should really start being a pre-bolus of about 20 to 30 minutes. This is especially true when eating foods that are primarily carbohydrates such as fruits, starchy vegetables (potatoes), breads, and any beverages containing carbohydrates. The biggest exceptions to the pre-bolus are foods that are tremendously high in fat as well as carbohydrates, like pizza, Chinese food, lasagna, and rich desserts (especially those containing buttercream frosting— watch out!). Refer back to our pre-bolus chapter in the preparation section to review your pre-bolusing guidelines!

- **COUNTING YOUR CARBS...NO, SERIOUSLY.** If you've lived with type 1 diabetes for a good deal of time (let's say, at least a decade), chances are that it's been awhile since you actually used a measuring cup when serving yourself dinner. "Eyeballing" it becomes the norm for us type 1s when we've been guessing the carbs in everything we eat for years and years. But when it comes to the 2nd and 3rd trimester of your pregnancy, you may want to pretend you were diagnosed, like, yesterday. Measuring things such as rice, pasta, fruits, and potatoes so that your insulin dose is truly as accurate as possible can have a huge impact on your post-meal blood sugars. Just think of it as a little refresher course in the art of measuring your food!

* *Remember: During pregnancy, you want to make a change in your doses after seeing a trend of higher or lower blood sugar levels over the course of two days rather than three or more days when not pregnant. It's also important to never make increases of more than 1 to 2 units in one day. Make an adjustment of up to 2 units, assess its efficacy over the next day or two, and adjust again as needed. Within each trimester, you will likely see a total increase in your insulin needs of anywhere between 3 to 7 units. Those with higher levels of insulin resistance and weight-gain will see the greatest increases in their insulin needs.*

"UM...HONEY, CAN YOU...HELP ME, PLEASE?"

Always been the independent type? Nobody's ever taken care of your diabetes except you? That's awesome...until...that blossoming belly of yours is complicating your diabetes technology needs.

You know you need the technological support of your partner when:

- **THE SKIN ON YOUR BELLY IS TOO TAUGHT TO PINCH:** If you can't pinch at least a little chunk, you shouldn't put your pump site there. This is different than general leanness or being a naturally thin person, because when your belly is growing, that skin on your belly is being pulled from all directions. This will actually interfere with the the cannula sitting properly in your skin, preventing the insulin from being effectively pushed into your flesh. Taught skin = not a good site for your pump.

- **WHEN YOU JUST CAN'T REACH:** Believe it or not, there will be a point in your pregnancy when you can't turn around enough to even place a pump or sensor onto your love handle! (Just wait, in the last trimester simply getting in and out of your car is going to feel like an olympic event.)

- Instead, there are two things you should consider doing now when you're still plush and twisty:
- TEACH YOUR PARTNER HOW TO SET-UP A NEW PUMP-SITE AND CGM SENSOR: Both of these things are crucial. Even if you normally put your pump or CGM on your arm, it's still important that your partner knows how to place them for you on any part of your body, because things change, or you might just suddenly decide you do want help.
- USING NEW SITES: Before you are forced to use alternative sites for your pump-site and CGM, it might be helpful to start using those areas earlier to figure out which work best for you. Additionally, having your partner place your sites means they can put your pump or CGM in an area you have never been able to reach, such as the middle of your "side-back." Or below the waist of your pants on your upper-glute (upper "tooshie" area). Basically, anywhere you can pinch at least a little bit of chunk is a place for a CGM or pump site. Love-handle, upper thigh, above the belt-line, below the belt-line, your lower back, your mid-side-back, and back of the arm.

Even though most of us have been managing type 1 diabetes on our own for years or forever, there comes a time when...it takes two. You never know, you might even enjoy being able to delegate one of the many chores that comes with this non-stop disease!

AT THE DOCTOR'S OFFICE

This month your check-ups will be pretty standard. By now you might notice that at every check-up, they are going to ask about swelling and puffiness, because type 1 mama's have a higher risk of developing pre-eclampsia. They should also be asking about your current insulin doses (which should be different than your doses at your last appointment), and what your fasting blood sugar has been, as well as your blood sugar two-hours after eating.

For those with a CGM, the "two-hours after eating" question doesn't quite make sense only because you are looking at your blood sugar 30 minutes after eating, 45 minutes after eating, 90 minutes after eating... you get the point. When you're wearing a CGM you aren't stuck with only being able to manage your insulin based on your two-hour post-meal blood sugar. With a CGM you can adjust how you dose your insulin to change your blood sugar within that entire two-hour period.

Depending on your doctor's familiarity with CGM technology and their experience working with type 1 diabetics, they'll either understand this or not understand this at all. In some cases you may just have to give them the information they want without trying to teach them about more modern methods of managing type 1 diabetes (and how much more information you have at your fingertips).

Hopefully, either way, you have a team who realizes you're working very hard!

GUILT-TRIPPING A MAMA-TO-BE AIN'T NICE

By now, don't be surprised if you've been guilt-tripped a few times for basically being in a body that doesn't produce insulin. The system is designed, unfortunately and hopefully not on purpose, to make you feel like this major thing that is greatly out of your control (we haven't heard of any preventative treatments for type 1 yet...have you?) is all your fault because of how it might impact that growing little baby.

The measurements, the A1C tests, the measurements...the looks in their eyes that say, "Your A1C isn't 5.0 percent? What's wrong with you? Just eat the diabetic diet and you ought to be fine!"

The guilt-tripping (again, that is mostly not on purpose) only gets thicker, which means your skin needs to get thicker, too. But don't hesitate to stand-up for yourself. If you're being scolded for a 170 mg/dL (9.4 mmol/L) blood sugar after eating even though your A1C is well within the recommended range of pregnancy, you might just need to take a deep breath and remind your team that you have type 1 diabetes. Even though they are medical professionals, that doesn't mean they necessarily understand just how many variables go into the blood sugar management of type 1 diabetes.

They don't know that you had to reduce your breakfast bolus because you knew you were going to be gardening with your neighbor shortly after eat, but then your neighbor ended up cancelling and you had all that breakfast without the normal amount of insulin you would have taken...yada, yada, yada. They don't know that this is just one of a million scenarios that complicated the "basics" of managing type 1 diabetes.

This is where record keeping with notes comes in handy—when questions like "Why is this blood sugar reading so high?" come up, you can easily respond and educate them about the adjustment that was made, etc. In the end, what you bring to the visits will also help educate your team, giving them less to question and helping them learn more about type 1 management in real life.

Don't be afraid to speak-up. You're working really hard, no matter what your A1C is, and you deserve a little credit for showing up every day in a body that doesn't produce one of the most important hormones in the human body.

MONTH 4: GINGER'S PREGNANCY DIARY

WEEK 13

I have conquered Chinese food! This was the second time since becoming pregnant that we succumbed to the easy allure of Chinese food on a day when cooking a meal seemed extremely unappealing (not because cooking bothers me but because I was just too damn tired). Pregnant or not, we limit our Chinese food indulgences to one night per month.

The last time we had Chinese food—the same exact meal as this time because the only thing I like are boneless spareribs—my blood sugar seemed to plummet an hour after eating and then it spiked tremendously high more than 2 hours after eating.

This time, I prepared for that super delayed pregnancy digestion process and took half my dose for the meal upon eating and then took the other half of that dose two hours later. For people on insulin pumps, there's obviously a variety of fancy settings you can program for your meal bolus to be extended over a lengthy period of time, but for those of us on injections, this is the next best thing. This same approach would work well for things like gluten-free pizza if I did decide to have that again at some point during this pregnancy, and possibly tacos, too, which is something I make about once a month that always makes my husband extremely happy.

I definitely still have a blood sugar at or above 200 mg/dL every couple of days, but for the rest of the day, I'm finding that while none of this is "easy," I am getting better at predicting what my body needs in order to stay in the tighter range. Believe me: I ain't perfect and neither are my blood sugars…but I feel as though I'm spending less time trying to figure things out and more time knowing what to expect. (On that note, remind me to never bother trying a fresh slice of freshly baked gluten-free banana bread again until post-birth. Not worth it!)

Although, I should add that I started having an obnoxiously high blood sugar after eating grapefruits in the morning. It took me several days and an email conversation with Jenny to realize that the difference about the carbs in the grapefruit and the carbs in my other breakfast options (toast with eggs, etc.) was that the grapefruit wasn't being eaten with any fat or protein! Yes, I was eating eggs maybe 45 minutes later, but by simply eating that damn grapefruit all on its own, it was digesting too quickly and spiking my blood sugar rather than digesting a bit more slowly like the toast with the eggs.

I have fallen deeply in love with my morning blueberry protein smoothie. It is the perfect combination of macronutrients (protein, carbs and fat) for the sake of insulin timing and gradual digestion! I can take my insulin dose for the smoothie merely 5 minutes before starting to consume it and because it it takes a little time to consume plus it digests at a medium pace because of the protein and fat, I can easily keep my blood sugar under 130 mg/dL and am back near 100 within about 75 minutes after consuming it.

THE RECIPE IS 4 SIMPLE INGREDIENTS:

In an individual-serving-sized blender, combine:

- 1 cup frozen blueberries
- 1.5 tablespoons peanut butter (or any nut butter of your choice)
- 1 scoop JayRobb Chocolate Egg-White Protein Powder (I prefer this brand because it's sweetened with stevia, not aspartame or sucralose. And egg-white protein as the source instead of whey just for the sake of reducing dairy intake in my diet)
- Fill with unsweetened vanilla almond milk

Blend...and enjoy!

I find that even though this recipe is barely 22 grams of carbs, I need insulin as though it's 30 grams of carbs because of the protein quantity.

In other news, my "diabetes staycation" (also known as my pancreas producing some of its own insulin) is clearly starting to be challenged by the placenta's increased production of progesterone. While I had worked my way down from 17 units of Lantus per day to 10 units of Lantus per day, over the past three weeks I've raised it up to 11 units and now up to 12.

I noticed I needed each increase particularly during the nighttime hours when my blood sugar kept trying to rise slowly above 150 mg/dL and my normal correction dose seemed to have zero impact on the number. Instead, I was take 2-3 times my normal correction dose just to get it to budge. Once I made the increase to 11 units, that worked perfectly for 2 weeks of keeping me between 70-100 mg/dL throughout the night. Then, this past week, I had the same stubborn numbers during the night, raised it to 12 units with Jenny's blessing, and voila, back in my ideal range of 70-100 mg/dL through the night.

Now that I know what to look for (in other words: that stubborn nighttime blood sugar), it'll be easy to spot when I need the next increase to 13 units at some point, most likely, in the next two or three weeks. Oh, diabetes is so much fun, sometimes I just can't stand it!

In other diabetes-pregnancy books, forums, and blogs, women are often saying they ate the same things every day for the sake of consistent blood sugars. And sure, that totally makes sense, and would absolutely make dosing and blood sugar goals simpler. When I was a competitive powerlifting athlete, eating the same things every day was pretty much one of the most important parts of your training and success.

But for me, I'm finding my tastebuds are just too flaky for such repetitiveness. I wanted nothing but toast and eggs during the first 2.5 months, and now I want only my blueberry protein smoothie.

In the beginning, I was all about peaches. Then one look at peaches in the store and I just felt "bleh." Then oranges and grapefruit. Now those citrus fruits are still enjoyable but not really especially appealing. The last few weeks, my fruits of choice have been apples with peanut butter for lunch, and a couple times in the last month I've made homemade whipped cream with sliced-up strawberries. Which is heavenly but obviously not something I'd eat every day!

Then there are avocados with tomatoes and black beans...which tasted just glorious for about a week until the smell suddenly made me totally repulsed.

For about two or three weeks I wanted greek yogurt, and now it just sits untouched in the refrigerator. (And then I threw it out, and I'm glad to report that I don't think I'll want it again! Something I always considered to be a lame source of sugar and not worth it!)

And vegetables are totally appealing if I'm getting a salad at a restaurant for lunch or a side of veggies on a meal...but I have absolutely no interest in cooking them at home. At home, my brain says, "Ugh, gross, please, not broccoli," even though I used to eat it almost daily prior to pregnancy.

The only true consistencies have been peanut butter, baby carrots, sugar snap peas, and starches, like rice or potatoes, and almost any type of salad from a restaurant. Mmm, and whipped cream with strawberries... (although I can't say I've had that more 2 or 3 times in the past 4 months so far...but I'm sure my taste-buds would never reject something so delicious).

Before becoming pregnant, I remember thinking, "Oh, I'll just follow the same consistency in my nutrition that I followed when training in powerlifting," but that simply doesn't feel possible now that I'm almost 4 months in and looking back on how many times my choices and tolerances have changed.

Instead, I'm trying to create consistency within that "phase," because consistency is definitely a good thing in the world of blood sugar maintenance. If I'm all about apples and peanut butter one week or two weeks, then I'll make the most of that and be as consistent as I can by making that my main meal for lunch or snack. Trying to find the consistency within all the inconsistencies!

In the end, I feel really good about what I've been feeding my body, but also hyper-aware of how often my tastebuds have been changing merely because I know how valuable consistency in nutrition is for blood sugar management.

WEEK 16

Stress. I feel increasingly stressed over the past couple of weeks, but this week I've become incredibly aware of it. It almost feels as though someone has been pouring "stress" into the top of my head like you might pour water into a vase, and it's been accumulating, starting in my toes, and they stopped pouring just two inches from the very top of the vase.

Partly hormonal, for sure. I know some women say they feel as though they're on the verge of tears all the time from the hormones. Instead, I feel like I'm on the verge of biting someone's head off or simply yelling about little things.

But of course, on top of the hormones, is the oh-so-fun non-stop task of managing type 1 diabetes. And while every part of my is fully committed to this for the sake of both my health and our growing little fetus (which my seven different pregnancy apps tell me is now the size of a tangerine or an apple or an avocado or a tomato or...), the amount of energy that goes into simply thinking and worrying about your diabetes all day is intangible but so huge and real and present at all times.

The funny part is that I feel as though my blood sugars have been awesome lately, as though my brain is getting better and better each week at staying between those tight little lines on my CGM. I'm finding several days can go by without my blood sugar going above 150 mg/dL after eating and staying under 100 mg/dL throughout the night, but it doesn't mean it's not stressful. If anything, the fact that my blood sugars have been staying in range so consistently isn't because anything has gotten "easier" but merely because I'm being extra diligent, habitual, obsessive, and thoughtful around every aspect of diabetes management. And while the results are pleasing, they don't lead to less stress.

While I'm not sure what I can do to truly subdue the stress (at least not for more than the time I spend exercising each day or more than the hour or so I might spend treating myself to a pedicure), I think being aware of it is helpful because I can try to "shake it off" every once in awhile. And, of course, I know when to avoid my husband to prevent scratching his eyes out just because he made a joke that I didn't think was funny (that behavior I'll blame on the hormones).

Regardless, this is supposed to be a stressful process. So taking deep breaths need to become a more consistent daily habit!

Like Jenny says, "...it's a labor of love."

NOTES

MONTH 5

POP! HELLO, YOU!

Dear Type 1 Mama-to-Be,

This is it! You're almost halfway thru one of the most arduous diabetes management experiences you'll ever endure. Halfway. Woooooooooooo...deep breath, mama. Ahhhhh.

A year from now (or even just 20-ish weeks from now), you're going to be so overwhelmed with love that there will be times that you really do want to say that overused adorous line, "Ohh, I could just eat you up!"

It may be overused and cliched, but people keep saying it for a reason: there's just no better way to express it! All your hard work is going to be worth it.

We promise!
Love, love, love,
Ginger & Jenny

MAMA'S MENTAL HEALTH

Pop! This is when things start to get really...cute. Enjoy it, mama! That little bump is not only an invitation for friends and strangers to say, "Oh! Congratulations!"...it's also going to make the reality of motherhood start to feel all the more real. And that's a good thing, because the more you feel that baby inside you, the more connected you'll feel to the baby, too. For women with type 1 diabetes, this can provide a much-needed boost of encouragement for the non-stop effort you'll be putting into managing your blood sugars during the next 20 weeks.

Don't hesitate to talk to your baby, to tell baby about your blood sugar levels...and don't be surprised if you find yourself apologizing to baby for those imperfect blood sugar moments, too. You can't prevent every high or every low, you're just doing the best you can in a body that isn't doing its entire job, but you'll likely still feel guilt for those imperfect numbers. Talk to baby, talk to your partner, talk to your friends. The guilt is something we're all going to feel some version of during pregnancy with type 1 diabetes, but you don't have to keep it bottled up. Let it out, brush it off, carry on.

SPEAKING OF BUMPS...

While most of us wait in anticipation to finally see the "pop" of that bump, most of us also all wonder, "What will my body be like after my baby is born?" During these next few weeks, your body is going to change every week—it's beautiful! And exciting!

And weight-gain, of course, is part of that process, but don't be alarmed that gained a little body-fat is also part of that process, and it has nothing to do with your cravings for ice cream.

In fact, the average woman gains approximately 5 pounds of body-fat during pregnancy for one specific purpose: this is the body's natural way of ensuring their are energy reserves for producing breast-milk once the baby is born.

Your body is taking on a whole new role in life...by creating a life. Enjoy every little curve. You'll have plenty of time to focus on "getting back into your jeans" after the baby is born, but it's important to remember that it takes months for the body to heal from pregnancy and delivery. The uterus alone takes months to shrink down to its near-original size.

Stay active. Eat mostly whole foods, and embrace those baby-making-curves.

"OUT OF THE OFFICE"...MORE OFTEN!

This month is also a good time to have a conversation with your employer and announce your pregnancy if you haven't already. Why? Starting later this month and thru your third trimester, you will be visiting your healthcare team far more often and you'll need an understanding work-relationship for all those appointments. Keep in mind that these appointments aren't always quick and speedy, some of them will take longer than others and trying to predict that length is nearly impossible unless your doctor's office runs a really tight schedule.

If you have additional health concerns during your pregnancy, that means you'll have additional doctor's appointments, too. Overall, every OB-GYN office operates slightly differently and has different protocol for how they care for type 1 patients.

Here's what you can generally expect in terms of OB-GYN appointments as type 1 mama-to-be:

- **WEEKS 20 TO 28**: 1 to 2 appointments per month
  (at least 1 ultrasound per month)
- **WEEKS 28 TO 32**: 1 to 2 appointments per month
  (at least 1 ultrasound per month)
- **WEEKS 32 TO DELIVERY**: 1 to 2 appointments per week
  (NST or BPP testing 1 to 2 times per week along with OB visit and possible ultrasound)

And of course, now is probably a good time to discuss with your employer your postpartum plan, as well. We hope for your sake and baby's sake that you'll give yourself plenty of time to rest and heal after delivery, and plenty of time to snuggle with that new little bundle. Keep in mind as well that diabetes management postpartum is a whole different ball game when you're adjusting to meeting the needs and demands of that new little bundle. Take as much time-off as you're offered to adjust to life as a mother who also happens to have type 1 diabetes. You won't regret it!

NUTRITION & FITNESS & SICK DAYS WITH DIABETES

Let's take a moment to talk about what happens when your nutrition and fitness are put on serious hold because of an illness.

Sick days (like, real people sick, not diabetes-sick) with type 1 diabetes are no piece of cake, but when we add pregnancy to that mix we need to take our sick days even more seriously.

IN A NUTSHELL: situations in which you might not normally think you need to visit the emergency room, like for a 24-hour stomach bug or the flu, can actually become far more serious in a type 1 pregnant woman compared to a type 1 woman or non-diabetic pregnant woman.

NEED TO KNOW ABOUT KETONES: Diabetic ketoacidosis (DKA) ketones are very dangerous and can easily develop during severe illness. Testing your ketones often with ketone strips during any type of illness is important, but do remember that urine ketone strips actually show what your ketones were several hours ago. If you can, ask your doctor for a prescription for a blood ketone meter. Precision Xtra Meter and Novomax Plus Meter are the only meters that measure both blood glucose and blood ketones, but you will need specific test-strips for measuring ketones. You won't use it very often, but it can come in handy a few times a year, even when you're not pregnant.

GETTING YOUR FLU SHOT: The real flu is much more than an upset stomach. Severe fevers and the inability to keep down fluids and foods can be easily fatal for people with type 1. This is why it's really important that you get your flu-shot as a woman with type 1 diabetes who also happens to be pregnant. Really important. If you suspect you have the flu, we absolutely recommend that you visit the emergency room.

WHEN & WHY YOU MIGHT NEED TO VISIT THE EMERGENCY ROOM:

- **VOMITING:** The difference between morning sickness vomiting and vomiting from an actual illness or food poisoning is that the vomiting is so severe it can easily (and usually) cause a person to be unable to eat or drink for over 24 hours. For a type 1 diabetic that means extra trouble becomes going to long without eating can lead to starvation ketones, even after only 6 hours. Not being able to eat or drink can also complicate your insulin needs. If you are unable to keep food and liquids down for more than 6 hours, or your blood sugar has become unmanageable, you should contact your healthcare team immediately to assess if you should visit the emergency room. (Note: food poisoning can be the result of simple things such as deviled eggs at a family BBQ that have been left out on the picnic table far too long. Undercooked meat or meat that has gone bad are also common culprits!)

- **FEVER:** A severe fever is very dangerous very you and baby. A persistent fever over 100 degrees means you should contact your healthcare team immediately.

- **ANY ILLNESS THAT MAKES YOU UNABLE TO MANAGE YOUR BLOOD SUGARS:** Simply put, if even a brutal case of the common cold is making it difficult for you to properly manage your blood sugars, stay hydrated and eat enough food, you should contact your healthcare team.

It's important to remember that just because you're okay during your bout of illness doesn't necessarily mean that your baby is okay. Simple things, such as dehydration, can cause baby's blood pressure to rise, so if you're not sure, contacting your healthcare team or just going right to the emergency room is always a good idea. Trust your instinct.

SPEAKING OF THE EMERGENCY ROOM...

Here's the thing about emergency rooms: the doctors and nurses there generally do not have much training around diabetes management. In fact, just to emphasize that point, Jenny recalls a client of hers who went to the emergency room with severe ketones, high blood sugars and vomiting...and the doctor said, "Since you're not eating or drinking, you need to disconnect from your insulin pump."

Umm...no. Wrong. Very wrong, doc. Fortunately, she knew this was wrong and she convinced the doctor they were wrong as well. (In other words, be prepared to speak-up and talk-back!)

Even if you've never found yourself in an emergency room during all your years as a woman with type 1 diabetes, pregnancy is different. You may be able to manage your blood sugar during a horrible streak of flu-induced vomiting, but that doesn't mean the baby is necessarily okay. When you're sick, baby can suffer, too. For example: you may be dehydrated from vomiting which can raise baby's blood pressure to unsafe levels.

Being prepared can go a long way if you do have a need to visit your Emergency room.

TIPS FOR MANAGING YOUR DIABETES DURING EMERGENCY HOSPITALIZATION:

Following these guidelines you can prep for an emergency visit to the hospital and avoid lengthy discussion about why you can't stop using your insulin in an emergency.

- Always wear a medical ID bracelet or necklace which can alert EMT and Emergency department staff that you have diabetes.
- Wallet cards may not be noticed on a timely basis.
- Many medical ID bracelets that are provided by a credible place also allow the option of having an ID placed on the bracelet/necklace. This ID, enabled with an interactive health record, connects with an online database that holds all your medical information – such as insulin doses, use of an insulin pump (and possibly a CGM), type of insulin used and other medications. It can also contain emergency contact info as well as a note about what to do/not to do with your insulin pump.

- Do not let anyone take you off your insulin pump unless they have a clear plan for delivering insulin through another method. You should never be without insulin, even an extremely small dose will always be needed.
- Do not let anyone take your CGM from you. It shouldn't interfere with their processes unless it is in a very inconvenient location (like your lower back when you're about to receive an epidural). Take time to explain what it is to them so they realize it's an asset, not a mysterious threat.
- Bring your own meter and test-kit with you so you can check your blood sugar between the times when they're checking your blood sugar. They're following a protocol of when they believe your blood sugar needs to be checked. You are following real life, knowing all too well that just because your blood sugar is fine before you eat lunch doesn't mean it's going to be fine an hour later.
- Do not let them give you any medications without confirming what those medications are. If you need to research that medication online to make sure it is safe for your blood sugar, go right ahead and do that. (*Hint: remember that Tylenol can cause inaccurate readings in your CGM.)
- If your voice isn't being heard, your concerns are being respected, and your medical needs aren't being cared for properly, call the Patient Advocacy Hotline within your hospital. Stomp your feet. Raise your voice. Do what you need to in order to keep yourself safe.
- Whoever joins you at the hospital—a partner or a friend—ask them to be your advocate, to speak sternly for you, to call the Patient Advocate Hotline within your hospital if they need to.

BEING PREPARED FOR EMERGENCY VISITS IF YOU USE AN INSULIN PUMP:

If you use a pump, plan ahead. A "Diabetes Emergency Bag" can be packed to carry in your purse, briefcase, gym bag or even stashed in your desk at work or your gym locker. This is really something you should carry with you everywhere because pump malfunctions are a real part of wearing an insulin pump.

PACK THE BAG WITH EXTRA SUPPLIES INCLUDING:

- extra reservoir cartridges and pods
- infusion sets
- batteries
- tapes and adhesives

- emergency glucagon kit
- Non-perishable food and/or glucose tabs/gel
- insulin vials/pens and syringes in case your pump is not working properly
- note card with pump settings including basal rates, ratios, targets and active insulin time (in case your pump settings get changed or deleted).
- printed prescription for each prescribed item in the bag for a backup
- record of and info including the names of your healthcare team

In the event you need to go to the hospital quickly, you'll have some supplies to last a few days as well as information to help the medical caregivers understand your plan of care. Carry a pump emergency card (given by most pump manufacturers), which gives treatment recommendations if something should happen to you.

There's nothing quite as "fun" as an emergency visit when you're uber-pregnant...hopefully it isn't something you have to experience!

INSULIN MANAGEMENT

That insulin-producing "vacation" you've been experiencing is really going to be a distant memory this month as pregnancy hormones increase, baby grows, mama grows, and blood sugars start gradually rising, due to increasing insulin needs.

This month (and the months to come), there are three things that are going to have a gradual yet noticeable impact on your insulin doses:

- **PROGESTERONE & OTHER PREGNANCY RELATED HORMONES:** The increase in this hormone causes an increase in insulin resistance...the major reason behind all of your increasing insulin needs throughout your entire pregnancy.
- **WEIGHT-GAIN:** That little bump is growing. Don't be surprised if you wake up one morning and suddenly feel like you've gained inches in every direction—it's normal! In fact, it's wonderful, but it will also cause your insulin needs to increase due to insulin resistance.
- **MORE CALORIES:** As your baby gets bigger, their caloric needs increase bit by bit, too, and your increased calorie consumption will lead to an increase in your background insulin needs, not just your doses for meals. Just remember, when thinking about that old phrase "eating for two"...one of those two people are very, very small. Resist the urge to over-do it.

EXPECTED INSULIN ADJUSTMENTS

Here are a few things to keep in mind when assessing your insulin doses this month:

- **BACKGROUND INSULIN DOSES:** Due to all of these gradual changes you can generally expect to see an increase in your background insulin needs every 7 to 14 days. For some, the increase may be small while for others that increase may be larger.
- **MEAL BOLUS DOSES:** This month, you'll will really see a clear need for a longer pre-bolus before eating. This means that instead of waiting 20 to 30 minutes between when you take your insulin and when you eat your meal, you may need to wait up to 30 to 40 minutes in order to prevent that post-meal spike in your blood sugar.

* *Remember: During pregnancy, you want to make a change in your doses after seeing a trend of higher or lower blood sugar levels over the course of two days rather than three or more days when not pregnant. It's also important to never make increases of more than 1 to 2 units in one day. Make an adjustment of up to 2 units, assess its efficacy over the next day or two, and adjust again as needed. Within each trimester, you will likely see a total increase in your insulin needs of anywhere between 3 to 7 units. Those with higher levels of insulin resistance and weight-gain will see the greatest increases in their insulin needs.*

AT THE DOCTOR'S OFFICE

This is the time in your pregnancy where your appointments will start to increase in frequency because your pregnancy is considered "high-risk." This month also comes with the coolest ultrasounds:

- **BABY'S GENDER:** At 20 weeks, you'll have your "level 2" ultrasound scheduled with a much fancier, more powerful ultrasound machine than you've used for all your regular check-ups. The pictures of your baby are vivid and real. Unlike the other ultrasounds where you can sort of see how what you're looking at could be a little human, this ultrasound is clearly your baby. And if you want to, you get to find out the gender!
- **BABY'S ORGANS:** Also at 20 weeks, during the same ultrasound to determine the gender, your technician will look closely at each organ in the baby to determine everything is healthy or pinpoint any concerns. This scan will also check for cleft lip and palate, and it ensures all organs are formed in the right location of the body. It will also check on the amniotic fluid quantity and for obvious issues such as a low-lying placenta.

- **BABY'S HEART:** This ultrasound will come a week or two after your baby's organs and gender scan. This ultrasound is looking for any concerns within the development of the heart. As women with type 1 diabetes, our babies are at a higher risk for heart abnormalities but remember this is still rare. Don't worry unless you're given a clear reason to, and just continue to do the best you can with your blood sugar management.

If you have any concerns or questions before, during or after these scans, don't hesitate to ask your doctor. These scans can be very nerve-wracking, especially before they happen. As women with diabetes we know all too well the reality of our bodies working against us. It's easy to imagine things going wrong, but the other reality is that abnormalities are still rare. Take a deep breath and try to face these extra scans with as much courage and positivity as you carry with you each day when you face your diabetes.

MONTH 5
GINGER'S PREGNANCY DIARY

WEEKS 17–20

The past month has been very consistent in symptoms and what-not: I have more energy for exercise but I'm feeling increasingly less energy for the day as a whole. I wake up the mornings with a raging headache and very groggy—nothing a ½ cup of coffee can't handle—but then within an hour or so I'm ready to rock 'n roll.

By 2 p.m., I start fading. By 4 p.m., I feel like a total couch potato. I just want to sit and stare. Most of the time I'm not tired enough to actually nap, but the need to sit and zone out is strong.

I decided during this past 4-week period that as I approached that half-way mark of pregnancy (week 20), it was time to start cutting back wherever possible on my work and duties. For me, this means cutting back all the extra freelance work and random freelance projects. I'd already been turning down extra work but I gave a heads-up to a company I make diabetes coaching videos for that I was going to be "out to lunch" starting October 1st until at least two months after the baby was born, because video production was getting to be particularly exhausting.

This leaves me with my daily work as Editorial Director at Diabetes Daily which is never stressful and always consistent in terms of how much time and energy it demands from me.

I felt a major sense of relief after letting the video company know I'd be checking out for a while. A decision I'm very glad I made now rather than trying to endure it and keep it up for several more weeks only to likely end in a puddle of exhausted tears mid-production. (Probably not the video performance they're looking for!)

I reminded myself: this is not just a normal pregnancy. A tremendous amount of my energy is being spent on trying to make it appear as though I'm not diabetic! To a non-diabetic, this may sound like a little side-hobby that you think about before you eat, but to those of us with diabetes, we know this is a constant, constant, constant mental effort. It isn't just the meals, it's everything. Getting the whole day to line up smoothly and beautifully so that our blood sugars look that much more non-diabetic.

With 20 weeks under my belt, this more intensive diabetes management has become a regular concern of each day, almost as if I've forgotten what it's like to see a 130 mg/dL on my meter and not feel annoyed.

But I cannot forget or underestimate how much energy I need to devote to my diabetes. Tight blood sugar management is just as important in the next few months as it has been during the past 4 months! (And on top of it, I'm definitely noticing my fibromyalgia muscle spasms are increasing during the second trimester! Dear Psychotic Neck Muscles, please relax!)

But I don't want to feel as though I don't have the energy I need for diabetes. I don't want to feel as though I'm trying to muster up more energy for diabetes. I want diabetes to be first in line for energy!

(I can only assume that women with diabetes who already have another child to care for have developed some sort of impressive motherly endurance that us first-timers have yet to experience.) *Spoiler Alert: Ginger is half-way thru her second pregnancy at the time of writing this... and it ain't easy!

CRAVINGS

On another note...vegetables and salads at home have a made a reappearance in my cravings! After a several months of not wanting vegetables or salads made at home, I have found myself craving them tremendously! Tremendously. Big salads. With spinach and red onion and cucumber and green pepper and tomato...and delicious Brianna's dressing.

Green beans. I'm feeling very into green beans suddenly.

My appetite in general has definitely increased this month, but I'm finding my intentions of ignoring cravings for junk continuing to be successful. The other day, around 10 a.m., I found myself thinking strongly about chocolate cake. Instead of hunting down a gluten-free chocolate cake or something else equally not so ideal for a woman with type 1 diabetes and tight blood sugar goals...I Googled pictures of "delicious chocolate cakes" for probably 10 minutes and found myself oddly satisfied.

And it further convinced me that I really don't want to feed my body a bunch of cake right now. Not that there isn't a time or place for chocolate cake during pregnancy, but I don't want it to be an impulsive thing that could leave me eating more than a reasonable serving. If I'm going to eat dessert, it's going to be thoughtful and planned, and ideally something I made myself at home.

Regardless, the goal is always 90/10: 90 percent of whole, fresh, high-quality foods...and 10 percent treats. Today, for instance, my treat was a coffee ice cream milkshake using Breyer's Coffee ice cream and unsweetened almond milk. Barely 300 calories and barely 25 grams of carbohydrate. Very low impact on the ol' blood sugar as far as treats go, never going above 130 mg/dL with 3 units of insulin properly pre-bolused.

INSULIN

During weeks 14 through perhaps week 18, I very consistently needed a 1-unit increase in my Lantus insulin every 10 days. By week 19, I had increased my Lantus dose from 15 units to 16 units after 2 days of feeling like a horrible person for seeing my overnight blood sugar stubbornly sitting between 130 to 150 mg/dL. But after just a few days at 16 units, I felt like I was back at 130 mg/dL all the time, even during the day it just seemed like my blood sugar wanted to rise up to 130 mg/dL.

And so, merely a few days after an increase to 16 units, I was making an increase to 17 units. I actually resisted this increase for probably two days because it just seemed too soon for another increase! Foolish of me to think that the body was going to be consistent! Hah!

After making this adjustment, though, I felt a huge relief because my blood sugar is now sitting more easily around 70 to 100 mg/dL between meals and overnight...and there was something so tremendously yet subtly painful and stressful about merely 1 week of sitting at or above 130 mg/dL! Again I found myself needing to be reminded that this was only this week. It's not that high all the time. It can't be, I know this from my A1C as evidence, and yet, I just felt like I was doing a horrible job! It's just a few days! Relax!

Regardless, the point is: insulin adjustments are not always consistent and simply paying attention to those stubborn blood sugars and simple patterns can make all the difference.

Wow, I am hungry. This hunger beats the hunger I felt after powerlifting training sessions. This hunger is like, "Love me! Feed me!" And every bite is like, "Ahh, yes. Perfect. Now do it again."

This week I've had to make major increases in my insulin doses, more so than any other week. Across the board: background insulin dose, insulin-to-carbohydrate ratios, and correction factor doses. Bump. Bump. Bump.

But, amazingly enough, my A1C came back at 5.1 percent—definitely the lowest A1C I've ever had. I don't know how...I mean, yes, I'm putting 90 percent of my energy into blood sugar management, but I always thought a 5.1 would be the result of perfection, and my blood sugars have definitely not be perfect. I really don't feel like I earned that, but again I know my brain clings to the numbers that were out-of-range and dismisses how much effort goes into spending most of the day in-range.

Ahhh, this is so much fun, I almost can't stand it.

NOTES

MONTH 6

WHOA, MAMA!

If you weren't feeling the glow last month, you'll definitely start hearing about it from everyone around you this month. This is it, mama!

MAMA'S MENTAL HEALTH

How are you feeling? No, really—think about the answer to this question. You have a lot on your plate as a woman with type 1 diabetes who is 6 months pregnant. It's an amazing thing that we can do this so successfully compared to what women in the 50s, 60s, and 70s had access to simply live with type 1 diabetes let alone become pregnant and create life inside themselves! It's an amazing thing. But with all this modern technology and modern insulin, there's a lot of work and stress, too.

If you're feeling up to your ears in stress, anxiety, and worry because of everything on your plate, now might definitely be a worthwhile time to schedule an appointment with a therapist of psychologist. (Or any other health practitioner whom you feel might help ease your stress! Massage? Acupuncture? Naturopath? Meditation? Or hiring someone to clean your house! Whatever would help you lighten the emotional and mental load.)

If talking with a professional doesn't sound like your cup of tea, then you might find benefit from simply carving out 8 minutes in your morning or during your lunch-break to meditate or to just listen to 3 songs that help you relax. The goal is to acknowledge your stress and manage it instead of trying to pretend it's not there.

At the very least, remember to just pause for a moment and give yourself credit for everything you're juggling right now. Deep breath, mama.

NUTRITION & FITNESS

Not only are you about to start filling out your maternity clothes more adorably this month, you're also going to start feeling more full earlier after each meal as baby grows and there becomes less and less space for your vital organs, like your stomach!

This can certainly be an issue if you dose your insulin for far more than you manage to eat.

Instead of trying to pack all your calories into 3 to 4 meals a day, eating every 4 to 5 hours, you may find it's much more comfortable to start eating smaller meals more often if that's not already a habit. (This is ideal for non-pregnant life, too!)

To make this switch, start think about every time you eat as a "small meal" rather than "meals vs. snacks." An apple with a handful of nuts is about 300 to 400 calories, just as a chicken salad with veggies and a drizzle of salad dressing is also about 400 calories.

SMALLER MEALS. MORE OFTEN.

One of the great things, however, about this month's growing belly is that many of you will find there's more belly to adore without really seeing an increase on the scale. Just because the scale doesn't go up, though, doesn't mean your insulin needs won't need a boost...but we'll talk about that later in the chapter!

TIPS FOR PREPARING WHOLE-FOOD SNACKS & MEALS

As things start to get bumpier, your energy might start to fade a little bit, too. Which might mean you're reaching more often for processed stuff or fast-food instead of whole foods.

Now might be a good time to do a little check-in on what your nutrition is looking like overall. Whether you track what you eat for a few days with pen and paper, or you enter it into a nutrition app, considering just "tuning-in" closely for a moment.

Is at least 80 percent of your diet whole-foods? If not, maybe you could pick one meal of the day that you'll recommit to making healthier, whole-food choices during. Remember, a satisfying meal is never just one macronutrient (like eating just an apple). Try to combine foods so you're getting protein and carbs or protein and fat, etc.

We've talked about clean-eating meals in the preparing for pregnancy sections of the book, but here are a few tips for making healthy meals easy to grab-n-go:

- Pre-package ¼ or ⅓ cup servings of mixed nuts into ziplock bags, so you can keep them in your desk at work for quick snacks.

- Buy 7 apples to start the week and keep them in your desk at work... to go with your mixed nuts! A perfectly healthy and easy snack.

- Prepare a pan full of sliced sweet potato or slice zucchini and yellow squash. Drizzle in olive oil and sprinkle with salt, then bake at 400 degrees for about 30 minutes or until done. Pack a reasonable serving into bags or containers for the week!

- Choose one day of the week to pre-cook your proteins. For instance, you could grill 20 ounces of steak on Sunday, cut it up and put it in small tupperware containers. Salt and pepper. Then pair it with bell peppers that you've chopped up and put into 5 separate ziplock bags to eat with your steak! A nutritious meal for the middle of your day!

- Choose a protein powder (our favorites include: Orgain's vegan chocolate flavor or JayRobb's egg or whey options), and use enough scoops to equal between 200 to 300 calories, made with unsweetened almond milk and water. Pair with a handful of nuts, a choice of fruit, or carrots! (Tip: even though protein powder is low-carb, you will likely find your blood sugar reacts to it as though it's about 10 to 20 grams of carbs because the protein is so broken down and isolated, some of it is easily converted to low-impact glucose.)

These are just a few ways you could prepare some of your healthy meals in advance. It doesn't take as much time as you'd think, just an hour one day a week (ideally Sunday), and it'll save you time and effort during the week!

PLAN YOUR TREATS IN ADVANCE

Do you feel like your sweet-tooth and cravings are already out of control? If so, let's reign this in now so you can enjoy your sweets and treats without sabotaging your entire diabetes management goals and overall pregnancy health.

The simple approach is to plan your sweets and treats. Here are a few tips for keeping those taste-buds in check:

- If you're desperate for French-fries the moment you wake-up in the morning, resist the urge to eat them in the a.m. by immediately eating something healthier for breakfast. Fruit and nuts, toast and eggs—whatever you can find that isn't loaded with grease or sugar.

- Choose a time each day or on certain days of the week that you will give yourself an appropriate serving of that treat. Maybe Mondays and Thursdays are your French-Fry days? Or 4 p.m. is when you get to enjoy some chocolate or ice cream with carefully dosed insulin and blood sugar checks afterwards?

- Make sure you're eating enough real food. If you're simply not eating enough real food each day, you're going to be hungry. And the first thing you might crave when you're really hungry is nutrient-poor yet calorie-dense foods like burgers, fries and candy bars. Sure, the baby "wants what it wants" but there's no way your baby really wants to spend its first 9 months of existence being fueled and developed by high fructose corn syrup and heavily processed oils. Give your body plenty of real food, clean and wholesome, and leave room for treats as appropriate!

THIS ISN'T THE FIRST TIME AND IT ISN'T THE LAST TIME WE'RE GOING TO SAY THIS: developing these healthier habits now will help you during pregnancy but they'll also benefit you throughout the remainder of your life as a mom with type 1 diabetes.

INSULIN MANAGEMENT

Your hormone production may have begun revving its engine last month but the real evidence of it will be this month. Remember, every little unit makes a difference—don't be afraid of making small changes in your doses!

EXPECTED INSULIN ADJUSTMENTS

Here are a few things to keep in mind when assessing your insulin doses this month:

- BACKGROUND INSULIN DOSES: This month, don't be surprised if you have to bump your background dose up once each week due to increasing hormones. Your body will be making a big shift this month and the proof will be gradually increasing insulin needs. If the tiniest increase in your doses can make a big difference.

- **MEAL BOLUS DOSES:** This month, you'll will likely see a need for a longer pre-bolus before eating. This means that instead of waiting 15 to 20 minutes between when you take your insulin and when you eat your meal, you may need to wait up to 30 minutes in order to prevent that post-meal spike in your blood sugar. Assess where blood sugar is with the pre-bolus about about 1 and 2 hours post meal—if you're in your target at one hour (<140 mg/dL or 7.8 mmol) but it stabilizes and doesn't come down to target (<120 mg/dL or 6.7 mmol) after this, then a decrease in I:C ratio by 1 to 2 grams may be needed to give enough insulin to cover the meal better.

- **CORRECTION FACTOR:** Until now, you may have not had to increase your CF at all, but this month that's going to change. If it used to be 1:50, you may find it becomes 1:40 or 1:30.

* *Remember: During pregnancy, you want to make a change in your doses after seeing a trend of higher or lower blood sugar levels over the course of two days rather than three or more days when not pregnant. It's also important to never make increases of more than 1 to 2 units in one day. Make an adjustment of up to 2 units, assess its efficacy over the next day or two, and adjust again as needed. Within each trimester, you will likely see a total increase in your insulin needs of anywhere between 3 to 7 units. Those with higher levels of insulin resistance and weight-gain will see the greatest increases in their insulin needs.*

WHERE TO PUT YOUR CGM & INFUSION SITES

As that adorable bump begins to grow, you're likely going to need new real estate for your CGM and infusion sites.

Remember these details when choose new locations for your CGM & infusion sites:

- You should be able to pinch the flesh so there is at least 1 to 2 inches of "chub" between your pinching fingers. Infusion sites are not going to work well if they are placed in skin that is pulled taut by your growing bump. And CGM insertions are going to hurt like the dickens in these areas, not to mention that the wire of the sensor itself may bend and no longer work correctly.

- If you can't reach it, ask your honey to help you! That's why we emphasized how important it is that your partners know how to place sensors and infusion sites early on when you can still show them and teach them. You may not require their help, but it'll be nice to have more options for placement by letting them help.

- Areas to consider: side-thigh, upper-glute, side-glute, love-handles, lower back sides, back of the arm tricep area)...anywhere with a good amount of adorably pinchable chub!

Ain't this fun? Ahh. Okay, now onto another quirky problem you may face with pump sites....

HIGH BLOOD SUGARS WITH NEW INFUSION SITES

You've probably experienced this problem to a certain extent prior to being pregnant, but when every ounce of your energy is focused on trying to maintain certain blood sugar levels, it can be pretty infuriating when a new infusion site is the cause of major highs.

As you approach the part of your pregnancy during which you'll have the highest insulin needs, this extra effort to prevent high blood sugars with new infusion sites may be particularly crucial.

WHY THIS HAPPENS

This doesn't happen to everyone but it does happy to many. When you place a new infusion site, inflammation can occur at the new site due to the "injury" of the tissue. Just because this puncture is being made to save your life by creating a location to deliver insulin doesn't mean the tissue of your skin necessarily loves the idea.

Assuming there isn't an actual technical malfunction such as a kinked cannula or blood blocking the insulin from pushing through the cannula, here are the primary reasons why your blood sugar might rise during the 4-hour window after setting-up a new infusion site:

- The old site is typically pulled out right away and insulin from that site has a tendency to leak out. If you have just bolused with this site, or if it only has basal insulin, the site will leak a bit of the unabsorbed insulin when it is pulled out of the skin. In pregnancy, if you have your sites on your abdomen after it has started expanding, this can also leak more since the "tunnel" the cannula sits in under the skin is stretched. Reminder: during pregnancy, it isn't recommended to use the abdominal area after the stomach has started stretching as it can cause leakage of insulin around the cannula completely unrelated to a new infusion site.
- The actual insertion of a new infusion set (via tubed or tubeless pump) actually causes a bit of irritation and inflammation in the tissue under the skin at that site. (Believe it or not, your body doesn't love getting stabbed and left with stuff in its skin! Go figure!) This irritation and

inflammation decreases insulin absorption, causing a bit of delay in your body actually getting effective insulin from that new site.

- The previous two issues above compound each other—as there is a lack of insulin from the old site (leaked out) as well as a slower absorption from the new site— overall insulin deficiency which can translate into higher post site change BG for hours post site change.

Especially as you approach the last trimester, where insulin resistance increases gradually, this lack of properly absorbing insulin from a new site-change can be incredibly frustrating and detrimental to your blood sugar goals.

TIPS TO PREVENT THE HIGH BLOOD SUGARS WITH NEW INFUSION SITES

Remember, when experimenting with this tips, try one approach at a time (preferably in the order they are listed) to determine what is the best fit for you without causing hypoglycemia.

- **KEEP THE OLD INFUSION SITE IN AFTER SETTING UP A NEW SITE:** When it's time to change your infusion site, keep the old site in (including those who use Omnipod) after you disconnect or disable that site/pod. While the pump will not continue to deliver insulin through that site, it will allow any insulin still sitting under that site to be properly absorbed and prevent it from leaking out.

- **INSERT A NEW SITE AND WAIT TO USE IT:** Another option is to insert that new infusion set (for those on tubed pumps, not Omnipod) a few hours before you actually need to pump insulin through that site. This can allow the inflammation at the new site to subside while you're still getting your normal insulin doses through your older site. When you are ready to use the new site, connect to it properly, prime the cannula, and you may see significantly better absorption right away with your new site. It is still important to keep the old site in for that 2 hours after you disconnect because of the remaining insulin that could leak out.

- **CHANGE YOUR INFUSION SITE AFTER A MEAL:** The worst time to set-up a new infusion site is right before you eat when your body is going to desperately need every drop of insulin it gets. Instead, bolus with the old site, start up the new site using the above tips, and then leave that old site in for a minimum of 2 hours. (Remember if you use an extended/combo bolus for a meal, you'll have to wait for that to fully deliver from the old site before starting use of the new site). The timing of your new infusion site could make all the difference!

- **INCREASE THE "PRIMED INSULIN" DOSAGE OF THE NEW SITE:** Tubed pumps require you to "prime" the cannula. The "prime" dose is a predetermined amount based on the specific cannula length you use. To learn more how many units you should be using to prime your cannula, after inserting it, is located right in the pamphlet that comes with your infusion sets. The purpose of "priming" is to fill insulin into the space filled with air that remains in the cannula once you pull out the insertion needle. This ensures that as it pumps your basal dose, the cannula is pumping insulin, not air. If you neglect to prime your cannula properly, you'll miss out on a good portion of your basal dose because units of air will be pumped instead. However, even with this proper prime of the cannula, many people find it helpful to take an immediate bolus of insulin with their new site to get the site more "saturated" with insulin, enhancing the absorption of your normal basal insulin. The recommendation is to take a bolus of the amount of basal that is running at that time of day. For example, if you take .6 units per hour in your basal at 12 p.m., then that is how many units you would bolus to "saturate" your new site with insulin. NOTE: This amount may vary person to person, so it is important to pay attention to what happens to your blood sugar in the hours after a site change and evaluate the best course of action. Evaluating the amount of rise in your blood sugar after a site change can tell you a lot about how much insulin might be needed.

AT THE DOCTOR'S OFFICE

No doctor's appointment will compare to the excitement of finding out your baby's gender last month. This month, it's a bit more mundane (which is kind of nice for those of us with high-maintenance chronic illnesses!).

CROSSING YOUR T'S & DOTTING YOUR I'S:

- If you haven't already, definitely check-in with your doctor again about getting approval for using your CGM and insulin pump during labor and delivery at the hospital.
- Have you thought about if you'd like to schedule a C-section or would you like to give induction a try? While we all wish we could let Mother Nature take its course, research says it's safer for both baby and mama not to go past 38 to 39 weeks. Do a little research and reading to see what you'd like your plan to be—and remember that a plan is really more of a hope. If you want to be induced but you exhibit preeclampsia symptoms or early contractions, etc., your

healthcare team may find that it's safer to scoot you right along for a C-section. It's all about keeping everyone safe. Nothing will take away from the experience of meeting your child for the first time.

- Keep in mind: When you feel comfortable over the next weeks or months, consider talking to your healthcare team more closely about being the one with final say over your insulin doses during labor and deliver—if you feel comfortable with that responsibility. You know your body best. We'll talk later in this book about expected insulin dose changes, but the main point is that you feel empowered during your labor and delivery, and part of the decision process.

ALL THOSE BABY MEASUREMENTS

In the upcoming months, your ultrasounds will become more and more frequent, and with each ultrasound comes measurements. With each measurement comes a percentile. These percentiles imply where on the range of "average" your baby is measuring. If your baby's head is in the 90th percentile, that means his or her head is larger than 90 percent of most other baby's heads at the same gestational age.

At the same time, you'll be constantly hearing about how "women with diabetes have big babies." And this is where a bit of confusion and concern can arise if you're not clear on what part of the "big baby" is really attributed to the higher blood sugar levels in a type 1 mother.

What you and your healthcare team will want to see is a steady and gradual growth of baby's head, belly, legs, and overall length throughout the second and third trimesters. If your baby measures at the 90th percentile and continues to measure at or near the 90th percentile through to your last trimester, that's good because that is consistent and gradual growth. The same would be true for a baby at the 50th percentile, the 45th, etc.

(In certain circumstances, a very small baby could be a concern and your healthcare team would identify this. For example, particularly in obese women, a small baby can potentially be the result of a uterus that has "aged" due to the strain and stress on the body of being obese. This can result in a very small baby for a variety of reasons we're not going to get into in this book! But if this concern applies to you, talk to your healthcare team.)

Now, where your type 1 diabetes comes into play regarding the size and growth percentiles of your baby is when there is a sudden increase in the baby's measurements, especially in the third trimester when baby is growing the most and putting on the most fat.

The particular area of the body where this extra growth will appear specifically from mom's high blood sugar levels is in the baby's belly. If the belly is suddenly growing larger but the other measurements of the baby continue to stay steady with earlier percentiles, this is a sign of a baby getting excess sugar from their mother's bloodstream. The official term for a larger than average baby, as we mentioned much earlier, is macrosomnia. The consequences of macrosomnia are simple:

1. Yes, it does increase your baby's risk for other complications, but it is by no means a guarantee or even a likelihood that your baby will experience other complications due to macrosomnia. Except for…

2. Most likely, a baby with macrosomnia will be born with lower blood sugars at birth and will need formula or glucose immediately. This is simply because the reason that baby has macrosomnia in the first place is because of higher blood sugars in mom. Higher blood sugars in mom during pregnancy means that baby is producing higher amounts of its own insulin to compensate for all of that extra glucose. As soon as baby is removed from mom's body and no longer getting all that excess glucose from her bloodstream, it can take several hours for baby's body to regulate its insulin production for normal glucose levels.

3. C-sections. If your baby is larger due to higher blood sugars (or due to pure genetics) you'll likely need a C-section for the sake of keeping everyone involved as safe as possible.

The best thing you can do to prevent macrosomnia is to keep your A1C as well below 6.5 percent as possible with steady blood sugars as much as possible. In the end, you're going to do the very best you can. You didn't ask for type 1 diabetes. You didn't do anything to cause it, and you couldn't have prevented it. Don't let anyone shame you for giving birth to a larger baby if that's the case. Do the very best you can and ask for help when you need it.

MONTH 6
GINGER'S PREGNANCY DIARY

WEEK 24

It would be so wonderful if your insulin needs during pregnancy increased exactly every 11 days or every 7 days or every anything. But the reality is that there's nothing consistent about it whatsoever! Not even the amount that it's going to increase by.

During the beginning of the second trimester, an increase by 1 unit in my Lantus insulin seemed to make all the difference for at least a week if not 10 or 11 days. But during the past couple weeks and especially this first week of month six in my pregnancy, the inconsistencies are getting even more inconsistent!

For instance, at the start of this week, I increased my Lantus dose from 20 units at night to 21 units at night. And that seemed to work wonderfully for a full week, keeping my fasting blood sugar in the 70 to 100 mg/dL range and helping me stay in that range between meals, too.

Then, this past Sunday, 6 days later, it was clear that I needed another boost, so I upped the dose to 22 units of Lantus. That worked well for about...oh...36 hours. It was clear by Tuesday at midnight that it was already time for another increase—two days later! But I was hesitant to make yet another change because it seemed so recent that I'd just increased to 22 units...surely my stubborn blood sugars last night and today are the result of a mistake I'm making with food and carb-counting, right? So I gave it another day before increasing to 23 units, and that extra day proved to me clearly that I needed more background insulin.

SO TONIGHT I WILL INCREASE TO 23 UNITS.

And that is my story about the inconsistencies of insulin dose adjustments in the second trimester. The best I can do is pay attention to the little details, think carefully before making another change (because even 1 unit extra of background insulin can leave me on a horrible roller-coaster of lows, (consult Jenny), and be patient.

On an amusing note, it almost seems as if those weeks where I need to increase my Lantus insulin dose twice in one week actually coincide with the same week where I can noticeably see my belly getting bigger. (Unfortunately, this is also unpredictably subtle because the number on the scale doesn't necessarily change and yet I know my stretchy cotton shirts aren't fitting me properly anymore. So it's not as though I can use this as a method for determining my next insulin dose change!)

WEEK 25

My recent A1C came back at 5.1 percent, and I was personally shocked. All I can ever remember are the "horrible" blood sugars. (Yes, I know we shouldn't label blood sugars, but in pregnancy, I find it helpful to just be honest about what that number feels like. A high blood sugar feels horrible, because it's not my goal and it's not ideal for the baby.) But all I can remember are the 170s and the 200s and the times where I only waited 5 minutes instead of 15 minutes before starting to eat a simple apple with peanut butter only to watch my blood sugar rise to 160 mg/dL and hang there for a while before finally coming back down. But I must be doing something right most of the day with a 5.1 percent, and only in "low blood sugar" range for 10 percent of the time according to my CGM's report. Don't get me wrong, I was ecstatic and very proud to see these numbers, but this is something I never thought I'd achieve. I'd read stories from other type 1 women who had been through pregnancy and remember in particular the one from the woman whose A1C was 5.1 percent throughout most of her pregnancy. I remember thinking, "Geez, that's crazy. I couldn't do that."

I'm realizing though, that the A1C was the result of a few things:

1. 200 mg/dL is no longer a regular "high" for me. Instead, thanks to proper pre-bolusing most of the time and diligently correcting rising blood sugars sooner than later, a blood sugar of 160 mg/dL is the new "horrible." And now 200 mg/dL is considered "super high" rather than just "high."

2. Despite the amount of intensity and thinking still involved on a daily basis to maintain "baby range blood sugars," the overall daily goals are the new normal. It's not "stressful," but instead it's just life. It's just the new standard.

3. Super clean eating. This would not be possible if I wasn't making a very clear choice every day to eat mostly whole foods, cooking my own meals, and avoiding temptation to eat junk foods.

Regardless of the A1C, I have to also mention that whoa this month also struck the beginning of significant changes in my insulin needs. The hormones needed for this stage of pregnancy are clearly causing more insulin resistance than the prior 4 months. In addition to recent increases in my background insulin, I have finally noticed a significant need to increase my meal doses. Also, I definitely need to pre-bolus sooner and wait longer before eating. 15 minutes used to be enough. Now it's looking more like 20 to 30 minutes depending on the food being eaten.

It's a labor of love! That part is easy to remember . . . every time she kicks me!

WEEK 26

Hello, appetite! There you are! I mean, I've been "hungry" during the first 5 months of this pregnancy, but I wouldn't say I was ever overwhelming hungry or wanting food even when I'm not feeling physically hungry in my stomach.

UNTIL NOW.

This past week I've found myself thinking about food all day long. Like those stereotypical scenes in movies with pregnant women where they seem to only want the greasiest, fattiest, heaviest foods.

And don't get me wrong: I certainly have had days here and there where all I thought about was a giant cake or French fries...but I started my pregnancy off firmly telling myself that not all cravings must be satisfied. Instead, I can just think about those foods. Look at pictures of those foods on Google. Pretend I'm taking a bite...and then go eat some green beans and steak instead. And sure, I save room for a little treat most days but that's usually a small fraction of my day's nutrition.

This past week, though, I gave in more than usual.

And this unfortunately coincided with my 29th birthday which means I accidentally celebrated my birthday with not-so-awesome junky foods for 5 days instead of just 1 day. Gluten-free pizza. Gluten-free strawberry cake. Cheese popcorn. Ohh, and a strawberry milkshake. (I've been thinking about real strawberry milkshakes for months. I mean months. And I finally indulged in one this past week and it was magical. Pre-bolused my insulin 40 minutes before eating it and it worked out pretty well considering the size of this amazing creation, and the fact that I was completely guessing the carbohydrate content. My blood sugar went up to 170 mg/dL momentarily and then back down.)

Anyways, the result of my 5-day indulgence excursion during which half the day's meals were clean, whole foods and the other half the day was junk lead to not-so-awesome blood sugars! During the day wasn't as much a problem as overnight. Almost every night in the past 5 days, my blood sugar sat stubbornly between 200 mg/dL to 250 mg/dL and took forever to come down. I always had it down under 100 mg/dL by early morning. but it took all night.

Needless to say, the birthday party is over. It's time to get back to business.

WEEK 27

If you're reading this and you're 27 weeks pregnant, please give yourself a hearty pat on the back. This isn't easy.

Most days I'd say it feels like my new "normal" (but that doesn't mean it's easy) and then suddenly, for a day or even just an hour, it feels so tremendous...even when it's going smoothly.

The combination of hormones (whoa, they weren't kidding) and a quiet moment in my recliner to sit and think about just how much mental and emotional effort goes into growing this little baby in this diabetic body every day has hit me especially hard and brought me to tears.

It's so much work.

All day. It takes up so much space in my brain and my thoughts, I can't possibly imagine what life is like for a non-diabetic pregnant woman. What do they think about all day if they don't have to think about all of this blood sugar bullsh*t?

If my insulin needs would just magically stay in one place for a consistent period of time, that would probably lighten the load. Instead, we work so hard to get everything fine-tuned (again), and then two days later it isn't working properly and you're feeling like you're doing something wrong until you fine-tune them (again) and things are smoother.

It's tremendous. The daily grind. In some ways, to an onlooker, it might look very gentle and steady with extra insulin doses and extra finger pricks. They can't tell that in our heads (and, oy vey, our hearts) we are thinking about our blood sugar non-stop. Worrying. Wondering. Hoping. Hoping that everything will be okay and that the "great blood sugar" moments will out-number the "not so perfect" moments.

They can't tell that 30 minutes before I was supposed to meet my friend for lunch I was trying to think about precisely what I would order so I could take my insulin 15 minutes before I arrived so that the pre-bolus would be kicking in 15 minutes after arriving when the food was being served.

They can't tell that my blood sugar has been sitting stubbornly at 155 mg/dL all day and I feel like I've done everything to get it down and it still won't budge. And that my mind isn't really thinking about lunch or our conversation but instead how this is going to affect my A1C, my baby, my average blood sugar estimate that week. Will this one freaking day undo all my hard work so far? Will an entire day stuck at 155 mg/dL make my A1C go up by...how much?

It's such an irrational line of thinking (that one day could ruin everything) but it's there, nonetheless.

I can't even make the 30-minute drive from home to downtown without looking at the number on my CGM at least twice. In a more rational state of mind, that seems really silly to me.

3 months to go, little chickadee baby. We can do it.

MONTH 7

THE JOYS OF
INSULIN RESISTANCE

Take a deep breath, mama-to-be, because while the "big day" is getting closer, you still have a lot of work to do.

This month is the start of a very different pregnancy experience for a variety of reasons. Sure, like any pregnant woman, you're going to start feeling far less "cute" in your curvy pregnant shape and far more uncomfortable instead. Gasping for breath while simply grocery shopping and struggling to get up off the couch are all typical parts of the next few months, but for women with type 1 diabetes, we have the added pleasure of hormone-induced insulin resistance that increases each week.

These last three months can be trying, particularly when it comes to keep your blood sugars in range and keeping up with the expected yet specifically unpredictable changes you'll need to make in your insulin doses.

Now, more than ever, it will be so important to be kind to yourself as you work hard to manage your blood sugars. You're doing the best you can. It's not easy! So remember, take a deep breath...you can do this!

MAMA'S MENTAL HEALTH

How are you feeling, mama? Have you had it up to "here" with the excessive pressure to be perfect? The constant finger pricks and extra doses of insulin? The non-stop obsession with your blood sugar?

It ain't easy. Many women enjoy the extra attention and care they receive during pregnancy, but for those of us with type 1 diabetes, we get enough unwanted medical attention when we're not pregnant!

If you're feeling stressed out—remember that you are not alone! This is a stressful process for us insulin-dependent gals. Try to remember that this is all very worth it. Take each day one at a time. Give yourself credit for every few hours of time that pass-by during which your blood sugars are "perfect" and take a deep breath when you're struggling to get them there.

> Oh, mama, it's gonna be so worth it! We promise.

NUTRITION & FITNESS

KEEP MOVING MAMA

It's going to become more and more tempting to sit on your tush, put your feet up, and skip the gym after a long day at work (especially if you don't already have a little kiddo vying for your attention and energy).

But a secret to your success will likely be letting go of the workout you used to do and embracing a lower intensity type of exercise. Here are a few simple suggestions for keeping active while also getting some well-deserved rest:

- going for a 15-minute walk twice a day after breakfast and lunch
- play your favorite 5-song playlist and dance in the kitchen when you get home
- while watching T.V., just get up and do gentle squats and upper-body exercises with a light pair of dumbbells (5 to 8 lbs. is plenty if that's all that feels comfortable!)
- at the end of your lunch-break, walk up and down a flight of stairs 1 to 3 times (or whatever feels comfortable)
- use your kitchen counter to do push-ups, a kitchen-table chair to do squats—rinse and repeat for 15 minutes, dancing between each exercise to your favorite songs

The idea is to just keep moving rather than becoming an adorably beautiful couch-potato. The urge to sit and stare the wall is only going to increase, so it's important to commit to staying active.

As you battle insulin resistance more and more in these final months, remember simply staying hydrated by drinking plenty of clean water can have a subtle but powerful impact on your overall blood sugars.

If you're used to drinking flavored waters that are loaded with artificial sweeteners and artificial flavors, now is a great time to focus on drinking clean water. Let baby motivate you! Ditching all those artificial sweeteners for a few weeks will actually help your tastebuds become more aware of how unnatural they really taste once you get more used to drinking clean water.

For a flavor-boost to water, you can also try adding a squeeze of lemon or lime juice to cold water or try a few drops of the Stevia liquid which comes in a host of flavors and is subtle as well as void of "artificial" additives.

INSULIN MANAGEMENT

The almighty pre-bolus will become your very best friend this month. Embrace it fully and completely, because it will save you a lot of stress and frustration after each meal!

EXPECTED INSULIN ADJUSTMENTS

Here are a few things to keep in mind when assessing your insulin doses this month:

- **BACKGROUND INSULIN DOSES:** Due to all of these gradual changes you can generally expect to see an increase in your background insulin needs every 7 to 14 days. For some, the increase may be just one unit while for others that increase may be an increment of 3 to 5 units. Pay close attention to times without active insulin from a bolus to fully assess if basal insulin changes are what is needed. If using a pump, evaluate the time of day, rather than just adding more insulin all day long to the rates or pattern.

- **MEAL BOLUS DOSES:** This month, you'll will likely see a need for the longest pre-bolus ever before eating. You may need to wait up to 45 minutes in order to prevent that post-meal spike in your blood sugar. This month, you'll also see a big change in your insulin-to-carb ratio, likely needing a decrease in your ratio of 1 to 2 grams from where you were last month. Even a couple slices of bacon may call for a unit or two of insulin despite that 0 gram carb-count.

LET'S TAKE A CLOSER LOOK AT EACH OF THESE EXPECTED CHANGES:

THE 45-MINUTE PRE-BOLUS

Starting this month, you will notice that your 20 to 30 minute pre-bolus isn't working as well. Hormones are in high gear helping your baby grow, but the flipside is that those hormones actually act as "anti-insulin" hormones! Just to keep you on your toes...we wouldn't want this to be easy, right?

Keeping your blood sugar in close to the ideal range after eating (under 140 mg/dL) during these last few months will be very challenging and will depend largely on your ability to take your insulin at least 45 minutes before eating. For some foods, you may find you actually need 60 minutes between injection and eating.

To the non-diabetic, that may not sound like a very big deal...but we are well aware that knowing exactly what and when we're going to eat isn't easy.

Not hungry now, but find yourself desperately hungry 60 minutes from now? You're gonna have to wait an additional 45 minutes before you can eat!

Headed to a restaurant where you can't predict your meal or how long it will take to be served after eating? Taking your insulin 45 minutes ahead of when you hope they will serve the food could mean having to know what you're going to order even 30 minutes before you get to the restaurant!

And of course there's always the potential for a total debacle like taking your insulin 45 minutes ahead of time for your pre-planned lunch but getting severely distracted by a coworker, an unexpected meeting or phone-call, your dog suddenly chasing the neighbor's cat requiring you to chase after him around the neighborhood.

In other words, these anti-insulin hormones don't just raise the likelihood of high blood sugars but can also become part of the recipe for tedious lows when you were trying so hard to do the "right" thing.

A FEW TROUBLESHOOTING TIPS
FOR YOUR 45-MINUTE PRE-BOLUS:

- Are you desperately hungry right now? After you take your insulin for the carbohydrates you'd like to eat in 45 minutes, start munching on fats and veggies, like carrots and cucumbers with dip, steamed broccoli, peanuts or cheese—any non-starchy vegetable and naturally low-carb fat source—to help curb your hunger. Yes, veggies have a few carbs but the impact will be far less significant especially if you pair them with a fat that will slow down the digestion of those few carbs. (Of course, don't forget to take some insulin for the small amount of carbs in your veggies if necessary!)

- Order a low-carb meal. If you're going to a restaurant you don't know well, committing to ordering a low-carb meal can help prevent a super-spike in your blood sugar by avoiding unpredictable carb-quantities and the inability to pre-bolus 45 minutes before eating.

- Eat your fats, proteins, and veggies first! You may have been able to get your insulin dosed 20 minutes before sitting down to eat but that remaining 20 minutes is still really important. Postpone eating the most carb-loaded things on your plate and focus on the low-carb veggies and the fats and proteins instead.

- Combine your carbs with a fat or a protein. Eating an apple all by itself, even with a 45-minute pre-bolus will spike your blood sugar more quickly than an apple eaten with a handful of almonds, some cheese, or peanut butter as well.

- Ugh...plan ahead and set a timer. This goes without saying, and is obviously not always very doable, but if you know you're not hungry now but you're due for a meal soon, determine what you're going to eat, take your pre-bolus and set a timer (on your phone, the oven, your watch, whatever) to remind you to stop what you're doing and eat that meal.

- Be prepared for lows if things go awry. If you're going to try something like...taking your insulin an hour before you hope to meet a friend for fries and burgers, and running a few errands between the insulin dose and the fries, but you find yourself derailed by traffic, you need to make sure you have enough carbohydrates in your car or your purse to take care of the whopping insulin dose you took for those fries!

It's gonna be tedious. It's gonna be frustrating. But the super-early pre-bolus is going to make your blood sugar easier to wrangle.

ADJUST YOUR INSULIN-ON-BOARD PUMP SETTINGS

In this third trimester, it may be helpful to adjust the setting in your pump for your IOB (insulin on board) from 3 or 4 hours down to 2 hours.

YOUR INSULIN-TO-CARBOHYDRATE RATIO

In addition to that ever tedious 45-minute pre-bolus, your insulin-to-carbohydrate ratio is going to make you feel like you'll use a whole vial of insulin in one day.

At this point, you will likely need at least a 1:6 insulin-to-carb ratio. Some of you may find you need 1:5 or 1:4 at some point during month 7.

Regardless, you're going to feel like you're taking a massive amount of insulin compared to what you used to take for things as simple as an apple or two slices of toast. During the first few weeks of taking these larger quantities with each meal, don't be surprised if you find yourself a little extra paranoid about low blood sugars that haven't even happened.

"How could I possibly take that much insulin and not go low in two hours?"

This paranoia can easily lead you to treating lows that haven't happened yet merely because you see that you're already down at 90 mg/dL on your CGM and you feel as though there's still an incredible amount of insulin on-board. To ease some of your worries, make a new habit of reminding yourself to wait and see if you actually do go low. You can have that juice box right by your side. You can set an alarm on your phone to wake you up 30 minutes after falling asleep to double-check. You can test your blood sugar on your meter a dozen times in 90 minutes. Whatever you need to do to feel safe.

And hey, at first, you might need to actually prove to yourself that you weren't going low by treating the almost-low with 15 grams of carbs and watching your blood sugar spike back up over 200 mg/dL. Do this two or three times, and the frustration you'll experience in wishing you hadn't will help you start to trust your new insulin doses a little more.

THERE'S NO SUCH THING AS A "FREE-FOOD" ANYMORE

Remember when you were first diagnosed, and the diabetes educator would give you a list of "free foods" that you could eat without worrying about your blood sugar? Well you can toss that list out the window at this point in your pregnancy.

Even a serving of chicken can raise your blood sugar 50 or more points and require several units of insulin.

In the past, you may have been able to eat a handful of carrots or a handful of almonds without any insulin, maybe seeing a rise in your blood sugar of barely 15 or 20 points? Not anymore! Every little thing, except perhaps a bowl of Iceburg lettuce, is going to need at least a little insulin.

The one good thing about those "free foods" is that they probably won't require much of a pre-bolus. Which means, as mentioned earlier in this chapter, you can use those foods to munch on while you're waiting for your pre-bolus to kick-in so you can eat your carbohydrates.

"Free foods" like cheese, nuts, clean animal proteins (ie: not breaded), eggs, and non-starchy veggies will come in handy when you find yourself starving in the middle of the night or right before bed, because taking a whopping dose of insulin to cover a peanut butter and jelly sandwich at 10 p.m., which means you can't eat until 11 p.m. is going to put you at risk of falling asleep with a whopping dose of insulin in your bloodstream... not to mention that you're hungry and you need your sleep, mama!

Think about what "free foods" you prefer that have real calories (in other words: sugar-free J-ELL-O isn't gonna cut it), and real nutrients (protein and/or fat) to satisfy your hungry growing baby, and be sure to keep a good supply of them in your the kitchen.

And of course, that leads us to other areas of insulin dosing that will inevitably need more tweaking this month...

GETTING ENOUGH BACKGROUND INSULIN?

Knowing when to increase your background insulin doses in these last few months can be particularly confusing because you're also dealing with the stubborn post-meal blood sugars and the super-early pre-bolus.

Is your blood sugar high after this meal because your pre-bolus wasn't perfect or are you due for another increase in your background insulin doses? Or is it both?

As a refresher, here are a few ways to tell the difference:

1. If a high blood sugar takes more than two hours to start coming down after giving yourself a correction dose of insulin, and especially if it seems to hover at, 200 mg/dL for example, for 3 or 4 or 5 hours despite your repeated attempts to get it down, then this is clearly a sign that your background insulin doses need increasing. While it can seem directly related to the meal, because the high occurred after you eat, the insulin should still do its job within 3 hours if you're getting enough background insulin.

2. If your blood sugar is sitting steadily overnight or between meals at 130 mg/dL instead of the ideal 80 to 100 mg/dL, a simple increase in your background insulin can make all the difference. For example, merely 1 to 3 extra units of insulin spread over the course of the day (via insulin pump basal rates) or 1 to 3 extra units of insulin added to your long-acting insulin dose (via lantus or levemir) can be enough to bring your blood sugar down to a cozy resting place of 80 mg/dL. Ideal for mom and baby.

3. Remember, back in the day (when you weren't pregnant), making a sudden 3-unit increase in your background insulin would only happen if you'd come down with the flu or taking part in an adrenaline-induced sporting event...but with pregnancy, your insulin doses can change that quickly as you hit each new phase of pregnancy.

  * *Remember: During pregnancy, you want to make a change in your doses after seeing a trend of higher or lower blood sugar levels over the course of two days rather than three or more days when not pregnant. It's also important to never*

make increases of more than 1 to 2 units in one day. Make an adjustment of up to 2 units, assess its efficacy over the next day or two, and adjust again as needed. Within each trimester, you will likely see a total increase in your insulin needs of anywhere between 3 to 7 units. Those with higher levels of insulin resistance and weight-gain will see the greatest increases in their insulin needs.

AT THE DOCTOR'S OFFICE

PRE-ECLAMPSIA: WHAT YOU NEED TO KNOW

You've heard the word pre-eclampsia mentioned a lot during the past 7 months—from every doctor you encounter, from every app you read, from every little voice in the back of your head that is handling the extra responsibility of being a pregnant woman with type 1 diabetes. Having type 1 diabetes makes us more susceptible to developing pre-eclampsia so it's important you're very aware of the signs and symptoms.

SIGNS & SYMPTOMS: Pre-eclampsia is a condition defined by dangerously high blood pressure (over 130/100 bpm) and swelling in the face. While swelling in the legs and feet are also part of pre-eclampsia, swelling in those areas can accompany any pregnancy, whereas sudden swelling in the face is a clear symptom of preeclampsia. The other tell-tale sign of this condition is protein in the urine which can be assessed through a "creatinine clearance" test.

If you notice persistent swelling in the legs and feet accompanied by swelling in the face and a headache, you should call your doctor immediately. If your doctor is unavailable you should visit an emergency room. Do not wait until Monday to talk to a healthcare professional if your symptoms appear Friday night and your usual OB-GYN team is unavailable.

When left untreated, pre-eclampsia can become eclampsia which is defined by seizures and strokes in the mother. In other words: don't hesitate to visit the emergency room if you are seeing signs and symptoms of this condition.

TREATING PRE-ECLAMPSIA: The most effective way to treat pre-eclampsia is to enable the mother to give birth to the baby so she is no longer pregnant. The goal will be to keep baby safely inside you until at least 35 weeks because their lungs are not fully developed prior to this time. Medication will be given to the baby to help ensure proper development of the lungs, and medication will be given to you to help lower your blood pressure.

As a mother-to-be diagnosed with pre-eclampsia you may be told to go home and be on "bed rest" so you don't contribute to your elevated blood pressure or you may actually be required to stay in a hospital bed for the remaining weeks until your baby can be delivered. The decision will really come down to just how high your blood pressure is, how much protein you're expelling in your urine, and the overall safety of you and baby.

It is very common for with with pre-eclampsia to deliver via C-section because vaginal labor, even when assisted via induction medications, can actually worsen your blood pressure, putting both you and baby at greater risk.

THINGS YOU CAN DO TO REDUCE YOUR RISK OF PRE-ECLAMPSIA:

There are a few things you can do to help reduce your risk of pre-eclampsia, especially during this last trimester where your healthy habits may start to slide.

- **STAY ACTIVE:** Even a little exercise counts as a lot when you feel like your belly is the size of a Mini Cooper. Walks. Walks! Short walks, longer walks—whatever feels comfortable to you—just keep moving.

- **KEEP YOUR SODIUM & PROCESSED FOODS INTAKE DOWN:** If your diet is currently loaded with fast-food and processed foods full of sodium, now is the time to minimize those foods as much as possible. Period. Eat more whole foods, prepare more of your own meals, use fresh ingredients! This is essential to long-term health even when you're not pregnant, but when it comes to pre-eclampsia, it could you out of the emergency room and prevent emergency C-Sections.

- **HYDRATE:** Drink your water, mama. Seriously.

- **MANAGING BLOOD SUGARS CLOSELY:** Above all else, the more in-range your blood sugars are, especially in this trimester, the healthier you'll be and the more safely you'll be able to deliver your baby when they are truly ready to come into the world.

It's everything you've already been encouraged to make a priority. The more you can think of these habits as lifelong choices, the healthier you'll be once your baby is born, too.

GINGER'S PREGNANCY DIARY

WEEK 28

3rd trimester is kicking my butt...not in relation to diabetes but just general pregnancy symptoms. Achey. Tired. Sore. Did I mention the word tired? The countdown to when I'm taking a break from work (1 month before her due-date, so I can rest, focus on blood sugars, and... rest) seems so far away, but I'll make it!

In a weird way, the insulin resistance that comes with this stage of pregnancy is almost making blood sugar management easier because I can take so much insulin, wait 40 minutes before eating (which is obnoxious), and not go low! At first this phenomenon was a little unnerving because I felt like I had so much insulin on board and my blood sugar is just hanging out around 90 after eating. Surely that insulin must drop me, right? But...nope! Instead, it just hangs out there steadily as my food is slowly digested and my insulin is slowly doing its job.

That's not to imply I'm not putting a heck-of-a-lot-of-effort into it. Waiting 30 to 40 minutes before eating is pretty crucial, and eating primarily clean, whole foods is definitely 2nd on the list of important ways to keep blood sugars in range around meals...but even home-baked gluten-free molasses cookies didn't spike my blood sugar with enough insulin on board and a proper pre-bolus.

One unfortunate bummer for this stage of pregnancy is that any form of real walking (like, walking for exercise) even at a pace of 2.2 mph on the treadmill or in the woods with my dogs, makes me feel like I'm about to give birth. The pressure in my pelvic area was so intense one day that I went in for an extra appointment to be sure I wasn't experiencing preterm labor. Thankfully, everything looked completely normal. But I've put my gym membership on hold until I'm back in action a month or two after the baby arrives. And walking in the woods with my dogs just means I walk really slowly while they run around freely. Considering I'll soon be walking in two feet of snow in the woods very soon will help make-up for the lack of gym workouts!

I'm just bummed because being able to get my heart pumping, getting a little sweat going, and truly exercising with a real power-walk would feel good in many other ways. But the pressure in my pelvis became unbearable and was lasting for hours after the exercise was over.

Regardless, everything else is healthy and going well, so I'm grateful for that!

WEEK 29

I think I've searched for the symptoms of "pre-eclampsia" almost every day this week. My symptoms don't seem to qualify and my last doctors appointment showed no abnormal levels of protein in my urine or high blood pressure...but oy vey, I feel lousy! Every day for the past week my heart has started racing. At least it feels like it's racing, beating, pounding. I feel light-headed and have to work so hard to breathe just through ordinary tasks. At first it was just happening at the end of the day, so I thought it was either the result of too much running around or having not eaten enough. (There were a few days where I had very little interest in food and definitely didn't consume enough calories). But now the pounding heart and light-headedness (even while relaxing late at night) is starting earlier in the day!

Meanwhile, I know this can also be a totally normal part of pregnancy, especially since I'm carrying the baby very high up on my torso, putting more pressure on my lungs.

But...I've stopped in at three different pharmacies in the past week to use those blood pressure cuff machines. The results always appear normal but I don't trust them. Am I really going to feel like this for the remaining three months? (Most likely, it's another case of Ginger The Hypochondriac.)

I have another doctor's appointment in two days...but perhaps I'll stop by the pharmacy on my way home today and just check my blood pressure again. Maybe. Okay, yes. Ah! (Update: My blood pressure was completely normal. Turns out I'm just pregnant.)

WEEK 30

Thanksgiving was a success thanks to 3 extra units of Lantus. I was expecting to fight highs all day, but on the morning of Thanksgiving I gave myself 3 extra units of Lantus. (I take my normal dose of Lantus at night, before bed.)

I was planning on serving dinner around 2 p.m. so I figured that would be enough time for the extra Lantus to get going in my system—and it did, because I had a mild low, 55 to 60 mg/dL around 1:30 p.m.

The carbohydrates I consumed at Thanksgiving were: mashed potatoes, cranberry sauce (homemade, which contains far less sugar than the canned version), gluten-free homemade gravy, and several hours later, homemade blueberry crisp with vanilla Ben & Jerry's ice cream (oh, how I've missed you, B&J!).

30 minutes before dinner, indeed at the same time I was going low, I took a pre-bolus of 8 units of insulin. When I sat down to eat, my blood

sugar was back up thanks to a glass of orange juice and sitting around 135 mg/dL. I took another 8 units of insulin when I sat down.

My thinking behind this split bolus was: 1. I didn't want to feel like I had to eat quickly in order to keep up with a mega-dose of 16 units of insulin all at once and 2. I expected the meal to digest a bit slowly considering it's a larger quantity of food than I would normally consume in one sitting.

During the couple hours after the main meal, I was hanging out just below the 130 mg/dL line on my CGM.

40 minutes before dessert (the blueberry crisp and ice cream), I took 10 units of insulin, and another 6 units when I started eating. Again my "theory" was that some of this meal would digest very quickly but some of it would take a few hours. (How did I guess the carbohydrates in blueberry crisp? I have no idea. I totally winged it. Totally. Maybe my brain has a sixth-sense for blueberry crisp carb-counting.)

Dessert was finished by 6:30 or 7 p.m. and I didn't eat anything else for the rest of the night. Before going to bed, I noticed my CGM was very slowly creeping up towards my 130 mg/dL line, and my meter confirmed that I was at 155 mg/dL, so I took another 5 units to cover the delayed digestion of all those calories, and went to bed. Much to my surprise, I stayed in range all night, between 70 to 130 mg/dL.

The moral of the story: I was totally winging it! A little strategy mixed with a lot of guessing, testing, and hoping. But mostly: effort. It wasn't stressful or frustrating. I just knew I was in this 7th month of mega-insulin-resistance and I was gonna need mega-doses of insulin to deal with it. I'd rather treat a low with a little juice than spend hours fighting highs. Lows are easy to fix. Highs take forever to fix. That's just the approach that works for me.

NOTES

MONTH 8

GETTING READY...

Okay, so if you're not sort of totally and completely exhausted by now... then you're quite a gal. Months and months of feeling like every single digit on your meter is either saying, "Awesome!" or "Uh...nope, you failed," can really weigh on the mind of any type 1 diabetic, let alone one whose body is growing a human inside of it. (You might have to remind your healthcare team of this!)

But you've made it this far. Take every wonderfully "winning" moment for what it is, and brush off the negative weight of the numbers you're not fond of as quickly as possible so you can get back on track. Each day. Each blood sugar check. Just keep doin' it.

MAMA'S MENTAL HEALTH

There is no shortage of anxiety in the life of a person with type 1 diabetes. If anxiety is already something you've faced in the past, then pregnancy—particularly this last trimester as insulin resistance requires you to work even harder and anticipation of how your entire life is about to change—could certainly stir things up for you.

For any first-time mother-to-be, we face this complete and total mystery: "What is life going to be like next? Will I be good at this? How will I even know when the baby is hungry? I've never given a baby a bath, what the heck do I do? I have no idea what's about to happen...." (Or maybe you grew up with 11 younger siblings and you're already a pro—good for you!)

When you place type 1 diabetes on top of it, that list of concerns might include: "What will I do if the baby is crying but my blood sugar is plummeting? What happens if I can't hold the baby because I'm so low? How is breastfeeding going to affect my blood sugar? What happens if I my milk doesn't come in because I have diabetes? How often is my diabetes going to totally interfere with being a mom? What do I do when my kid is 3 years old and rips my insulin pump infusion site right out of my skin?"

If these questions are just stirring around, that's one thing, but if they are keeping you up at night and cause mild, moderate, or severe anxiety attacks, that's something you should address head-on. The first person to report this to would be either your OB-GYN team or your primary care team. Ideally, they would talk to you about anxiety medications safe for pregnancy or they'll refer to work with a therapist or an alternative medicine speciality that can treat anxiety. The important thing is that you address it.

Secondly, schedule an appointment with your CDE or a diabetes pregnancy coach like Jenny so you can actually pose your questions to someone who knows what life with a newborn is going to be like for you as a woman with type 1 diabetes. Sure, we're going to talk about this later in the book, but sitting face-to-face with someone who can really have a conversation with you about it is going to do more for your anxiety than just words on a page.

Lastly, an important step you could take is to reach out to other moms with type 1 diabetes and ask them about their experience postpartum! (The great part of this is that you have instant proof that it can be done... because they are doing it!)

Here are a few communities where you could easily post a question like, "What was life as a mom with diabetes like for you after your first child was born?"

- DiabetesDaily.com
- BeyondType1.org
- Facebook: "Type 1 Diabetes and Pregnancy" Group with over 3,000 members

Mingle and chat with other moms who have been there and done it. You'll find relief in seeing just how well a woman with type 1 diabetes can handle motherhood. In fact, having type 1 might even make us better moms!

NUTRITION & FITNESS
MOVIN' WITH THE BUMP

So aside from the occasional power-house-mom who runs marathons in her third trimester (I once saw one pregnant with twins running on the treadmill with total ease, trying to induce labor), you're going to need to lower the intensity of your workouts this month. This is simply because a) you're gonna be really tired and b) your belly is going to get in the way, whether you like it or not.

The weight of that darling bump can really cause a great deal of back pain and strain. Some women find a lot of relief from wearing a pregnancy band/belt. Some women love it (like Jenny), and some women hate it (like Ginger). Some women just wear maternity exercise pants with a full band that is a little extra snug in order to get a little more support. You may also consider wearing "support hose" to help with compression for your legs and feet, especially if swelling or varicose veins have become a concern.

The most tempting thing is to go home and sit on the couch. That honestly is going to feel best. But as type 1 mama's we need to keep active because we need to do everything we can to compensate for those rising hormones and rising insulin resistance levels.

Remember, every little bit counts! Walking slowly on a treadmill while you watch Netflix on your cell-phone or waddling back n' forth at home while your partner smiles at you adoringly counts as movement.

Every little bit will make a difference. In a few months, you'll be nearly 30 pounds lighter and able to get up from your chair without rocking your bodyweight forward! Until then, keep moving as best you can.

SMALLER MEALS & MORE FREQUENT INSULIN DOSES

You're going to feel fuller sooner this month and the next thanks to baby pressing firmly into your stomach—and all of your other vital organs. This means your meals will likely need to be smaller, but for a type 1 mama this means you'll likely be taking doses of insulin very close together, also known as "stacking" your insulin.

In an ideal non-pregnant world, we aren't supposed to take large doses of fast or rapid-acting insulin closer than about 3 to 4 hours apart because insulin stays in your system for 4 hours.

However, in this last trimester this won't be as much of a concern as it has been in the past. Your insulin is going to actually be processed more quickly and your raging levels of pregnancy hormones are going to require you to need every last drop of each dose—even if the last dose was merely 2 hours ago.

If you do find that taking your insulin doses so closely together is causing you low blood sugars very shortly after eating the next small meal, a strategy would be to take insulin for the meal and then split the meal into a 70/30 amount. Take the full dose of insulin for lunch now—let's say 30 grams, but only eat 70% of this 30 grams now and save the other 30% to eat about 1.5 to 2 hours later. This will help you avoid stacking your insulin and help your blood sugars stay in range after eating.

Another strategy is to establish regular meal and snack times and adjust your I:C ratio for the snack to avoid too much stacking. For example, if your I:C ratio is 1:7 for lunch, then use a ratio of 1:10 for the snack that you eat 2 hours later. This will cover the snack with less insulin – assuming there may be a tail end of the insulin from the lunch left hanging around and will help prevent lows. This is again something to test and see how it works for you.

Mostly likely, at this time in your pregnancy, "stacking" won't be an issue because your body will need every last drop of insulin you dose.

PREPARING FOR BREASTFEEDING: JUICE BOXES & JELLY BEANS

Now is actually a good time to start preparing for life after baby as a type 1 mom. Specifically, it's time to buy a good supply of the glucose you're going to use to treat low blood sugars after baby is born. And then, placing that glucose in the different areas where you will be breastfeeding, and of course, sleeping.

Will you need to treat a blood sugar every time you nurse? Definitely not, and the low may not even be related to nursing, but it'll give you great comfort to know that you're not "stuck" in an area of the house when your blood sugar is dropping. Being prepared for lows with stashes of glucose thoughtfully placed around the house will simply make life easier and less stressful.

Here are a few suggestions but of course you should swap in your own glucose sources for treating lows based on what works best for you. These are merely suggestions to help you think about preparing for your own management of low blood sugars after baby is born.

WHERE & WHAT: STASHING GLUCOSE FOR LOW BLOOD SUGARS

- **NEAR THE ROCKING CHAIR:** In the middle of the night, when baby is nursing and hopefully falling asleep, you won't want to move a muscle for fear of startling them. Keep juice boxes within arm's reach of the chair.
- **NEXT TO YOUR BED:** You likely already have these in place, but again, make sure you have a good supply of glucose to treat lows when you're nursing baby in bed. Remember that you may be

lying down on your back or on your side while nursing baby in this area, so you'll want a glucose option that can be eaten while you're horizontal! (In other words, juice boxes probably aren't a good idea.) Raisins, jelly beans, glucose tabs, etc. would all work well here.

- **NEAR THE COUCH:** It seems silly that you wouldn't be able to just hop up and grab some glucose from the kitchen if you're in the living-room, but again, there will be times that you simply won't want to move and you'll need that glucose right there, within arm's reach.

- **IN THE GLOVE COMPARTMENT:** Make sure that the glucose you put in this area isn't going to freeze, rot, or melt due to severe temperatures. (That means no juice boxes!) Glucose tabs, gummy candy or fruit snacks work well here.

- **IN THE DIAPER BAG:** This is a big one. You're going to be at the grocery store, at the pediatrician's office, and wherever else, and your arms will be more full than they've ever been before! You don't want to find yourself halfway through the doctor's appointment when you realize your blood sugar is plummeting and your glucose source is in the car. Prep your bag with smaller sources like jelly beans, where a small bag can actually treat many lows because 5 jelly beans equals 5 grams of carbs (at least with JellyBelly brand).

- **IN THE PANTRY:** This seems obvious but you'll likely have more lows than usual in the first few weeks following your baby's birth simply because your insulin needs are going to need some gradual fine-tuning. You'll also be adjusting to the production of milk and baby's appetite potentially causing low blood sugars until you get into a hopefully smoother rhythm. Get yourself a really good supply of 3 to 4 things that you'll use specifically to treat low blood sugars so you don't have to go to the grocery store after 5 days of being home with your adorable baby! (And while you're at it, relish the simplicity of going to the grocery store with just your purse, because soon grocery store trips will always involve carrying some very precious cargo with you!)

We'll talk more about balancing blood sugars during breastfeeding in the **DELIVERY & POSTPARTUM** chapter.

INSULIN MANAGEMENT

For most of you, this is the last month during which insulin needs will rise. After month 8, you'll either find yourself holding steady or possibly decreasing your doses. Keep in mind, though, that these last two months are extra important when it comes to staying within your goal blood sugar ranges.

Even though your baby's organs are fully formed, this is the month where baby could potentially put on the most unnecessary chub (ie: macrosomnia) due to mama's higher blood sugar levels. (It's also easy for mama to put on extra weight during this month, too.)

It's also crucial to be within your goal ranges as much as possible because baby's own insulin production at birth is directly impacted particularly by the last month of mama's blood sugar levels. The higher your blood sugars are, the more insulin baby will produce to compensate for that excess sugar, which means the more likely baby's blood sugar will be low after being born when it's no longer receiving that excess glucose from your bloodstream.

▌ Keep your eye on the prize, mama.

EXPECTED INSULIN ADJUSTMENTS

Here are a few things to keep in mind when assessing your insulin doses this month:

- **BACKGROUND INSULIN DOSES:** You'll see a small rise again in your background insulin doses this month, but it shouldn't be any more significant than previous months. The rise in your basal needs will be greater if you gain excess weight during this last month—which is easy to do if you're giving in to your ravenous appetite and spending more time on your toosh from exhaustion. Be mindful while being sure to eat mostly clean and getting some real activity each day.

- **INSULIN-TO-CARB RATIO:** You'll likely see a big jump in the amount of insulin you need to cover your meals this month. It may actually be a little startling to take so much insulin for a very small amount of carbs. You'll be taking an amount at one meal that you may have used to take over the course of the entire day. But the sooner you can pinpoint what you really need, the easier time you'll have staying within your goal ranges.

- **MEAL BOLUS TIMING:** Your pre-bolus needs will likely take another jump, going from around 45 minutes to 50 or even 60 minutes between when you take your insulin and when you begin to eat. Remember to consider the factors of your meal—the more carbs there are, likely the more committed you'll need to be to that 50-minute pre-bolus. But carbs associated with a lot of fat (like pizza) will likely need a combination of a lengthy pre-bolus combined with a much further delayed bolus for the second half of your dose. Tip: If you're having trouble managing your blood sugar after meals this month, try splitting your meals. Take your full bolus dose, wait at least 45 minutes, eat 2/3s of your meal and save the rest of the meal for an hour or so after that. This will help the meal digestion coincide with the peak of your insulin.

* *Remember: During pregnancy, you want to make a change in your doses after seeing a trend of higher or lower blood sugar levels over the course of two days rather than three or more days when not pregnant. It's also important to never make increases of more than 1 to 2 units in one day. Make an adjustment of up to 2 units, assess its efficacy over the next day or two, and adjust again as needed. Within each trimester, you will likely see a total increase in your insulin needs of anywhere between 3 to 7 units. Those with higher levels of insulin resistance and weight-gain will see the greatest increases in their insulin needs.*

AT THE DOCTOR'S OFFICE

Do you have questions about your baby's birth? Goals or hopes for how you'll deliver your baby? Write these things down this month and bring them to your next appointment. Don't wait until you're two weeks from giving birth. By now, questions about what your baby's birth will likely be all consuming.

Some doctors will have a very friendly, casual way of talking about delivery, and others may sound much more clinical—which can feel overwhelming or even scary. Ask your questions—anything that comes to mind. Show them your birth plan, talk about what you hope happens, but keep in mind (no, seriously) that your baby's birth may very likely be completely opposite of what you planned.

There are so many variables and factors that play into how a baby is born and the primary goal is keeping both baby and mama safe. Adding type 1 diabetes to that mix only increases those variables. The very best thing you can do is have a clear idea of what you want and what you'll aim for, but keep your mind very open to the reality that nobody has full control over how their baby enters the world.

Both of us (Jenny and Ginger) wanted and planned on delivering our babies as naturally as possible. And we both ended up delivering our babies completely differently than that plan. But you know what? It didn't take away from the experience one bit. It was just as special, just as overwhelmingly amazing. Well...you'll find out. Keep reading!

CREATING A BIRTH PLAN
DOCUMENT & DISCUSSING WITH YOUR OB-GYN

Your OB-GYN team may already have a Birth Plan form they ask you to fill out, or you may want to create something entirely different.

Things to talk about clearly with your OB-GYN team when looking at your birth plan:

1. USING YOUR OWN INSULIN AT THE HOSPITAL: If you already have permission to wear your pump and/or CGM during delivery and postpartum in the hospital, that's great, but there's still one more step. Especially for those taking injections via syringes or pens, most hospitals require that any medications brought into the hospital to be used during an inpatient visit must be sent to their pharmacy to be approved by the pharmacy (to make sure it is what it says it is), and then they'll be returned to you. Even if you are on told you'll be on a glucose and insulin drip via an I.V., you'll still want to get your insulin approved for use. (You'll read in Ginger's delivery story why this can be awfully helpful!)

2. YOU ARE #1 IN CHARGE OF YOUR DIABETES DURING DELIVERY AND POSTPARTUM: Talk about this with your doctor sternly and seriously. Let them know how important it is that you are involved in every single insulin dose adjustment, and that you do know your body and your diabetes better than anyone else. This is your body. You've been managing nearly non-diabetic blood sugar levels for over 9 months in order to keep this baby healthy, and you continue to do so during delivery and postpartum.

Okay, let's take a look at sample birth plan so you can create your own! The following is merely one way to approach a birth plan document.

SAMPLE BIRTH PLAN

CURRENT INSULIN DOSES AT 33 WEEKS PREGNANT:

- CORRECTION FACTOR: 1:40
  (1 unit drops BG by 40 mg/dL)
- INSULIN-TO-CARBOHYDRATE RATIO: 1:5
  (1 unit for every 5 grams of carb)
- LANTUS: 32 units—
  (must be given all at once, patient develops ketones within a few hours when dose is split by 12 hours)

PRE-PREGNANCY INSULIN DOSES:

- **CORRECTION FACTOR:** 1:100
  (1 unit drops BG by 100 mg/dL)
- **INSULIN-TO-CARBOHYDRATE RATIO:** 1:15
  (1 unit for every 15 grams of carb)
- **LANTUS:** 14 units—
  (must be given all at once, patient develops ketones within a few hours when dose is split by 12 hours)

LABOR AND DELIVERY:

- Labor MAY cause lower BG due to the "activity," but hourly BG checks and CGM will help determine if/when adjustment to insulin drip is needed.
- BG target during labor 70-130 mg/dL.
- If Lantus insulin is taken in full dose prior to labor, evaluate BG and use IV glucose for BG maintenance OR clear liquids with glucose to stabilize BG (apple juice, glucose tabs, etc).
- If BG's running low (consistently less than 80 mg/dL) insulin IV drip should be decreased by 25% of current dose for 12 hours and continue to monitor hourly to assess need to change rate further—only applies if patient has not taken Lantus dose.
- Insulin corrections during labor/delivery should be given not more than every 3 hours.
- Decrease doses by 50% of what the calculated correction dose to prevent hypos.

INSULIN DRIP:

If an insulin drip is planned, this will take the place of your basal insulin (Lantus). Ensure the doctor knows your current dose of Lantus to enable the accurate dose to be calculated for the insulin drip.

- **CURRENT LANTUS DOSE:** 32 units—
  Given in full dose at 8 p.m.

POST-PARTUM: FIRST 24 TO 48 HOURS:

- After delivery, expect your basal insulin needs to drop back to at where it was "pre-pregnancy."
- As soon as you deliver baby/placenta switch to the lower/pre-pregnancy basal insulin dose. BG's will drop significantly as soon as all those "baby" hormones are gone.

- You may find you need an additional 10-20% reduction in basal insulin dose from the pre-pregnancy dose for the first 24-48 hours after delivery.
- If patient has pregnancy dose of Lantus in system post-partum, IV glucose or carbohydrates will likely be needed.
- Check BG every 3 hours to assess need for adjustment (this should coincide with your nursing which should be every 2-3 hours after delivery).

NURSING/BREASTFEEDING:
- BG may drop during or right after each nursing session.
- 5 to 10 grams carb before each session can be helpful to prevent the drop (simple carbs like juice, fruit chews, fruit leathers, etc.) along with a bit of protein can help prevent drops later—peanut butter, cheese, nuts.
- Keep food or treatment for lows in arms-reach of nursing areas in your home.
- Chronic high BG when nursing can hinder lactation.
- Try to aim for target BG <150 mg/dL (8.3 mmol/L) when nursing to decrease the amount of extra glucose going to baby in the breast milk.

MEDICATIONS IN THE HOSPITAL:

I, Ginger Patterson, will be bringing the following medications to the hospital with me to have approved by the pharmacy as soon as I arrive:
- Lantus Insulin
- Novolog Insulin
- Syringes
- BG test strips - FreeStyle Lite
- Dexcom continuous glucose monitor with sensors

I plan to use these medications as prescribed and waive the use of the medications that may be prescribed as comparable replacements here in the hospital.

While creating your own birth-plan, remember, it's mostly a source of information for both you and your healthcare team during delivery and postpartum. Print out several copies and give one to each new staff-member (nurse or doctor or resident) that is assigned to you. Tack it to the wall if you have to! And above else, remember a birth-plan is a hope.

NON-STRESS TESTS

Hopefully your commute to your doctor's office isn't a long one because this month you'll start visiting your OB-GYN team for non-stress tests (NSTs). These sound far more intimidating than they actually are.

An NST involves sitting in a cozy chair (hopefully your docs sprung for the recliner) with two different small monitor strapped around your belly. One of the monitors is testing the baby's heartbeat and the other is testing for any possible early contractions. The tests usually last for about 20 minutes. Your job is to relax, sit still, and drink water while catching up with celebrity gossip magazines.

Depending on your OB or MFM clinic's protocol, you'll be going in for an NST starting at week 32. These tests will most often be once a week combined with an OB visit or they may be twice a week with one of the visits including an OB visit. They can be boring but we've all gotta do them, so it's best to just embrace the tediousness of it! In a way, it's nice to see what your baby is up to you, and when everything goes well, it's a nice little reassurance that baby is doing well!

GINGER'S PREGNANCY DIARY
WEEK 31

I am counting down the days. As I start this 8th month of pregnancy, my fibromyalgia is rearing its adorable head. Not necessarily in pain, as that's usually triggered by repetitive exercise which I simply avoid, but in terms of insomnia, fatigue, and muscle fatigue. My leg muscles feel like they're made of pudding with just a few steps in the woods on my very short walks with my dogs. I stop every time, because it surprises me how exhausted they feel, and then convince myself to ignore it and keep walking. Every step feels like one climb higher up Mount Everest.

And the nighttime sleep, oh, the sleep. It's taking 3 to 4 hours now to fall asleep. I'll get into bed early, at 8 p.m., feeling totally tired and ready to sleep, but within 30 minutes of lying there, I'm alert again. Within 3 to 5 hours, I can finally fall asleep. Occasionally, I sleep well once I've dozed off, but mostly I just sleep for a couple hours, then I'm awake for another 2 or 3 hours and then I fall asleep again from 4 to 6 a.m. Last night, however, I didn't fall asleep until 1 a.m., woke up at 3 a.m. and was awake until I got out of bed when my husband woke up at 5 a.m. (He makes really great coffee...which is more appealing, even at 5 a.m., than lying in bed staring at the ceiling.)

The only thing that's even remotely helped combat the insomnia is playing Hunt for the Red October every night. I know every single line and image so well, I can watch it with my eyes closed and it distracts me from my insomnia frustration, often putting me to bed. I've "watched" this almost daily month in the middle of the night for the past couple weeks.

I suppose this lack of sleep is all great practice for when Lucy arrives, right?

And not to my surprise, my A1C has gone up from 5.1 to 5.6 percent. Not horrible, I know. Totally great, I know, but getting this news on the morning when I slept only 2 hours wasn't helpful. But I had a feeling it would be higher because I feel like I spent most of Month 7 getting used to 3rd trimester insulin resistance and was hitting 200 mg/dL once every day. I feel like this coming month will be better, at least in terms of avoiding 200 mg/dL spikes, because I have a better sense of just how much insulin I really need with certain types of foods. And I know, in my body, that the sign I need more background insulin is when it takes too long for correction doses of insulin to take effect on high blood sugars. 5.6 is a number I should be happy with—it's safe and sustainable.

So, anyways, that's my Week 31 Pity Party. Now I'll get back to appreciating the amazing thing my body is doing: making this baby who I'm just sure will be the cutest thing I've ever seen. (Spoiler alert: I was right!)

WEEK 32

With intentional focus and a little more insulin, things are going really well in terms of keeping blood sugars down mostly in that lovely non-diabetic range. I'm finding my appetite took a big jump this week because I'm getting hungry (like stomach-aching hungry) within 1 or 2 hours of eating. And because I'd really rather not have to be eating every 90 minutes, I'm trying to make my meals more hearty. For instance, I'm eating gluten-free bagels (ah! Bagels! I can't remember the last time I ate a carb-loaded bagel) and putting an egg on top of each half of the bagel so I'm getting a good dose of carbs, fat, and protein...and it seems to be helping me make it to at least 3 hours before my stomach starts demanding more food!

And foods like Ben & Jerry's ice cream have reappeared in my life once or twice a week! Oh, how I missed thee. But it's actually really "easy" to keep my blood sugar under 140 mg/dL with...gasp...half a pint of Ben & Jerry's ice cream as a treat, because the combination of slow digestion with the longer pre-bolus waiting time seems to add up perfect. I know I have a 1:5 insulin-to-carbohydrate ratio, so I take half my dose for the ice cream about 15 to 20 minutes before I start eating, then as soon as I'm done with that serving of ice cream, I take the remaining half of the dose. It's worked like a charm.

In the end, I think the "secret" to keeping blood sugars in range during these last two months really just comes down to getting enough insulin on-board and not being afraid to take more. Yeah, it's freaky to take 10 units of insulin for just a large apple with peanut butter when I used to take 2 to 3 units, but that's what my body needs right now! Every little unit makes a huge difference.

WEEK 33

My hat goes off to you ladies who work right up until you go into labor. I don't know how you do it. In addition to being severely sleep-deprived, my brain just feels like it's made of mashed potatoes, and these last few weeks of work (until I begin my planned—and early—maternity leave) have been truly difficult. Trying to stay focused and motivated to finish the day's work is...I don't even have the words for it.

A good chunk of my physical energy goes into walking my dogs in the snowy woods 4 times a day (10 to 15 minute-long walks don't seem to cause pelvic pain at all like the longer power-walks I was doing before). Those walks are good for me, too, of course, and I'm grateful to have the motivating needs of the canines to ensure they happen! And simply a few hours of running errands has me totally wiped and exhausted.

When I get home from running several errands, and then take the dogs on a short walk, I just need to sit and stare and breathe! Trying to be productive and work, actually using my brain to produce something seemingly intelligent...it's barely happening.

I'd been warned that the last two months were truly uncomfortable and challenging...and those warnings were accurate! It's nothing in particular that's uncomfortable or challenging, it's just everything. And when you add diabetes management on top of it all, it's a lot.

So again, to those of you who work right up until the day you pop...I think you're incredible!

WEEK 34

Christmas was quite generous this year: I celebrated the end of Christmas night with the worst gastrointestinal virus I've ever experienced. Not the flu, but a "stomach bug" that is making its way through society...and through the variety of families with whom I ate Christmas dinner.

By 11 p.m. on Christmas night my blood sugar had been below 50 mg/dL for an hour and despite two juice boxes and handful of dry cereal, it wasn't budging, and I couldn't bring myself to eat another bite of food because I was so queasy. I knew something was wrong, and I knew I shouldn't be by myself in bed while my husband had fallen asleep on the couch in front of the T.V. (Honestly, there isn't enough room in this bed for all of us right now anyway!) So I went downstairs to find him.

"Roger, I need you to stay up with me. Something's not right. I don't feel right."

He woke from a very deep slumber and encouraged me to drink more orange juice.

I wanted to lie down on the couch but he wouldn't let me, forcing me to sit upright on the edge of the couch. The orange juice went down very slowly. I also poured a small amount of cereal into a coffee mug, drenched it in almond milk thinking that would help it go down more easily...but I couldn't take more than one bite. Roger was getting annoyed with me because he was so worried about my blood sugar now sitting at 40 mg/dL despite all of the carbs I'd already eaten. And then, my firm refusal to eat or drink anything more really set-off a bit of mild panic in him.

"I need a bucket. I need a puke bucket," I said.

"No, no, you're not gonna puke. Ginger, you need to eat," he begged me.

I ignored him and fetched the largest plastic tupperware I own from the kitchen and sat down on the couch. About 5 minutes later, I puked 6 times, filling the entire container to the brim with everything I'd consumed starting since the appetizers of Christmas dinner.

No wonder I was so low...I had all that insulin in my system and none of the food I ate was being digested. The food was just lurking and bubbling, and creeping and crawling...waiting for its revival! Bleh.

Then I puked several more times into the toilet. As soon as my body took a break from puking, I looked up at Roger and said, "We need to go the E.R."

He drove 100 miles per hour on the highway to get there. This man does not like severe hypoglycemia. He likes it even less when it's consuming the woman who is carrying his baby girl!

The E.R. hooked me up to an I.V. of saline and gave me some "D5"—a liquid dextrose that they can pump into an I.V. They also gave me Zofran, an anti-nausea medication, some tylenol, two juice boxes and some peanut butter. I reluctantly drank the juice and had a smidge of peanut butter off my finger, but I couldn't keep going.

Sure enough, 30 minutes later I was puking again. 6 more times, at least a 2 liters of fluid.

I had a fever of 100.7 degrees, my resting heart rate was 150 bpm (normally my heart rate is in the 70s or 80s), but fortunately my blood sugar was finally stable in the 90s mg/dL along with my blood pressure around 100/65 bpm. However, the baby's heart rate was 200 bpm (she's normally around 150). Too high for baby!

It was clear that baby and I would be spending the night.

I was transferred to the Labor & Delivery department to be officially admitted and observed. (Mind you, I wasn't having contractions, but it's the policy at this hospital that all pregnant ladies who aren't getting a quick-fix from the E.R. be admitted to L&D so both mom and baby can be properly cared for and monitored.)

Sometime around 2 a.m., they tried giving me another type of anti-nausea medication, Phenergan, and asked me to try eating a popsicle. I took one little bite and knew it was a horrible mistake. 30 minutes later I was puking again, filling another glorious puke bucket to the brim with fluid—all because of one chomp of a popsicle.

To make the rest of this long story short, I was finally given the most painful injection I've ever received directly into my adorable heiny—an injection of Phenergen rather than taking it orally to guarantee it got into my system.

Despite the digestive chaos, my blood sugars were sitting steadily around 90 to 120 mg/dL throughout the night and all the next day thanks to the I.V. of slowly dripping glucose and an occasional sip of juice along with an eventual appetite by late morning for canned pears.

The constant drip of glucose helped counteract the full dose of Lantus insulin that was in my system from my usual evening injection (that I'd given myself shortly after Christmas dinner, before I knew I was so sick).

I spent the rest of the weekend at home, mostly sleeping. I reduced my Lantus by ⅓ (from 32 units to 22 units) per Jenny's suggestion. And I ate an occasional can of pears and a couple homemade almond-milk strawberry milkshakes over the course of the weekend until I was able to chew and eat real food 4 to 5 days after it all began.

Oddly enough, now a week later, I'm still only taking 25 units of Lantus and my blood sugars have never been easier to manage. I don't need to pre-bolus by more than 10 minutes and I'm eating plenty of carbohydrates. I have a little hunch my body is preparing for labor...but your guess is as good as mine! Or maybe my body is just still horrified from all the puking!

Dear Santa, feel free to skip my house next year!

NOTES

MONTH 9

THE FINAL STRETCH

Take a deep breath, mama, because while the "big day" is getting closer, you still have a lot of work to do. We're not saying that to overwhelm you but to simply remind you that even though you're nearly at the finish line, your blood sugars still matter now more than ever.

MAMA'S MENTAL HEALTH

You know, mama, that is one lucky little baby. When he or she is born, they will be laid in the arms of someone who worked remarkably hard to bring them safely into the world. Certainly, all mothers' bodies work remarkably hard to create life and endure pregnancy, but the journey you've been on is something your child will someday learn was a tremendously challenging experience. Every day, you essentially worked to keep yourself (and thus your baby) alive for another day. That is no small feat.

By now, it's likely crossed your mind, "Will diabetes interfere with my ability to be a good mother?"

It's a natural question and concern, because we all know how much diabetes slithers its way into every part of our lives. But we also have to remember how much we've accomplished in spite of our diabetes, or perhaps even because of our diabetes.

The following letter is from by Sysy Morales. Sysy is a type 1 and a mother of twins, a boy and girl, and you'll read in the "Type 1 Mothers Share" chapter that her pregnancy was beyond challenging. (It's jaw-dropping, to be quite frank! She is admirable for surviving it.)

But Sysy has captured something very simple and clear in the following story about how type 1 diabetes will affect your ability to be an amazing mother, and we want you to keep her message in mind during this last month of pregnancy and the months to come as you adjust to life with your new little bundle of love.

Dear New Type 1 Mama,
Here Are 5 Ways Diabetes Makes Me a Better Mother

There are days when I think my diabetes is a huge disadvantage for my entire family. I feel guilty about the extra medical expenses our budget needs to accommodate, I feel wimpy when I can't help my husband get the groceries in the house because of a dropping blood sugar, and I don't like my blood sugars stalling a game as I tell the kids, "Sorry, mommy needs to fix her low blood sugar."

And then I ask myself, "How does diabetes actually make me a better mom?"

1. Parents with diabetes can teach their kids gratitude. It takes a lot of strength to wake up with a 240 mg/dL on your glucometer, push through the sluggish sensation of a poor night's sleep and still greet the day with a smile. People with diabetes often celebrate a reading that is in range, because well, it is something worth celebrating! But we have to move forward even when there are blatant challenges in our way. Life can always be a little easier when we look on the bright side and children learn this by watching us cope with our diabetes.

2. Parents with diabetes model perseverance. Children watch us work and struggle to manage our blood sugars within a ridiculously narrow window, and they probably can't help but notice how we try over and over to hit the best numbers we can. They see us eat in a disciplined way, exercise regularly, go to the doctor, and take our medications. I hope my kids learn that hard work and getting up each time they fall down is the only way to accomplish anything worthwhile.

3. Parents with diabetes show their kids that they don't have to be perfect. Parents with diabetes know that perfection is an illusion. We know that we can't be perfect diabetics or perfect parents. There is

a great lesson here for children. We can show them that they, too, don't have to be perfect. I don't hold my children to unreasonable standards because I know what that feels like! It's super frustrating and not at all helpful. Instead, I'm showing them how to stay positive and continue working hard even when it isn't easy and the results aren't perfect.

4. Parents with diabetes demonstrate supportive empathy. Living with diabetes can be heartbreaking and frustrating. As a result, people with diabetes tend to have large reserves of empathy for others. Parents with diabetes may have an easier time empathizing with their children and listening to their concerns. We know what it is like when we don't have an outlet for all our emotional diabetes baggage, and we naturally become better listeners as a result. We know that support doesn't always mean having answers or solutions, but sometime it's simply about saying, "I know this is hard."

5. Parents with diabetes live in the now. People with diabetes worry a little more than the average person about their health and mortality. I've heard various parents living with diabetes say that they are extremely aware of the precious time with their children, because they live with a sense of urgency fueled by their diabetes. We know that blood sugars can sometimes make us extremely vulnerable, and we know that time increases our risk for complications. We want to embrace the time we have with our kids and make sure we don't put anything off for later. Our kids will learn to seize the day the same way we appreciate each day we're given.

Sincerely,
Sysy Morales
TheGirlsGuidetoDiabetes.com
DiabetesDaily.com

———

NUTRITION & FITNESS

How do you feel about preparing multiple meatloaves, huge containers of chili, and lasagnas? If food-prep isn't really your thing, you might want to ask a friend who does love cooking and prepping meals in advance to do you an awesome favor, because nothing will be more helpful after your baby is born than being able to grab a container from the freezer that is full of healthy dinner!

Even if you just prepare 6 or 7 dinners to help you get through that first week of postpartum at home with your new family member, it'll help. And it'll be better for your blood sugars than eating pizza and take-out every night! (Plus a well-fueled partner/husband/wife means a partner who has more energy to support you and the baby!)

If you do ask a friend to help you prepare some meals in advance, you might want to ask them to include the carb-counts if possible. Or at least the ingredients, so you can try to estimate for yourself.

YOU WANT ME TO...MOVE?

You might feel like curling up in bed and never leaving this month. For those of you with particular health concerns, especially high blood pressure, exercising may be completely out of the question.

For the rest of us, the reasonable goal will be to get at least a 20-minute walk each day. If you can do more, that's awesome. If you can't, so be it. Do what you can to keep your muscles and bones moving. Your blood sugars will thank you, even if it's just a tiny bit!

INSULIN MANAGEMENT

This month, things will eventually start to "lighten" up and actually feel a little easier compared to the battles with insulin resistance you've had during the past couple months. That increasing climb of insulin resistance will actually start to gradually walk itself downhill.

EXPECTED INSULIN ADJUSTMENTS

- BACKGROUND INSULIN DOSES: Overall, you'll likely see a decrease in your background insulin needs by about 10 to 15 percent. Reasons why you might not see this drop would definitely include overeating and excessive weight-gain, so remember to be mindful with your nutrition this month just as you have been during any other month.
- MEAL BOLUS DOSES: Fortunately, this month you'll likely see a drop in the amount of time you need with each pre-bolus for meals. Instead of 45 minutes to an hour, you may likely reduce your pre-bolus to a mere 20 minutes! If you were using a 1:6 insulin-to-carb ratio, you may be able to change this to 1:8.
- CORRECTION FACTORS: These may actually stay relatively the same during these last few weeks, but some of you may see a slight decrease in these doses. If you were using a 1:50 correction factor, you may find you can go up to 1:60 or 1:75.

* *Remember: During pregnancy, you want to make a change in your doses after seeing a trend of higher or lower blood sugar levels over the course of two days rather than three or more days when not pregnant. It's also important to never make adjustments* *of more than 1 to 2 units in one day. Make an adjustment, assess its efficacy over the next day or two, and adjust again as needed. Within each trimester, you will likely see a total increase in your insulin needs of anywhere between 3 to 7 units. Those with higher levels of insulin resistance and weight-gain will see the greatest increases in their insulin needs.*

PREPARING YOUR INSULIN PUMP FOR POSTPARTUM...NOW.

This will save you a lot of headache in the hours after your baby is born: setting up your Postpartum Basal Profile.

At least one week before your delivery, set-up (but do not use or activate) a new pattern in your pump at least one week before your due date or your scheduled induction or C-section. with the following post-partum basal profile.

This profile should be about 50 percent less than your basal settings at the end of your pregnancy. If the time segments of your basal profile are not different than they were pre-pregnancy, some women are able to simply go back to their pre-pregnancy profile.

BASAL RATE:
  12A.M. =
  (**50%** of all your WEEK **38** basal rates)

INSULIN-TO-CARB RATIO:
  12A.M. =
  (return insulin-to-carb ratio back to pre-pregnancy
  ratios, or about double what they were at the end of
  pregnancy. For example, if you used a **1:5** ratio at the
  end of pregnancy, you'll need at least a **1:10** ratio
  post-partum.)

CORRECTION FACTOR:
  12A.M. =
  (return correction factor back to pre-pregnancy factor,
  again paying attention to any time differences for
  factors throughout the day.)

TARGET BLOOD SUGAR:
  100mg/dL (**5.5**mmol/L)

ACTIVE INSULIN TIME:
  4hours

AT THE DOCTOR'S OFFICE

Your appointments this month will definitely be frequent with twice-weekly NSTs and blood pressure checks, as well as constant questions about whether you're noticing any swelling in your face. All for the sake of making sure you're not displaying symptoms of pre-eclampsia.

Here's your last month checklist as this grand adventure winds its way to the grand finale!

1. Have your doctor sign-off on your birth plan and create several copies of this to keep with you at the hospital, handing it to anyone who needs a reminder that you're actually the one in charge.

2. Create your hospital bag! This bag should include:
   - All your insulin pump supplies—bring extras!
   - All your CGM supplies—bring extras!
   - Your own glucose monitor
   - Extra test-strips, lancets, etc.
   - Non-perishable snacks (if you know you C-section date, you could stash some apples and nuts, etc. in here when the timing is appropriate)
   - Treats for postpartum lows that you prefer
   - Nursing pillow if you prefer that over a normal pillow
   - Baby nail clippers and emery board
   - A going-home outfit for baby that is warm and cozy
   - A going-home outfit for mom (that is loose and very comfortable)
   - Sweatshirt, nursing bra, sweatpants, underwear that are comfortable for while you're still lying in bed at the hospital—you may or may not want to stay in your gown, and you may or may not like the hospital underwear after the first day or two!
   - Warm socks or slippers
   - All the copies of your birth plan
   - Magazines, books, phone-charger. Do yourself a favor and leave your laptop at home! You'll have your arms full and you'll be doing plenty of sleeping between nursing sessions. Email can wait!
   - Extra bags to bring home the extra stuff you'll leave the hospital with: gifts from visitors, baby supplies from the hospital, etc.
   - All your essential toiletries (and possibly your partner's,) such as toothbrush, toothpaste, face-wash, etc.

This is both an exciting and exhausting month. Physically and emotionally, you're probably quite ready for the next stage of motherhood to finally begin and this one to finally end!

GINGER'S PREGNANCY DIARY

WEEK 35

I ended up losing 8 pounds initially from that Christmas stomach bug, and then 2 more in the second week following...which is frustrating because I feel like I'm eating as much as I can eat! There were really only 4 days of not eating more than a few cans of pears, so the fact that I can't seem to put on weight is irritating. I was expecting to spend my last month of pregnancy eating very clean and carefully but instead I'm trying to get as many calories as possible in the least amount of food possible (because I get full so quickly that I can't really eat much).

Oddly enough, my insulin needs are still quite low since they were reduced for the stomach bug, and I don't need to pre-bolus for my meals by more than 5 or 10 minutes at most! Most likely, this is due to the weight-loss but it's still bizarre! I can eat gluten-free french toast, covered in syrup, take my insulin using a 1:10 insulin-to-carb ratio (rather than 1:5 like I was using before the stomach bug), and I don't go over 130 or even 120 mg/dL. So bizarre!

Now that I'm down 8 pounds from where I should be ideally, putting me at a total of 22 pounds weight-gain, I feel like every meal needs to consist of really dense calories! This is not a time in my life when I'd like to lose weight! Seriously! But the doctors say the baby is totally fine and they aren't worried, as long as I keep eating regularly.

I had several calorie-dense treats this week. I ate French fries. Some ice cream. And even gluten-free pasta with alfredo—something I usually avoid fully and completely! Thank goodness I'm experiencing such bizarre sensitivity to insulin to go along with this otherwise keeping blood sugars in range would be much harder! But it's totally all working with me instead of against me. For that, I am grateful!

WEEK 36

At last, by the end of this week the scale has finally gone up. I've gained back all 8 pounds that I lost from getting sick, but my insulin needs, specifically my Lantus dose, is still down. I was at 32 units before I got sick, then I was at 22 units while recovering, then made my way up to 25 units. I briefly went up to 27 units but started having tremendous lows, so it's safe to say that I'm in the period Jenny warned me about where insulin needs start to back down.

I continue to be grateful I was able to take this last month off from work in order to rest, focus on blood sugar management, and keep stress to a minimal level. Simply going to the grocery store can feel exhausting. Add walking 3 dogs, house-chores, and 5 degree winter in Vermont to the mix, and there's still plenty to get done in a day. (How do people with other children manage their energy and sanity during this last month of pregnancy?)

The only times I've thought "this would be easier with an insulin pump" are on the days when I realize I actually need to reduce my Lantus dose because of the recurring lows. Recurring lows are exhausting and knowing that I have to work around them or try to prevent them or endure them for another __ hours until my next Lantus dose can be frustrating.

Anyways, they really should have couches or beds in the grocery store so people can stop to take a nap.

WEEK 37

So my induction date has been set for next week, at 38.5 weeks! Baby is measuring at the 85th percentile and considering I "don't have a large pelvis," my OB team doesn't want to wait much longer. Part of me feels like, "What?! How can she be so big! My A1C has been in the 5s the whole time, what more does a girl have to do?"

But then I need to remind myself that my diabetes is just one part of what determines the baby's size. Apparently all 6 of my mother's children were on the bigger size, between 8 and 11 pounds! My nieces and nephews were also 8+ pounds. And my twin brother and I were a month early and still weight 6 ½ pounds! And my husband is no tiny cupcake, either.

Regardless, I'm totally cool with being induced and relieved in many ways to have the date set and an endpoint in sight. Obviously the first most exciting reason is that we get to meet her! And yes, the baby's needs are far simpler when she's in the womb, but I'm looking forward to walking without the pressure of a bowling ball between my legs, of going up and down the stairs without pain, of being able to loosen up a bit on blood sugar management. (To be at 130 mg/dL and not feel like a horrible person!) Oh, and it will be nice to have more than 6 items of clothing to choose from!

Just a few more days, baby! We're almost there.

WEEK 38

▎ And now it's time to meet this baby . . . .

DELIVERY & POSTPARTUM
GOOD MORNING, BABY!

THIS IS IT.

Whether you go into labor naturally or you're scheduled ahead of time for an induction or C-section, there are a few things you can do to help prepare your blood sugar for the next part of this life-changing adventure.

PREPARING YOUR DIABETES FOR DELIVERY

The day your water breaks or you arrived for your scheduled induction or C-section...that can be a rather nerve-wracking day. The stress and excitement just from getting ready to get in the car can send your blood sugar spiraling upward.

So...if you can, try to keep your cool, mama. Keep your thoughts simple. Just think about the next little step rather the big one. The last thing you need right now is an adrenaline rush sending your blood sugar up to 300 mg/dL (16.6 mmol/L). If that does happen, dose carefully and thoughtfully...and listen to some Enya! Or whatever it is that calms you down.

Here are important steps to take and things to consider depending on the method of delivery used to welcome your baby into the world!

BEFORE YOU LEAVE FOR THE HOSPITAL

An important thing to remember when you're headed to the hospital is that you're not going to be eating again for a while. Once labor begins, you likely won't want to eat, and you won't be allowed to eat as soon as you're hooked up to induction medications, therefore you do want to get a reasonable meal into your belly before you leave. Eating a low-carb meal (like eggs, sausage, non-starchy veggies, cheese, etc.) that requires very little insulin is helpful because it means you'll have less bolus insulin in your system by the time you're hooked up to an induction medication or being prepped for a C-section.

FOR PUMPERS:

- For those on tubed pumps, it can be helpful to insert an extra site before you head to the hospital that you don't actually connect to. In the case that the old site gets accidentally pulled out during labor/delivery – having an accessible and ready-to-go site to connect to can be a time and situation saver. It's also important to head to the hospital when you have plenty of insulin in your pump. You don't want to realize you're nearly out of insulin when you're about to receive your epidural for a C-section.

- Inform your nurses and entire team where your on your body your pump is connected when you get to the hospital and you are going over your diabetes plan. It's important that everyone in the room understands what your pump site is, what it looks like, and why it's there!

- It's important to make sure your pump site and your CGM site are both in areas that are least likely to be disturbed during delivery via vaginal birth or C-section. If you are planning a c-section, having the CGM and infusion site on the back of your arm or your lower back, or the side of your thigh is often the best option, rather than your love-handle area which could be affected by the surgery.

FOR INJECTIONS:

- Even though you won't be eating during an induction or C-section, you will be hooked up to an IV of glucose because your body still needs fuel. If you take your background insulin dose at night, and your C-section or induction is the next morning, you'll want to cut back on your dose by ¼ to ⅓ to account for the reduction in calories. You'll also need to make sure you inform your delivery team how much long-acting insulin is in your system, and when it will be out of your system so they know when to set-up an IV of insulin for the remainder of your induction. While it's disturbing to imagine your blood sugars being managed by strangers and IVs of glucose and "regular" insulin, this is often the smoothest method of insulin delivery for those on injections because it can be stopped and changed quickly, unlike a dose of long-acting insulin.

- If you're going in for a scheduled C-section, you'll simply take your background insulin the night before but again, a reduced dose by ¼ to ⅓ to keep you stable during the C-section. Refer to the "postpartum insulin doses" section for further instruction on your next background insulin dose after your baby is in your arms!

- If you wear a CGM, remember to explain what it is to your team, and make sure it's located on an area that will not be affected during the C-section: such as the back of your arm, your side thigh, or your lower back. It is not recommended to wear your CGM on your love-handle area during a C-section.

FOR EVERYONE:

- Above all else, your goal is enter the hospital with an in-range blood sugar and very little insulin on-board besides your basal rate or background insulin.

- If your blood sugar is high on your way to to the hospital, don't let your nerves cause you to over-correct just so you can get down as quickly as possible. Use good old fashioned logic and thought and take the appropriate dose that you've been using for the past week or two. Remember to wait at least 2 hours before taking any further correction insulin. You don't want to find yourself on a roller coaster.

- If you're low on your way to the hospital, treat the low with fast-acting carbohydrates (rather than something containing fat or protein). Treat it thoughtfully and reasonably, bring yourself up to an in-range blood sugar. Remember to wait at least 15 minutes before testing again to determine if you need to treat with further carbs.

- If you arrive at the hospital and you're very concerned about your blood sugar level because it's too high or too low, express your concerns to your team. But most of all, try to relax and let your actions take effect before reacting again.

LABOR AND DELIVERY

The hardest part about knowing what will happen to your blood sugars during delivery is that you don't know how your baby is necessarily going to enter the world until it's all happening. You could find yourself in labor for 12 hours and then your team will decide the safest option is a C-section because another issue making a vaginal birth unsafe.

And of course, no one can truly predict how your body will react to labor. Some people give birth quickly, others take hours or even days. Some people eat ice chips and are relatively "well" aside from the tremendous work and pain of labor. And others might find themselves very unwell, sick with vomiting, or any of the other long list of variables that can play into the delivery of a baby.

The best you can do is prepare yourself for pregnancy by knowing your insulin needs really well, being thoughtful in the moment, and continuing to be the courageous type 1 mama you've been this entire pregnancy.

HERE ARE GUIDELINES AND TIPS FOR MANAGING DIABETES DURING DELIVERY:
FOR PUMPERS:

- **LABOR MAY CAUSE LOWER BLOOD SUGARS DUE TO THE EXERCISE**—like "activity," but hourly blood sugar checks will help determine if or when basal rate changes need to be made.

- **IF YOUR BLOOD SUGAR IS RUNNING LOW**—consistently lower than 80 mg/dL (4.4 mmol/L) on your CGM—then set a temporary basal reduction of 25% to 50% for 12 hours and continue to monitor hourly to assess if additional changes need to be made.

- **FOR HIGH BLOOD SUGARS,** take 50% of your calculated correction dose. Correction doses of insulin during labor and delivery should be given no more than every 3 hours.

- **IF YOU'RE HOOKED UP TO AN IV FOR YOUR INSULIN,** keep your pump infusion site on your body so you can easily reconnect to it after the baby is born and you're disconnected from the IV drip of insulin.

FOR INJECTIONS:

- Labor may cause lower blood sugars due to the exercise-like "activity," but hourly blood sugar checks will help determine if or when you need to increase or decrease the dose of your insulin IV drip and/or your glucose IV drip.

- If your blood sugar is running low—consistently lower than 80 mg/dL (4.4 mmol/L) on your CGM—ask your team to reduce the insulin IV drip by 25% to 50% for 12 hours and continue to monitor hourly to assess if additional changes need to be made.

- If you are not on an IV of insulin or glucose, but instead using background insulin alone, sip juice to manage lows.
- For high blood sugars, take 50% of your calculated correction dose. Correction doses of insulin during labor and delivery should be given no more than every 3 hours. Always aiming for an in-range blood sugar and preventing any roller coaster swings.
- If you are hooked up to an insulin IV drip, ask the nurse to inform you in advance when you'll be disconnected from the drip after delivery. Take your basal insulin dose about 1 hour prior to disconnection from the insulin drip, to ensure that you have active background insulin on-board when the IV drip is disconnected.

BLOOD SUGAR TARGET RANGES FOR VAGINAL BIRTH OR C—SECTION

GOALS: Higher than 70 mg/dL (3.8 mmol/L) and lower than 140 mg/dL (7.7 mmol/L)

CORRECTION DOSES: Corrections during labor/delivery should be given no more than every 3 hours. Doses should be decreased by 50% of what the suggested/calculated correction dose is via the pump to prevent low blood sugars during delivery. (Example: If 3.0 units is suggested by your pump or calculated manually, take only 1.50 units for the correction.)

Remember, call the Patient Advocacy Hotline in your hospital if you feel as though your voice as a patient is not being respected or heard, and you are not getting the insulin you need to manage healthy blood sugars during delivery.

POSTPARTUM: The First 24 to 48 Hours After Your Baby is Born Congratulations! In an ideal world, all you'd have to do now is snuggle with your newborn baby. In a type 1 world, your blood sugars still need to be managed.

If you're looking for motivation to care about your blood sugars once your baby is out, remember two things:

1. Your body needs to heal and high blood sugars will absolutely interfere and slow down your body's ability to heal.
2. Look at that beautiful baby! That little creature needs a healthy mama to feed them and kiss them and swaddle them and kiss them again.

Okay, so let's look closely at what to expect for your postpartum insulin needs and adjustments. Keep in mind, again, everyone is a little different, so you will need to watch your blood sugars closely and adjust as needed.

FOR EVERYONE:

- As soon as the baby/placenta is delivered switch to the lower/pre-pregnancy pattern. Your insulin needs will drop significantly as soon as all those "baby" hormones are gone! This is an important time to beware of low blood sugars, because the drop in insulin needs will happen within hours after delivery. Work with your healthcare team to ensure you have access to glucose either via an IV or juice within arm's reach of your hospital bed in the maternity ward at all times. While the number on the scale will take longer to adjust as your uterus shrinks and extra fluid retention is released, your body will be impacted most significantly by your body simply no longer being pregnant.

- Based on how much your insulin needs increased during your pregnancy, the postpartum plan may be about 30 to 60 percent less insulin than you were using by the end of your pregnancy. For example, if you were taking 30 units a day in your total basal rate or long-acting insulin dose, you may only need about 15 units total in your basal rate or long-acting insulin dose for the next day or two.

- For some, your insulin needs following a C-section can remain a little higher compared to a vaginal birth because the stress and inflammation and healing that is a normal part of an major surgery can cause more insulin resistance than usual, and thus require higher insulin doses than you might need if you'd had a vaginal birth. Again, many people don't experience this, so you may find it's most comfortable to start with a reduced rate of 30 to 60 percent, and then increase if your blood sugars remain high postpartum.

- Based on your pre-pregnancy insulin doses, you will find you likely need a reduced rate of about 20 to 40 percent less insulin for that 24 to 48 hour postpartum window.

- Check your blood sugar every 3 hours to determine if you need more or less insulin, more or less juice. This timing should coincide with your breastfeeding schedule which should be every 2 to 3 hours after delivery.

The "hard part" is over. Now all you have to do is take care of that gorgeous baby while being a powerhouse mom who just happens to live with type 1 diabetes. Piece of cake, right?

Take a deep breath, and remember to be flexible and forgiving with yourself. Over the next several weeks and months, you will be adjusting physically, emotionally, and constantly to this new life. And so will your diabetes. Give yourself plenty of room to make mistakes, make adjustments, reflect, breathe, sleep, rinse and repeat.

BREASTFEEDING WITH TYPE 1 DIABETES:
THE MYTHS, THE FACTS, AND THE CHALLENGES

If you've decided and are able to breastfeed your children, that's a wonderful! For babies with family members who have type 1 diabetes, breastfeeding is one of the many things we can do to help further reduce their risk of developing type 1 diabetes themselves one day.

But you've probably heard a lot of myths and warnings about breastfeeding as a woman with type 1 diabetes. And these things you've heard may have really left you with further worry and concern: type 1 diabetes is going to complicate this, too? Really?

Here are three very common concerns and questions you might have because of common misconceptions about breastfeeding and type 1 diabetes:

1. "Will I have trouble producing breast-milk because I have type 1 diabetes?."

2. "Do I have to 'pump and dump' my milk if my blood sugar is high?"

3. "Is my blood sugar going to plummet every time I breastfeed my baby?"

So let's tackle this immediately.

CAN WOMEN WITH DIABETES PRODUCE BREAST-MILK PROPERLY?
ANSWER: YES.

In the end, if you're managing your blood sugars to attain an A1C at 7.5 or below during postpartum, type 1 diabetes shouldn't interfere with your body's ability to produce milk for your baby. It is true that insulin and blood sugar levels plays a key role in the production of breastmilk, so persistently high blood sugars (over 200 mg/dL / 11.11 mmol/L) that remain high long enough to leave you with an A1C near 8 percent or higher can certainly interfere, but it'll also interfere with your body's ability to heal properly, too. So aiming for reasonable blood sugars after your baby is out of your uterus and in your arms is very important.

The best way to establish and maintain a strong milk supply is to feed your baby 'on-demand' which means as frequently as they ask for it. You can't nurse a baby too often but you can nurse a baby too infrequently and this can interfere with your milk production. Newborn babies should be nursed at least 10 to 12 times a day.

The reality is that if you're managing your blood sugars reasonably well and you're having trouble producing milk, you may simply be one of many women (diabetic or not) whose body has difficulty producing milk. While this can be disheartening, frustrating, and heartbreaking, we are fortunate to live in a world with formula so your baby can still flourish, and grow, and get the nutrients they need.

Women with type 1 diabetes are able to safely take nursing supplements such as fenugreek which is said to help increase milk production. Hydration is also key in ensuring adequate milk production, since breastmilk contains a great deal of water! Be sure to stay hydrated, drinking water regularly throughout the day.

DO I HAVE TO "PUMP & DUMP" MILK IF MY BLOOD SUGAR WAS HIGH? ANSWER: NO.

It isn't ideal to have persistent high blood sugars when you're breastfeeding, because again it will interfere with your production, and it isn't healthy for you as a healing new mother. However, breast-milk is naturally sweet and is largely made-up of glucose and galactose, two types of basic sugar. On top of that, the sugar in your bloodstream has actually very little impact on the sugar content of your breast-milk. Only about ⅓ of the glucose in your blood will make its way to your breast-milk.

And on top of it all, the milk you produce was likely "made" several hours before your baby drinks it, so the mere idea of trying to figure out when to pump and dump the milk that might have slightly more glucose in it is just crazy. Ridiculous, even.

And it needs to be said that asking a mother to pump and dump her breastmilk—when so much energy and effort goes into breastfeeding and milk production in the first place—is cruel and is more likely only going to cause tremendous burnout and exhaustion in this new mom who is working very hard to feed her baby!

IN OTHER WORDS: if your A1C is at or below 7.5 percent, don't worry about the occasional high blood sugar. If your blood sugars are persistently high, adjust your basal needs to bring yourself down to at least a 150 mg/dL (8.3 mmol/L) average. It's hard to loosen the reigns after the baby is born and feel "okay" with blood sugars that aren't "near perfect" all the time. The result can mean you end up going sky-high from burnout and you give up because you know you can't maintain 90 mg/dL (5 mmol/L) as often as you did while pregnant. It's okay. Aim for 150 mg/dL if that helps you adjust to new life with your beautiful new bundle!

If your doctor gives you a hard time about this, just turn to this page and hand them this book. You're a new mother with a very intense chronic illness and you're simply amazing for having come this far in this journey, given birth to a beautiful baby, and for now attempting to breastfeed it for both your own benefits. Don't let anybody give you a hard time just because you still don't produce insulin, and you still aren't the perfect diabetic.

WILL BREASTFEEDING MAKE MY BLOOD SUGAR DROP CONSTANTLY? ANSWER: YES AND NO.

The fact is: breastfeeding can cause your blood sugar to drop. The tricky part is when. On average, the drop occurs during or immediately after the nursing session, and is usually managed by one reasonable treatment of carbs (15 grams, an apple, a small box of raisins, 15 jelly beans, or a small juice box, etc.). However, some women experience low blood sugars when their body is producing breast-milk rather than when their baby is actually nursing.

This will be the hardest part of breastfeeding.

Determining how breastfeeding impacts your blood sugars will take some time.

It takes approximately 3 months for your milk production to "regulate." This means that your body is actually going to be adjusting to the "work" of producing and delivering milk to your baby. If you can get through those first 3 months, you'll likely be able to find more consistency in how to manage your blood sugar around nursing sessions.

The frequency and length of those nursing sessions will also change. At first, your newborn may want to eat every 2 or 3 hours for 10 or 15 minutes at a time. When they are three months old, they may nurse every 4 hours, for 20 to 30 minutes at a time. Every baby is different! But you're both going to be working hard to get to know each other and establish something resembling a "routine" with some degree of predictability.

Fortunately, you likely won't need glucose for every nursing session. Instead, you may eventually find that your blood sugar is only affected at certain times of the day. This is where a little note-keeping can come in handy. Keep it simple: the time of day and the low blood sugar. Of course, trying to pinpoint if this low blood sugar was the result of a nursing session or the result of too much insulin for your lunch is always a challenge, but if you can try to be as thoughtful with your nutrition intake as you were during pregnancy, that will help tremendously!

Mostly clean foods, include treats once a day, and eat smaller meals more often.

You may also find, once you know what time of day your breastfeeding lows typically occur, that you can reduce the amount of insulin you take for a normal meal that is going to happen right before/during/after a nursing session, so you don't end up having to eat extra carbohydrates.

Complicating this learning curve are the other changes you'll need in your insulin doses simply due to your body recovering from giving birth. While you'll likely have returned to a total background insulin dose that is either at or near your pre-pregnancy dose, your body is going through a lot. Your uterus is working hard to contract and shrink back to a non-pregnant size. Your body is naturally going to drop some of the weight it gained during pregnancy. Within two weeks postpartum, the number on the scale will likely be dramatically different, whether you tried to make it change or not—and those changes mean you'll need gradually less insulin.

IN OTHER WORDS: your body is adjusting to a lot of things right now.

TIPS & REMINDERS FOR BREASTFEEDING WITH TYPE 1 DIABETES

- Basal adjustments may be needed due to fluctuation in sleep patterns—pay attention to your blood sugar overnight to determine if you need to adjust your basal rates or long-acting insulin dose.

- 5 to 10 grams carb before each session can be helpful to prevent the drop (simple carbs like juice, fruit chews, fruit leathers, glucose tablets, etc.). A bit of protein can help prevent drops later on if that is a consistent issue for you. Snack ideas might include peanut butter, cheese, nuts, etc.

- Nursing right after a meal may cause a low blood sugar due to loss of glucose from your system in the breast milk. If nursing time is typically after a meal, take the pre-meal bolus dose down 10 to 20 percent to decrease your risk of lows after nursing.

- Keep food or treatment for lows in easy access in the nursing areas in your home: baby's room, your bedside, next to the rocking chair or chair/couch, etc.

- Chronic high blood sugars when nursing can hinder lactation and will provide more "calories" to the baby than needed. Healthy blood sugar levels postpartum is the goal, even if they are a smidge higher than your pregnancy target ranges, you're still aiming to keep your A1C under 7.5 postpartum. Ideally, your blood sugar will be below 150 mg/dL (8.3 mmol/L) when nursing to decrease the amount of extra glucose going to baby in the breast milk, and to keep you, the new mama who is still healing, healthy.

- Drink at least 10 glasses of water daily to ensure proper hydration and to keep up milk supply. (Keep a water bottle at your bedside for as long as you continue to nurse your baby during the night. You'll be thirsty, and trips to the kitchen for more water won't be convenient!)

- Do not cut back on food intake – nursing takes a lot of calories out of the body. Nursing mothers should consume about 1800 calories per day when nursing—more may be necessary if you get back to active lifestyle quickly. Eating too little will interfere with your body's ability to produce milk. Eating too few carbs will also make it harder for your body to produce milk. Aim for all three macronutrients (protein, fats, carbs) and adequate calories coming from mostly healthy sources.

The moral of the story is that breastfeeding is a wonderful gift you can give to your child, but you're a woman who is also juggling the demands of a very intense chronic illness, too. If you can give your little one a couple weeks of breastmilk, that will give them a good dose of the many incredible long-term benefits breast-milk provides for a newborn. Their immune system in particular will thank you!

If you can't, or if you need to stop after a couple of weeks, that is your decision. You need to do what is best not just for your baby but for you as a new mother, and for your family overall.

POSTPARTUM DEPRESSION

You've read about it, you've heard about it, and you've probably had a friend or two who've experienced it. Postpartum depression is real, but as a mom with type 1 you're simply at an increased risk for facing postpartum depression because you have significantly more on your plate of responsibilities than the average mom.

We aren't going to dive deeply into this, because the real treatment for postpartum depression can't be found in a book.

If you are struggling, if you are crying on a daily basis (and not just over how adorable your child is), please reach out. First, tell your partner how you're feeling. Secondly, tell a trusted friend. And thirdly, tell a professional. You may find it easiest to tell your OB-GYN at your next appointment, and they'll likely have a great list of people to work with, but the important part is that you acknowledge it and get the support you need.

Even one session a week with a therapist could do wonders.

You've been through so much in the past year as you prepared for pregnancy with type 1 diabetes, endured pregnancy with type 1 diabetes, and now you're managing type 1 diabetes as a new mom. Yes, that is one beautiful baby, but adjusting to life as a new mom is not easy or straightforward. It's okay if you're overwhelmed, if you're feeling like your head is barely above water. Ask for help.

A KISS FOR YOUR BABY

Remember, mama, that is one lucky baby. It was born into this world with a mother who fought long and hard, for 9 months and more! Some women just walk down the street producing insulin, effortlessly managing perfect blood sugars all day long without ever stabbing their body with lancets or syringes or infusion sites.

You are walking down the street doing something incredible: you're keeping yourself alive every day, and you did so while growing a life inside you! You're already an amazing mother. And your little one is going to grow up knowing this about you, too.

A kiss, from us to your baby. And a hug, from us to you.

CONGRATULATIONS!

POST-PARTUM
GINGER'S PREGNANCY DIARY

GIVING BIRTH TO LUCY

We were scheduled for an induction on January 27th, bright and early in the morning, when I was 38.5 weeks pregnant. Why? Because my OBGYN was following the protocol of not allowing women with any type of diabetes to go beyond 39 weeks, and in her words, "You don't have a very large pelvis and the baby is measuring on the larger side."

SO AN INDUCTION IT IS.

The size of the baby is such a touchy subject for those of us with diabetes... at least, I find myself defending it because a big baby for a woman with diabetes feels like a failure. But at the same time, I know my blood sugars were in extremely tight control! I know I couldn't have done it any tighter than I did without my brain exploding. Lots of women have "larger than average" babies who don't have diabetes so why does the size of our baby always have to have be mentioned in connection with our diabetes, especially when we demonstrated and maintained excellent blood sugar control with A1Cs in the non-diabetic range? My mother had six "larger than average" babies and my husband was apparently a "larger than average" baby, too. So...maybe I'd have a baby in the upper 8-poundage area whether or not I had diabetes, right? And yet, it's always mentioned, "Well, she's larger than average because of your diabetes."

Okay, that's the end of my rant...for now. Anyways, my point is, the constant emphasis on this bothered me because she was still within the range of "normal," just on the higher end. Okay, now, truly, my rant is over.

I should warn you, though, that the following pages are going to be laden with frustration and resentment for the medical system and how they manage and think about type 1 diabetes. The way the hospital took care of me as a pregnant woman and my baby was wonderful—we always felt safe and so cared for every step of the way—but my type 1 diabetes management was only successful because I was hard-headed, stubborn, and well, moderately bitchy every step of the way.

So...here we go:

TUESDAY

My insulin needs prior to Tuesday had been plummeting daily. I took 12 units of Lantus insulin the night before the induction began (2 units less than my pre-pregnancy Lantus dose) and my blood sugars were steady in non-diabetic range all night and all morning.

My doctor and I had agreed I would eat a zero-carbohydrate breakfast because they don't want you to eat once you're on the induction medications, and she didn't want me to go a day or more without having been able to eat. So I had two eggs and two breakfast sausage links, took 1 unit of insulin, and my blood sugar stayed around 100 mg/dL without any issue.

It wasn't until I was out of the hospital and looking back on the six days I spent there when I realized the hospital is terrified of patients experience low blood sugars. I've been putting all my energy into preventing high blood sugars for the past nine months and during the hours when it is just as crucial—right before she's born—I found myself battling the hospital staff over every insulin dose because they wanted to cut back every dose much more than I felt was necessary.

During the first morning and afternoon of eating zero carbs while on the pitocin drip, the nursing staff never seemed to even wonder if I needed insulin for the eggs and the avocado and the almonds I was eating. Meanwhile, I was taking very small doses of fast-acting insulin because despite that those foods are extremely low carb, they still of course require some insulin. They never asked, so I never told them, and my blood sugars continued to hang out in non-diabetic range, a beautiful steady line around 90 to 100 mg/dL.

By the way, I went to bed that night in the hospital still at zero centimeters dilated.

WEDNESDAY

Still no dilation. (Have I mentioned just how fun it is to have your cervix examined several times a day?)

No eating all day, sipping on clear liquids, mostly just water.

By Wednesday evening, when my body was clearly still not in labor, and I hadn't eaten since the afternoon before because they don't want you eating close to when you might go into labor, they decided to take me off the pitocin drip for a bit so I could eat a real meal. They didn't want me to be too hungry and under-fueled because of the expected work of labor and delivery! It's a major workout, and just like a workout at the gym, you don't want to do either on a totally empty stomach.

But that's where the real insulin-dosing battle began. When I ordered the sweet potatoes, pork chop and vegetable dinner from the hospital cafeteria, I told the very sweet and very competent nurse that I'd like to take 6 units of insulin when the meal arrived. By this point, I was on an IV drip of regular insulin (the only kind that works in IV drips, apparently), and I was getting .5 units of insulin per hour (This is the lowest amount that endocrinology decided was allowed for a woman in the delivery floor...why? Who knows. I don't think they know either. And later on, I really would've benefitted from a rate of .3 per hour, but again, that wasn't allowed because some idiot decided that's too low! Really insane.)

The nurse was terrified by the idea of giving me 6 whole units of insulin. I explained to her the estimated carb-count of the sweet potatoes and the sauce on the pork chop but she was still extremely nervous about it. We went back and forth for awhile until she convinced me that regular insulin in a IV drip was going to get into my system much faster than my injected insulin. I honestly couldn't remember what taking regular insulin was like, and I hadn't received insulin via IV since my diagnosis, so I relented, and she only gave me 2 units of insulin.

Just 2 units.

Ugh.

Sure enough, my blood sugar rose to 200 mg/dL and took 3 hours total to slowly come down. The nurse was in tears because she knew how perfectly I'd maintained my blood sugar for the past two days around 90-100 mg/dL. I assured her it was okay, especially since the baby was obviously not anywhere near being born, but it was stressful nonetheless to have to worry about the high blood sugar.

My doctor knew that my blood sugar was high as a result of the nurse's judgment and funnily enough, had no real reaction to it despite having scolded me once during an appointment several months prior when she saw a similar high blood sugar reading on my CGM printout. The irony of this—it's not a big deal when it's the nurse's fault, only when it's my fault—is too frustrating to do anything but laugh about.

Throughout the next night, I sipped clear liquids (grape juice mixed with apple juice) to compensate for the fact that they weren't allowed to lower my IV drip rate to anything below .5 units per hour. My blood sugar was constantly trying to drop because, like I mentioned, what I really needed was probably .3 units per hour.

Meanwhile, by the way, my body had still not responded the pitocin at all except for gradually swelling of my ankles and feet as expected.

THURSDAY

Still no dilation. Three days of pitocin and my cervix was dilated zero centimeters! Zero! Zero!

They kept checking (again, not the kind of exam one would like to have repeated 2 to 3 times per day for 3 days…) and it never changed. This meant they couldn't even try other methods of getting me into labor, like breaking my water, because I wasn't even dilated 1 centimeter.

I must note here that these three long days in the hospital would've been so much more stressful if it weren't for my best friends Tara and Tanya who stayed with my husband and I almost all day each day we were there, and even during one of the nights. They helped get my whale-like (at least I felt like I whale) body out of bed, kept my water bottle filled, supported me in every insulin dosing battle. They were wonderful. My family.

By this point, none of the nurses or residents on the birthing floor argued with me about insulin doses. Every time a new nurse was assigned to me at the start of a new shift, the previous nurse would tell them, "She knows what she's doing with her blood sugars," and that was that.

Also by this point, the swelling in had made its way up to my knees and my blood pressure was starting to register as "pre-eclamptic" despite having been lower than normal throughout my entire pregnancy. Fortunately, my blood pressure never really escalated past a measurement of 95/140, so they didn't have to do anything about it besides continuing to check it regularly.

By Thursday at 4 p.m., my doctor came in and announced that if I still wasn't dilated, we would do a C-section.

Now, prior to all of this, I had always assumed a C-section would feel as though you missed out on the experience of giving birth. I assumed that you as the mother would be so out of it and separated from the experience of the baby coming out that it wouldn't feel the same as giving birth vaginally.

Fortunately, I was well aware before going into this part of the process that a "birthing plan" is really just a hope, and the most I could do was go with the flow and do what's best for the health of both baby and me.

And sure enough, I was still zero centimeters dilated, so when she said we would schedule the C-section, I was actually totally thrilled. We were ready. Let's get this party started.

My doctor finished her discussion about the C-section and asked if I had any other questions.

To which I quickly said, "I would like 9 units of Lantus tonight, after the C-section."

As soon as the baby was out, I would be taken off the IV of insulin because you can't be on IV insulin in the maternity ward. I knew that I was going to be really disoriented, on drugs, and exhausted after the surgery, so I wanted to put forth my moderately bitchy diabetic needs while I was clear-headed.

She furrowed her brow and thought for a moment.

"What about 6 units? 9 seems like too much."

"I need 9," I insisted. I can't tell you why I knew this, aside from my experience in fasting, going days with very few calories from my preparation for powerlifting competitions, but I just knew 9 units was the right amount.

"Okay, I'll think about it and get back to you."

I don't know what she thought about or who she talked to, but she came back 30 minutes later and told me she had instructed the nurses to give me 9 units of Lantus after the surgery. Victory is mine.

Now, it's showtime:

Oh, how wrong I was about a C-section feeling any less special than a vaginal birth. I was so wrong. And this is the part where my frustration and stress with the hospital protocol goes away for a bit because my doctor, the nursing staff, and the anesthesiologist were so swift and calm and wonderful with every step of the C-section.

I've honestly taken many Lantus injections and felt many CGM sensor insertions that were much more painful than the injection in my spine to numb my lower body. The only uncomfortable part was the incredible trembling and shaking I experienced throughout the entire surgery. My teeth and my entire body were chattering and shaking so severely, even my husband was a bit concerned.

As I lay on the table with a sheet blocking my view of my torso, I waited while my husband glanced over occasionally and finally said, "This is it! I can see her head!"

That's when I very quietly burst into tears, at the anticipation of her arrival. I expected to cry when we first met eye-to-eye but no, these tears, I think, were more about relief. The final home-stretch of the unrelenting stress of aiming for blood sugar perfection for 9 long months. Sure, carrying around that big belly with the sore back and the sore feet, that's not fun, but the building stress from the daily pressure of managing diabetes so tightly in a body that makes none of its own insulin finally left my body in the form of tears as she was slowly pulled out of me.

I heard the nurses say things like "Whoa, her head is huge! Look at all that hair!" and "She's beautiful!"

But there was no crying!

"Roger! Why isn't she crying? Is she blue? Is she breathing?"

"Just wait," he assured me. He later explained that she was still sort of asleep and stretching quietly as she was removed from her cozy little den. She wasn't crying because she hadn't just spent several hours being pushed down a tight tunnel! She had no idea she was being evicted!

And then I heard her tiny little cry.

It was all worth it. She was actually here, crying, out in the real world.

Every ounce of effort, every day of obsessive blood sugar management...it was all worth it.

At 9:28 p.m. on January 29th, Lucy was born, weighing 8 lbs. 12 oz.

I still hadn't laid my eyes on her myself. They took her over to a cleaning station, and my husband stood with her where she held tightly to his finger while they cleaned her up. Then, after what felt like 15 minutes but was actually only 3 or 4, they finally brought her over to me and lay her on my chest. I was no longer crying, but simply in a calm state looking at her. I really don't know how to write the sentence that describes how I felt during that moment. There's simply no way to describe it.

This little being came from me?

You? Lucy! You've been inside me all this time? You're perfect! I made you?

Look at you!

We made it!

You and me, kiddo, we made it!

Her blood sugar was checked at 1 hour postpartum, 2 hours postpartum, and 3 hours postpartum. If mom's blood sugar is high throughout pregnancy and particularly right before the birth, baby can have very low blood sugars during the first few hours of life. The hospital wants anything above 45 mg/dL. Lucy passed each test with a blood sugar around 57 mg/dL.

Her blood sugars were normal, her eyes were bright, she had ten fingers and ten toes. She was perfect. Perfectly healthy.

And pretty damn gorgeous, too.

There's nothing less special about a C-section. She's here, it doesn't matter how she got here. The moment you lay eyes on that little creature, all those ideas about what you hoped your delivery would be like disappear. Screaming in pain for 12 hours isn't going to make this moment any more incredible. It doesn't matter. What matters most is that you and baby are safe and healthy.

We made it, together.

Even as I write this, two months after she was born, I am still filled with awe and overwhelmed with gratitude that while my body can't make insulin, it can make Lucy.

FRIDAY, SATURDAY & SUNDAY

Most of what I want to share about Friday, Saturday and Sunday is about diabetes frustration, because I hope it helps you in your own delivery story. But I want to start this section by saying again that the nurses who took care of me as a woman who had just given birth and who took care of my newborn baby girl were wonderful. Attentive. Wise. Sweet. Compassionate. Wonderful.

And Lucy continued to be beautifully adorable and cuddly and amazing.

It's just diabetes management that continued to be a major headache and a major battle between the hospital and me.

A whole new floor in the hospital—the maternity ward—means a whole new set of nurses and residents who are going to argue with me over every single insulin dose. This ongoing nonsense was almost more exhausting than recovering from a C-section!

To make a long story short, they continued to want me to limit my insulin doses further than I was already limiting them—even though I had had no low blood sugars. Instead, I'd been in non-diabetic range the entire time except for going up to 145 mg/dL once! And I continued to be moderately bitchy about each requested insulin dose until I got what I wanted. And my blood sugars continued to hang out in non-diabetic range because of my bitchiness! An endless lesson in trusting your gut because we do know our bodies, especially our diabetes, better than anyone else ever will. Period. Trust your instinct, trust your knowledge, trust yourself...and don't be afraid to be a little unfriendly if you need to in order to be heard.

Unfortunately, once the catheter was removed and I could walk to the bathroom on my own Saturday morning to pee, it was discovered that the narcotics they were giving me were making me incredibly sick. I vomited every time I stood up to walk to the bathroom. So I wasn't allowed to eat, which means I'd basically eaten a total of two very small meals during the past 4 days.

By Saturday evening, I asked the nurse for my Lantus dose of 9 units. Now, had I been actually eating a normal amount of food that day, I knew I would've been taking 11 or 12 units of Lantus by this point after giving birth, so a dose of 9 units is actually a reduction despite that it is the same amount I was given the night before and the night before that. And I hadn't experienced any low blood sugars all day despite not eating, so 9 units was clearly working well.

The resident on duty that night said she wanted to give me 6 units because I wasn't going to be eating and hadn't been eating all day.

When the nurse told me this, I couldn't help myself, I rolled my eyes like a teenager and groaned loudly.

"Are you serious?" I was just so tired of all the insulin arguing. "I need 9 units. 9 is already a reduction. I'd be taking more than that if I were eating."

"I'll talk to her," said the nurse.

While she went to discuss the dosing with the resident, I sat in bed and started boiling over with frustration and diabetic rage. Get. Me. Out. Of. Here.

Why do I have to work so hard to keep myself healthy in a hospital? Why can't the staff on this floor talk to the staff on the birthing floor so they know I am an informed patient and should be at least part of the discussion when it comes to dosing rather than just being told what I need by someone who doesn't know one single thing about my diabetes management needs?

The nurse came back in the room—two hours later—and said, "She wants you to take 6 units."

To which I said, "Listen, if you only give me 6 units, I'm going to sneak 3 more units from the Lantus pen in my purse!"

The nurse's eyes widened as her eyebrows almost lifted right off the top of her head.

I am officially unleashed. I'm no longer making any effort to be cordial or polite. Watch out. I'm done with this. I'd been trying so hard to play by their rules, trying to not take more of my own insulin secretly in the bathroom—particularly the Lantus insulin—so that they knew how much insulin was really in my system...but this was getting ridiculous.

"I'll talk to her," the nurse said.

She came back 15 minutes later and said, "Okay, we're going to give you 9 units of Lantus...but you need to give us the insulin in your purse. You're not supposed to have that."

"Sure, no problem," I said, only because I knew I was getting 9 units I wanted.

"Do you have any other medications with you?"

"No," I lied—I'm not giving her my Novolog. She gave me 9 units, and I spent the next two hours that night packing up everything in my room so I could leave as soon as the sun started shining Sunday morning. (By the way, despite their fears, my blood sugar was steady throughout the night, and I stopped puking as soon as the narcotics were out of my system.)

SUNDAY MORNING

The resident came into my room at 7 a.m. She looked at the stitches in my abdomen, and said, "Okay, so I think you'll stay until tomorrow morning?"

"Tomorrow morning?" I said. I had already packed every single item in my room. All that remained was putting clothes on the baby and calling my husband to come help us escape.

"I would like to leave today," I said.

"Oh...okay," she said, very surprised. "Let's make sure you can eat breakfast and keep it down...then you can go."

"Okay," I agreed.

Breakfast was delicious. And I digested it properly. They gave me permission to leave.

And so...we escaped with a deep sigh of relief, back to the land where I am Queen of my own diabetes...and where Lucy continues to be adorably beautiful.

15 MONTHS LATER

Her name is Lucy. Just thinking about her silly, beautiful face is just... ugh...I can't describe it. Right now as I type this, she is upstairs sleeping— she just started truly walking yesterday at about 15 months old. She has become her own person, with quirky habits, and silly faces, an extreme love for bananas, and this personality that makes her suddenly no longer just my babygirl but actually this real human-being on the planet! I made her and she actually exists, and sometimes I still can't believe it.

As cliched as it sounds, I can't remember who I was before I became Lucy's mom.

I don't care that I can't get a pedicure whenever I feel like it. I don't care that I can't spend an entire day watching Sex and the City and baking cookies. I don't care that the skin around my belly button has a funky-looking wrinkle to it, and that even though I fit in my pre-pregnancy jeans, my belly still has an extra "poof" to it that I'd happily do without. I don't care that we've only gone to the movie theater twice in the past two years even though we both love movies. I don't care that I can't travel to various diabetes conferences, have to turn down extra freelance work, or that this book took me about 5 times longer to write and publish than every other book I've written because the only time I have now to write outside of work is between 9 p.m. and midnight.

I do not care.

What I care about most is being Lucy's mom. Everything else needs to support my role as Lucy's mom, and if it doesn't, then I don't do it.

What I'm trying to say is: all the stress and work you'll endure during pregnancy as a woman with type 1 diabetes is worth it. Every finger prick. Every CGM insertion that hits a really sensitive spot and hurts like whoa. Every tedious low and infuriating high. It's all worth it.

BREASTFEEDING

I breastfed Lucy for almost three months before having to stop. Unfortunately, I started having extreme flare-up in my fibromyalgia pain at about two months postpartum. It was so bad that I could barely pick her up in the morning and I was wrapping my hands in flexible ice-packs whenever I wasn't holding her. And when I wasn't wrapped with ice-packs, I was wearing compression gloves and looking online for something better than whatever I was wearing to see if something would help more.

Quitting breastfeeding didn't help at all. It was only several months after that that I realized my pain was coming from the IUD my OB-GYN team had suggested I have inserted for birth-control. I hadn't used hormonal birth-control in nearly a decade, but the idea of getting pregnant again anytime soon was enough to "scare" me into starting real birth-control again.

Within 1 week of having the IUD removed, my pain disappeared.

The moral of the story? I don't even know, but I won't be going back on birth-control again ever.

It is frustrating that that caused me to give Lucy only 3 month's worth of breast-milk when I likely could've gone much longer, but there's nothing I can do about that now. She got a very good dose of healthy, healthy stuff from my milk. (And heck, I was breast-fed until I was practically talking, and I still got type 1 diabetes!)

I will say, breastfeeding was a real pain to balance my blood sugars around. I was never able to find any real consistency in how it impacted my blood sugars, but then again, I never made it to that "regulated" stage after 3 months of nursing.

When I did fully stop, and my milk-production really stopped within 7 or so days of that, my blood sugars were remarkably easier to manage and I actually lost more weight because breastfeeding made me so hungry that I was eating more and had actually gained 5 pounds postpartum!

Regardless, it didn't go as I planned (to breastfeed for the first year), and that's just how life goes.

I can tell you about the rest, though, that it has gone very much as planned: I love this silly little girl to the moon and back. To the moon. And back.

NOTES

STORIES FROM
TYPE 1 MOTHERS

There is nothing more powerful and encouraging and eye-opening than hearing about pregnancy, miscarriage, delivery, and postpartum from other women with type 1 diabetes who have been through this journey.

As you read this stories, please keep in mind that everyone's body is different. These stories are not meant to serve as medical advice but to give you a glimpse into the many challenges and successes that any of us could face during pregnancy with type 1 diabetes.

And of course, we'd like to express a very special thank you to these wonderful moms who were willing to write their stories down and share these vulnerable and life-changing moments with us.

MELISSA HOLLOWAY'S STORY

FACING THE LEARNING CURVE OF PREGNANCY & D-MANAGEMENT

Pre-pregnancy, my target range on my CGM was 80 to 160 mg/dL (4.4 to 8.9 mmol/L). During pregnancy, with Jenny Smith's coaching support, I changed my range to 90 to 130 mg/dL (4.9 to 7.8 mmol/L). Yes, that's a high number for a low alarm, but it gave me more time to consider whether to treat a slow downward trend with carbs, or to reduce my basal rate and see if I could ride it out. And yes, my high alarm went off a lot. I got used to it and it didn't stress me out.

One thing I didn't expect to find out from using CGM during my pregnancy was how much progesterone could slow down my digestion after meals in the second and third trimesters. I could have a practically flat glucose level for just over an hour before the post-meal rise would start. If I had been using finger-sticks alone and checking 1-hour post-meal (per guidelines), I would have thought I had nailed my mealtime bolus—when my meal had not yet begun to fight! Dang!

And by the third trimester, after my glucose level went up after a meal, sometimes it got stuck at about 160 mg/dL (8.9 mmol/L) for a couple of hours, while my pump told me I still had some insulin on board. When I got to the point where I would just give myself 2 or 3 more units, and it worked, despite the pump saying I didn't need any, I ran the situation past my diabetes educator. She sort of shrugged her shoulders and had no real advice.

However, Jenny told me she'd worked with a few people who experienced the same thing I was going through. She suggested I chop my duration of insulin action time down from 3.0 hours to 1.5 hours, because it appears that insulin can clear through the body faster in pregnancy. This suggestion made so much sense to me, and it gave me 'permission' to do what I was doing anyway and take more insulin 90 mins-2 hours post-meal, when my body was actually dealing with the upswing from the food. Combo bolus (a.k.a. dual-wave) bolus became my favourite pump feature.

I got a bit grumpy when I thought harder about the situation: had I not been pregnant, I am pretty sure that my diabetes educator (not Jenny, but someone local) would have said my duration of insulin action time was too short. But because I was pregnant, that common-sense point didn't come up. The lesson I learned from this is that a healthcare provider may see pregnancy as something that alters the 'ground rules' of type 1 diabetes to such an extent that they miss an obvious solution. Sometimes the simplest solution still applies, even in a complicated pregnancy.

DATA, DATA, DATA

Glucose monitoring, whether CGM or finger-sticks just gives me data to help me make good decisions. The number on the screen is never a judgment of how hard I'm trying or my worth as a person. I had to remind my diabetes care team of this a couple of times though. My diabetes educator (not Jenny, someone local) had very few patients using a CGM. She wanted to focus on the blood tests logged in my pump memory when we reviewed my data on Diasend.

I uploaded my pump and CGM data to Diasend on a weekly basis for both Jenny and the hospital team to be able to have a look. With all of us able to see the same data, I was better able to explain to my team things Jenny suggested and why I thought they sounded good.

Jenny and I also worked up a birth plan that my team had only minor feedback on. I was terrified of being pushed onto sliding-scale IV insulin during labour, so we wrote it into my birth plan that I needed to agree with the team that I could no longer deal with my own glucose management, or be unable to communicate, for them to be able to institute this. I trained my husband on what to do with my CGM receiver, when to prod me if I should do something, etc. When the big day came, the hospital team didn't even bother following their hourly finger-stick protocol because they could see how flat my CGM trace was throughout my (induced) labour and emergency C-section.

DEALING WITH DIABETES EDUCATOR CRITICISM

One day in my second trimester, as we stared at a screen with a number of values in red boxes (to indicate above-target levels), my local diabetes educator said flatly, 'Your high blood glucose levels are damaging your baby.' I was wounded. I knew she was wrong and what she really meant was, 'I don't understand how to interpret the CGM data you're trying to share with me, so I'm going to make a statement based on what I can understand.' I challenged her back: 'So, looking at these numbers, what A1C would you predict?' She said about 7%. I said, 'Let's see if the finger-stick analysis is back from the lab.' She refreshed her system and, would you believe it, my A1C was 5.5%! She backed-off after that.

I realized that day that having more data to share could make me more of a target for criticism. If I only checked my blood sugar 6 times a day and all those numbers were in-range and my HbA1C had come back at 7% that day, the same diabetes educator probably would have leapt into action to help me. But whatever. Several months after I had my baby, the same diabetes educator asked me to speak at a diabetes education day for all the general midwives in the hospital, as an expert patient. I graciously accepted and gave a talk that was rated as the best of the whole day by all the participants. Ha ha. (That's the sound of the last laugh).

I also learned in my second trimester that increasing insulin resistance can be less of a steady climb and more of a cha-cha (two steps forward, one step back).

Having heard that the first sign of a problem with the placenta could be a decrease in insulin requirements, I panicked the first few times I needed to use a decreased temporary basal rate. Surely if I needed a temp basal it ought to be more and more only? But I dug into the literature and found out that this isn't necessarily the case. There can be more and less insulin sensitive days in a given week when the overall trend is 'more insulin resistant,' it's just that until relatively recently we haven't had technology to help document this phenomenon. [That said, a sudden decline in your insulin needs of 20% or more is a reason to contact a doctor.]

MY PERSONAL STRATEGIES
FOR MANAGING DIABETES DURING PREGNANCY

Before becoming pregnant, I had a pretty high level of physical activity for someone who sits at a desk for work all day. While I kept an eye on calories, I didn't deny myself a treat if I really wanted one. I maintained a pretty solid US size 6-8P (UK10-12 Petite) this way.

When I found out I was expecting, I was determined not to eat for two. Many of my college classmates put on a lot of weight during pregnancy and few have ever lost it. I thought a goal of returning to my pre-pregnancy jeans within 6 months of having my baby seemed reasonable.

What I didn't know when I set that goal was that I would develop postpartum thyroiditis 5 months after my baby arrived, or that it would be so very difficult to get myself to the gym during maternity leave!

That said, setting a research-based calorie goal of +200 during my first trimester and +400 during the second and third seemed to work well for me not to gain excessive weight, nor to feel hungry. Sometimes a craving for a cookie would strike and I'd declare, 'Baby wants carbs!'. I kept little packages of not-too-unhealthy snacks and fruit on hand so I didn't always succumb to the cookie craving.

In trying to reach my calorie goal, I had to factor in alcohol calories as a 'debit' on the baseline. I had 2 glasses of wine most evenings before finding out I was pregnant, so I really had 250 extra calories + my pregnancy amount to consume! A handful of heart-healthy nuts, some cheese and crackers, or an apple with peanut butter tended to satisfy me and help me reach my target intake.

For blood glucose control, I tried hard to eat no more than 45 grams carbs in one meal. I found that 60 grams carbs or more made it a lot harder to get my bolus dose right, and increased the time I spent out of my target range after a meal. I aimed to have about 200 grams carbs per day (vs. 130 grams pre-pregnancy), so I rarely had a carb-free snack during my pregnancy.

When all was said and done, I had about 15 lbs. to lose post-baby, and I felt fine about that.

STAYING ACTIVE THROUGHOUT MY PREGNANCY

I continued going to the gym around 3 times a week until I hit 34 weeks of pregnancy. At that point, my hands and feet got all swollen and I was put on blood pressure medication. I also just didn't feel like it anymore!!

When I was still exercising regularly, I found that increasing levels of insulin resistance made it less likely I would have a hypo at the gym, which was useful, I guess.

I had to remind myself that the extra weight I was carrying was going to make things challenging. Using my own body weight for resistance was probably safer than using free weights for my upper body and to make lunges harder.

I loved the book, "Exercising Through Your Pregnancy," by James Clapp and Catherine. It even has pictures to illustrate how to modify a number of types of exercise in pregnancy. Further, I was really motivated by the book's coverage of research into the benefits of staying active while pregnant. Several times when I felt like skipping the gym, I told myself to get over it and go for my baby's sake.

PREPARING MY HUSBAND FOR PREGNANCY WITH DIABETES

My husband and I talked a lot more about my diabetes during my pregnancy than in the previous 5 years we'd lived together. We were both aware of the potential risks: my mother-in-law is a midwife who has seen a lot of women with uncontrolled type 1 diabetes who had poor outcomes. I assured both my husband and my mother-in-law that I was in the 'shallow end' of the 'high-risk pool' thanks to my tight control and generally sharp medical team.

I didn't ask my husband to accompany me to every hospital appointment, just the important scans and the 36-week appointment where we discussed my birth plan with the doctors. After the 36-week appointment, my husband thanked me for prioritizing and not asking him to spend more of his Wednesday afternoons in the overcrowded waiting room with me. I was so bored and annoyed when I had to wait ages for appointments, I could not in good conscience have asked him to join me.

As I got closer to the end of pregnancy, my husband and I agreed that he needed to get more comfortable with my diabetes vocabulary and my decision-making process in order to support me well during labor and delivery. For several days running, would show him my CGM trace when I was pleased with the result, when I was upset, when I was perplexed, and talk him through my thought process on how to deal with the situation. Then one Saturday, I just showed him the CGM and let him try to problem-solve. He had been listening! I felt like we would be okay on the big day.

On the Sunday morning I went into labour (after 2 rounds of induction hormones since the Friday night), my husband did things like pour the coffee he had just bought me down the sink (I couldn't stand the smell), hold my CGM receiver for me and let me know if I needed to take action, and ask the medical team questions I couldn't as I was signing the pre-op paperwork for my emergency C-section. By 6pm that night, as I struggled to stay awake with our newborn baby on my lap and IVs in both my arms, he alternately put food in my mouth and poked me with the fork to make sure I didn't nod off before swallowing. He's a keeper.

POSTPARTUM THYROIDITIS

When my son was 5 months old, I started losing weight without trying. I couldn't complain about that! But within a few weeks, my hair started falling out, I woke up hot and sweaty despite sleeping under only a cotton sheet, and I could barely keep my concentration long enough to put together a simple meal. I had just returned to work part-time so I put all these symptoms down to 'new-mom-back-at-work' stress. Only when I noticed my blood sugars soaring after meals did I start to suspect something else might be at work. I reflected on the speed of the weight loss, and the continuing hair loss and inability to focus. I started to get worried: was I vitamin or mineral-deficient? Could it be a serious illness? Would I have to stop breastfeeding my son because of something outside my control?

By the time I went to see my family doctor, I Googled enough things to develop a hunch that I had postpartum thyroiditis, which affects around 15% of women with pre-existing diabetes who recently had a baby. My doctor ordered lots of blood tests. A few days later, she rang me at 7 p.m. to say I was not just hyperthyroid, but thyro-toxic, and we needed to consult my diabetes specialist ASAP. Via email, my diabetes specialist recommended I start taking carbimazole to knock down my thryroid hormone production and propranolol (a beta blocker) to reduce the anxiety symptoms. She also squeezed in an appointment for me a few days after I started the drugs. She reassured me that as my son was nearly 6 months old, she felt he would not be at high risk of anything untoward if I continued to breastfeed.

At the appointment, my specialist told me I was really not well and advised me to avoid all unnecessary activities or events for the next few weeks. I pulled out of speaking at a conference, which I was disappointed to have to do, but it was true that I didn't feel up to it. She ordered more blood tests to check for immune system markers, which would help determine whether I had Graves' disease or postpartum thyroiditis. A couple of weeks later, the results were in and she confirmed the postpartum thyroiditis. We agreed that I would have blood drawn every few weeks for the next few months to catch the onset of the hypothyroid phase, where the thyroid switches from over-activity to under-activity. Oh joy! (Not!!!)

On the plus side, postpartum thyroiditis can resolve within a year of onset, while Graves' is a chronic disease that can require radiotherapy to destroy the thyroid gland and then thyroid hormone treatment for life. On the minus side, I learned that while around 80% of non-diabetic women who get post-partum thyroiditis are back to normal in a year or so, women with pre-existing type 1 diabetes have about an 80% chance of staying on thyroxine treatment for life. That's the camp I'm in now. Since the onset of my postpartum thyroiditis, my diabetes has definitely been harder to control than it was before I got pregnant. Now that my thyroxine dose seems to be correct, I think things may be settling down, thank goodness.

However, I do wonder if my immune system's attack my thyroid sort of 'broke' my diabetes. I tested positive for C-peptide 12 years after I got type 1, I never experienced dramatic high blood sugars, and I have very healthy retinas and kidneys despite 22 years with type 1. Do I still have that C-peptide? Is my risk of complications now higher? It won't be easy to find answers to these questions, so I am living with them as best I can. At least my thyroid can't go haywire again if I have another baby, right?! (But if I get another autoimmune condition after baby #2, that will be no laughing matter.)

MY SON'S BIRTH STORY

"Don't worry," said the diabetes nurse during one of my diabetes appointments in the last few weeks of my pregnancy, "If you can't keep your glucose level under 110 mg/dL (6.0 mmol/L) according to hourly finger-stick checks, we will put you on a sliding scale. We do that a lot." I really hoped this would not be necessary, having heard of a lot of cases in which sliding scale turned out to be more like a blunt instrument for diabetes control. In consultation with my diabetes care team, I compromised on having it in my care plan that a sliding scale would be initiated if we mutually agreed that I was not managing well with my pump at any point during labor.

I wondered if with the help of my pump, CGM and husband I might be able to avoid both a sliding scale and formula being given to my baby. In case my baby needed glucose in the first day after birth, my diabetes and pregnancy team advised me to start expressing colostrum at 37 weeks. It took a couple of tries to get the hang of it, but by day 3 I felt like a pro.

On the morning my son was born, I started having contractions at 4:30am, about 26 hours after the first dose of hormones for my induction and 2 hours after the second dose. I sipped both coconut water and water for hydration and scarfed down a few nutrition bars with small boluses for energy. By watching my glucose levels like a hawk and judiciously using temporary basal rates, I kept my glucose levels between 85 and 95 mg/dL (4.7-5.3 mmol/L) throughout labor—despite an emergency C-section because of the umbilical cord being wrapped around my baby's neck. And his glucose levels were normal in the 24 hours after birth, without supplemental feeding. I used the expressed colostrum to augment his feedings in the first three days.

Despite all the things I would have liked to control about my son's entry into the world at 11:47am on March 22nd 2015, at least my diabetes was under control.

BREASTFEEDING & D-MANAGEMENT

The first few weeks of life at home with my newborn, I kept both a bowl of seedless grapes and a jar of glucose tablets within easy reach. I found that a 20 to 30 minute feed had a similar effect on my blood glucose levels to a brisk 20 to 30 minute walk. And because my son James' motto could have been 'Just because I just ate doesn't mean I'm not hungry again,' I could not proactively reduce the basal rate on my pump ahead of an anticipated feed. It was grapes and/or glucose tabs to the rescue— several times a day!

By week 2 of breastfeeding, anything that touched my nipples made me squeal in pain. I was overjoyed to discover the compresses sold by Multimum.com, which made me feel like a new woman. (Or at least like a cow with less sensitive udders.)

4.5 months after James was born, I returned to work two days a week. I pumped every morning before breakfast, before lunch and again just before I went home at the end of the day, both to maintain my supply and to ensure there was enough milk on hand for the time we spent apart. I didn't see much of a drop in my glucose level during feeding or pumping: the composition of my milk was definitely changing as my son's needs shifted.

When James was 6 months old, I increased my working days to 4.5, with Thursday mornings as time off with him. We started baby-led weaning, letting him feed himself finger-foods, rather than spoon-feeding him purees. I stopped the late-afternoon pumping sessions when James was about 10 months old, because he wasn't drinking all the milk I sent to daycare. I continued to pump first thing in the morning and at lunchtime until he was 12 months old. At that point, I was comfortable with James having cow's milk at daycare. I was glad to make it to his first birthday without giving him formula, but it was nice to put the pump into storage. I did dig the pump out for an overnight business trip shortly after James turned 1, so that I could 'pump and dump' while we were apart. (I would have been very uncomfortable without it!)

Now, at 17 months old, James eats plenty of solid food at mealtimes and has at most 4 oz. of cow's milk as a snack during a day at daycare. He expects a milk feed when I get home from work, he dream-feeds a couple of times overnight, and he has a feed as we wake up for the day (we still co-sleep with a cot attached to the bed). It's rare to see a feed impact my glucose levels these days. At weekends, he sometimes goes for the booby because it's there, which is usually fine. But if I can't stop to feed him (say, we are mid-way through a journey), a rice cake will usually suffice. If I'm out for an evening after work, James will eat dinner and my husband can usually get him to sleep without milk. That said, I am prepared to continue breastfeeding when we're together for a while longer.

━━━━━

JENNIFER DEAN'S STORY

THE DOCTOR'S APPOINTMENT I WOULDN'T WISH UPON ANYONE

I've always wanted to be a mom and knew I'd want to have children. I was diagnosed with type 1 diabetes at the age of 20. Two years later, I was married and I promptly began working with an endocrinologist who would help me prepare for pregnancy. Pregnancy with type 1 is considered high-risk. There's a lot of hard work, dedication, and diligence that goes in to being pregnant with type 1.

For about 3 years I worked to lower my A1c to a level that was considered healthy for a growing baby. For me, I started out my first pregnancy at about 6.5%. My second pregnancy was 5.8% at conception. Throughout pregnancy I worked to keep the A1c as well as every single blood glucose test at a normal rate. I had an average blood sugar of 95 for almost an entire year with both pregnancies.

For my first pregnancy, I didn't wear a CGM, they weren't yet widely used and available on the market like they are today. I used an insulin pump to mange my diabetes and tested my blood sugar about every two hours (10 to 20 times per 24 hours). I'd often check my blood sugars in the middle of the night.

For the second pregnancy, I wore an insulin pump and a CGM. This made keeping an eye on my blood sugars so much easier because the CGM does a lot of the testing for you. I still found myself testing about 6 to 10 times per day. The CGM kept me up a lot at night but I found comfort in knowing my sugars were under control. Both of my pregnancies were very similar but I definitely learned a few things from the first one.

My first trimester brought a lot of low blood sugars. I had to always be ready to treat a low. I didn't have much morning sickness, but I definitely had nausea that was eased with eating a little. Sometimes I felt like I was constantly eating.

During my second trimester, I felt better than I'd ever felt in my entire life. My sugars were so "normal" that I'm sure it had something to do with it. I love the second trimester because the queasiness of the first trimester has passed but my body wasn't as large and uncomfortable as I was in the third trimester.

During the third trimester, baby grew a so rapidly that I was constantly making adjustments to my insulin doses. By the end of my pregnancies I was taking at least 100 units of insulin. I used an insulin-to-carbohydrate ratio of 1:2 by the end of the pregnancy. I found myself watching my carbohydrate intake just to avoid taking more massive amounts of insulin.

Throughout my pregnancies I worked with a team of doctors who helped me manage my "high-risk" pregnancy. I had kept my regular endocrinologist at a diabetes center 35 miles from my house. I saw a "regular" OB/GYN at the hospital 5 miles from my house that agreed to take me on as a high-risk patient. I also went to the larger hospital in the city (about 25 miles away) for non-stress tests and to see a maternal fetal medicine doctor. Appointments started out every three weeks and got closer together as the pregnancies progressed. Toward the end of both pregnancies, I was seeing each of the four doctors once a week. So you'll believe me when I tell you that begin pregnant with type one diabetes is basically a part-time job. I suppose you could say it's a full time job if you factor in the middle-of the night glucose tests.

In my first pregnancy I had an experience I'd not wish on anyone. I was 37 weeks pregnant, things had been going great, and I had my final appointment at the large hospital in the city with the maternal fetal medicine doctor. The doctor was different every time I went in. I just saw whoever was there that day. They'd take an ultrasound and assess the baby, take my vitals and give my OB/GYN and me council and instruction.

At this last appointment the doctor measured my baby. He told me some things that were grossly misinformed and downright upsetting. He told me that my baby was "macroscopic," or big, and that I could kill him with one high blood sugar. He doubted my ability to manage my diabetes and pregnancy. He advised me that I never should have gotten pregnant. He asked me to send him my logs of blood sugars, food, and insulin. He told me I'd no doubt have to have a C-section and that I'd need to come back and see him again in a week.

When I left his office and made my way to the waiting room I was absolutely a complete wreck. I was sobbing uncontrollably and could barely make the appointment to come back. I called my husband and drove to his office where he consoled me and then I made the drive back home. I faxed the doctor my logs, and he simply wrote back saying that I was doing a great job and everything looked fine.

I suppose it's difficult seeing a patient you've never met before at that stage of pregnancy. I just wish that he had gotten a little more information about me, my baby, and my pregnancy before treating me in such a cruel way.

I was so upset from this experience that when I found out I was pregnant the second time I told my doctor I would agree to go to the MFM department at the large hospital only if I could arrange to see the same doctor for every visit. As it turned out, the doctor could meet me at my regular hospital and do the appointments on the second floor. I was so grateful for this change and it was a much better experience.

My doctor decided to induce me in my 38th week with my first child. I was admitted in the evening and began the process of cervical softening. This started contractions, but not hard contractions typical with active labor. My son was in some distress with the contractions. By the morning the nurses came into my room and asked if they could please take my baby out. I didn't know that his heart rate was dropping with each contraction. My doctor had been watching my labor at his home and when he arrived at the hospital early that morning he ran down the situation with us.

He told us that our son was in distress and it was time to either decide on a cesarean or give Pitocin a try. I was not interested in having both regular labor as well as a cesarean. I had the chance to try for a regular labor but risked not being able to deliver vaginally due to an emergency C-section. Since my son was already in distress, I opted for the C-section.

Our son was born about an hour later. He was 8.5 pounds and completely healthy.

Both of my sons weighed about the same at birth: 8 pounds 8 ounces and 8 pounds 10 ounces. Neither one of them had any issues with blood sugars after birth and both of them had a little bit of jaundice at about 3 days old.

I am so grateful that I was able to deliver two healthy boys. I know that without my team of doctors I wouldn't have been able to have such successful births. Pregnancy with diabetes is hard work. It requires dedication. It takes a lot of time to make all of those doctor appointments. But, having children, and especially having happy, healthy, intelligent children is all worth it. It is so completely possible. I know it is easy to generalize and tell women with type 1 diabetes that pregnancy isn't safe. But it most certainly is possible to have a normal, healthy pregnancy.

━━━━

NIKI BEDSON'S STORY

TYPE 1 DIABETES 3 MONTHS
BEFORE LEARNING I WAS PREGNANT

"I was diagnosed in September of last year, and it had been a huge shock to me. Diabetes was the ultimate insult to the lifestyle I'd always chosen to live, and accepting that for no apparent reason I had suddenly been struck down by the Gods was a lot to handle. I'd done my best to get a handle on it, but I hated it. I begrudged every second of my time I had to give it, I still ate what my friends ate when we went out: clueless on how to manage an all you can eat Chinese, I drank a lot of alcohol on nights out and was too hung-over to care about my blood sugar the next day.

All of that changed when in December of that same year I discovered I was pregnant.

All of a sudden, alcohol and cigarettes were out the window because I wanted them to be. I got rid of every vice, until the last one left was looking diabetes square in the eye. I was working on a luxury yacht in the Caribbean at the time, and poolside reading became the glycemic index as opposed to 'Glamour.' I worked out exactly what certain foods did to me, how to carb-count, and how soon before eating I should take my insulin.

I gave up my beloved crumpets, as they seemed to cause a spike in my blood sugar no matter what I did. I read everything about diabetes I could get my hands on, including the awful stuff people have written online about being diabetic and pregnant. But I didn't let it get me down. Instead, I was filled with a new resilience. Yes, diabetes had knocked me down momentarily, and challenged everything about my previous life. It had brought out the worst in me, threatened my health, my career and the happiness of my friends and family, not to mention my own emotional stability. But it was not going to harm this baby as well. Not on my watch!

I'd had two A1Cs by the end of my pregnancy and they were 4.7% and 4.8% because I was still "honeymooning," producing some insulin since I was so early in my diagnosis. I remember a doctor at the hospital telling me that I was controlling it better then his own non-diabetic body. My diabetic nurse (who was just the most awesome person) kept saying to me there is room here to let up a bit if I needed to...but I didn't want to. Obviously when you're running such a tight ship there are more lows to be aware of, but my trusty jelly beans were with me everywhere and it only takes a minute to feel right as rain again if you have a bit of a miscalculation. By getting to know the condition and myself so intimately I was taking the fear out of diabetes, and that was half the battle right there.

I got my diabetes under control because I had to—it wasn't just me anymore—but more importantly because I wanted to. My mindset changed from being dragged kicking and screaming to check my blood sugar and eat appropriately to me sprinting towards those goals by myself. And in that process I learned that, yes, being diabetic is a pain in the arse, but it is manageable if I put in the grueling effort. And more importantly I have this beautiful, healthy, tiny bundle of awesomeness to look after, and diabetes is not going to get in the way of that.

CHRISTA SMITH'S STORY

PREGNANCY WITH DIABETES IS A LOT OF WORK!

Pregnancy with diabetes boils down to a lot of work! My experience with pregnancy was very positive, but I worked so hard before becoming pregnant, doing the things they recommend healthy women do as well as the round-the-clock pursuit of stable, decently normal blood sugars. My goal for my A1C was under 6.0, and I used an insulin pump, a CGM, and a low carbohydrate diet to help me achieve that goal before and throughout my pregnancy! It was one of the most intense times in my life.

Once I was pregnant the work continued, knowing I was affecting my child at every moment. I had always wanted to be a stay-at-home-mom, but my husband and I decided I would go ahead and quit my job before becoming pregnant instead of just before delivery so that I would be able to give my full attention to taking care of myself and managing those blood sugars!

Thank goodness for the Internet. It was online from other Type 1 mamas that I read about the hypoglycemia common in the first trimester—not from my endocrinologist. In forums and blog posts I found tips about inserting my CGM sensor a full night before turning it on, and taking a ten minute walk before every meal to pre-empt that post prandial blood sugar spike.

In peer-reviewed medical journal articles published online, I found information about diabetes-related pregnancy outcomes that motivated and encouraged me to maintain tighter control than my maternal-fetal-medicine specialists thought necessary.

I really wasn't able to ever find anything online (or from any of my doctors) that spoke authoritatively about the issue of having nutritional ketones in my urine while having super controlled blood sugar. It seemed that everyone knew ketones plus high blood sugar was dangerous for type 1s, but didn't know what to say about ketones resulting from a low-carb diet with perfect blood sugar.

All in all, I felt a little alone, and like the information available to me as a pregnancy type 1 was scattered and disorganized. It was especially tough realizing my OB, endocrinologist, and CDE didn't have the nuanced information I was seeking to help me really understand what changes were coming and how to anticipate them.

I was fearful of gaining a tremendous amount of weight, of course for myself, but more for the safety of my growing son. I had read how diabetics can have big babies, which presents certain risks. For me, minimizing this risk boiled down to two things: lots and lots of low-to-moderate impact exercise, and eating on the lower end of carbohydrate spectrum. Of course, I didn't have a no-carb diet, but I mostly refrained from bread, pastas, potatoes, cereal, desserts, and any foods that packed a carbohydrate and sugar punch! I focused on nutrient dense fruits and veggies, meat, fish, nuts, eggs, protein shakes and smoothies, and different forms of dairy. I walked about 4 miles every day during the pregnancy. Toward the end that took about 2 hours!

I tried to stay on the go, on my feet, doing anything that would help my insulin sensitivity. My insulin needs in the final trimester were sky-high regardless. Pre-pregnancy, I would take 0.5 units of insulin to cover 3 eggs and 1 piece of toast for breakfast. In my last trimester I needed between 8 to 10 units for the same meal. I ended up gaining a normal amount of weight, and my son weighed 8 lb. 11oz at 38 weeks and 2 days. Despite these fairly normal numbers, I was borderline "polyhydramnios" during that final semester, having almost 95 percentile of amniotic fluid, too high, which brings its own set of risks. My doctor said it was from excess blood sugar. My son had measured only slightly ahead, but I was measuring 43 weeks when I was 37 weeks pregnant, and feeling incredibly uncomfortable due to all that extra fluid.

Some of my other fears concerned labor and delivery, and subsequent care of my son. My maternal fetal medicine specialist educated me about how babies of diabetics typically have low blood sugar after birth, and how my child would need to spend at least 4 hours in the NICU while his blood sugar was monitored.

He stayed in the NICU for 3 days being monitored, with an IV line and a feeding tube. I only got to hold him and begin breastfeeding about 30 hours after he was born—which isn't the norm at most hospitals.

Meanwhile, my blood sugar kept dropping as my insulin needs continued to decrease after delivery. I don't think the postpartum nurses knew what to do with me! Our arrangement ended up being that I was going to test, take insulin, and eat whatever and whenever I thought it was necessary, and they were going to trust me and accommodate my choices. My OB and endocrinologist would check-in of course, but my perception was that neither of them was specifically educated about immediate postpartum care of type 1 diabetic women.

I am very thankful for the care I received, thankful for my son's health, and thankful that we both left the hospital at the same time in great shape. However, those three days were definitely not the experience I was expecting, both for him and for myself. If I had to do it again, I would specifically ask about guidelines of infant blood sugar monitoring, what determines the length of a NICU stay, and if my doctor has an altered insulin dosing strategy for postpartum women.

Two years later, looking back at pregnancy, I feel incredibly thankful to live in this day and age! I feel like the inventions of rapid-acting insulin, continuous blood sugar monitoring, and the internet allowing information to spread has enabled me to achieve a goal that was not possible not so long ago. It has been a joy to watch my son grow over the past two years knowing I worked my hardest to bring him into the world kicking and screaming and healthy.

———

SYSY MORALES' STORY

HONESTLY, I FELT LIKE I WAS IN HELL

In 2008, I got married…and two months later found out I was pregnant. Two months after that, I found out we were having twins. I checked my blood sugar all the time, stayed on multiple daily injections, and didn't leave the house much.

I didn't gain much weight except in the belly. I got so big there that I outgrew maternity clothes—I literally did not fit in maternity clothes!

I craved salads and especially artichokes like they were ice cream and chocolate! I didn't consume any caffeine, not even in chocolate.

I will be honest, I felt like I was in hell the entire time.

When I 4 months pregnant, I fell down an icy set of stairs at work and popped my tailbone out of place. I had to carry a hemorrhoid donut ring to sit on everywhere I went. I had physical therapy for some pelvic floor muscles that were so tight during pregnancy they were causing me pain and not allowing me to hold my bladder well.

I finally left work at 6 months because my head was no longer in the game.

I remember making some mathematical calculations at work that normally took me about an hour and realized they had just taken me 4 hours. My boss at the time was also pregnant, and this was the first time in my life that I wanted to rip someone's head off (normally I'm eternally nice and get along with everyone so this was upsetting).

I developed some bleeding in my left retina at 7 months that really freaked me out. I developed preeclampsia a month before my due date and after many hours on labor inducing medications, with no pain medicine, I finally had such high blood pressure I had to have a C-section.

The kids came out perfectly and I remember bugging the doctor to tell me what their blood sugars were—fortunately, they were perfect and healthy. I'm told that as soon I heard this information, I finally passed out on my heavy pain meds for a half-hour.

All those months of working to give my kids great blood sugars truly paid-off. I'd done my job, and now I needed to rest!

I couldn't actually see my children very well for two days due to a medication I had to take to avoid seizures from my high blood pressure—the medication gave me double-vision!

I also couldn't hold up my arms or even hold my babies. A nurse got angry with me because I wasn't breastfeeding. The truth is that I couldn't move or see! Plus, almost immediately I developed multiple breast and nipple infections making it hard to get my sleepy preemies to latch-on and making me feel like I had the flu. I was in too much pain with my C-section healing to go to the doctor about anything.

I ended up pumping breast milk for 45 minutes every 3 hours around the clock for 4 months because I couldn't nurse them directly.

A few days after the babies were born I developed severe joint pain and sores on my skin that a dermatologist later described as autoimmune related and probably triggered by the intense stress of the pregnancy and birth. They never went away. Well, the joint pain went away mostly after about a year.

For a year, I had to wake up and first run my hands under hot water to get my fingers to move so I could pick up the babies—which I did almost all day because I had a strong feeling that I needed to hold them all day.

I couldn't wear them with one of those slings or anything to assist because my breasts swelled to size 34J from 34D and my back was killing me already.

My A1c during my pregnancy and during the first year after the kids were born was 5.3%. I was strongly compelled to start a blog a few days after the kids were born and did so by writing while pumping breast milk.

I wanted to tell other women with diabetes what was possible. Before doing it, I didn't think I could have healthy twins with my type 1 diabetes. I had additional challenges that first year after the kids were born like my husband being laid-off work, and depression, and the fact that I only slept 3 to 4 hours a night. But if you fast-forward forward seven years: The twins are healthy and happy. I'm healthy and happy.

I don't know how I survived.

I did decide before getting married that I was open to pregnancy and my A1c was good and I had a great partner, so if it happened I would be willing to tough it out. I think this is important, because realistically it can be difficult, especially without the right support. My mom and my husband were instrumental in helping me survive the pregnancy and first year with the babies.

My life hasn't been the same since—but that is a good thing. I look at my kids and know that they were worth it. But they definitely aren't going to have any other siblings. Fortunately, they have each other.

READ MORE FROM SYSY AT **WWW.THEGIRLSGUIDETODIABETES.COM**

MARIA MUCCIOLI'S STORY

IT'S HARD TO LIVE AS IF YOU ARE PREGNANT BEFORE YOU ACTUALLY ARE!

I think it's hard to live as if you are pregnant before you actually get pregnant—it was for me anyway! Prior to the start of this pregnancy, my A1C was 7.3%, which I knew I wanted to improve, but somehow had lots of excuses for why it was where it was and why it was fine to stop preventing pregnancy anyway.

If anything I read about being pregnant with diabetes was true, it was that once I learned I was actually pregnant, a switch flipped in my brain that increased my diligence towards blood glucose management drastically.

By the 11th week of my pregnancy, my A1C was down to an all-time low of 5.7%, and more recently, at 21 weeks, it was 5.4%. Amazingly, I was able to achieve this without an insulin pump, relying solely on my Levemir and Humalog (using a pen that delivers half-units for more precise dosing). I do give a lot of credit to my Dexcom CGM, which allowed me to become much more comfortable with routinely running numbers in the double digits, overnight in particular, as well as correct any highs very quickly.

I always thought before that achieving an A1C in the 5s would either be impossible for me, because I lacked the self-discipline, or if I ever did that it would be at the expense of extremely low frequent blood sugar readings. Much to my surprise, I found out that I was in fact able to do it without many lows (in fact, my lowest low this whole pregnancy was a 53 mg/dL), and although it did take (and continues to take) a lot of self-discipline and frequent adjustments, it somehow seemed easy to keep doing the work when seeing the reward of flat-line results and normal-range averages on my CGM and meter data downloads.

Here are a few tips from my own experience:

1. BE CONSISTENT

This applies to food (types of meals, carb counts and timing) as much as it applies to how much sleep and exercise you are getting. For example, I been eating the same variation of breakfast for months now: a small amount of toast, 2–3 eggs with cheese, and 1 cup of coffee; occasionally, I would switch that up and have a lower carb variation, where I would have some tomatoes or something like that with my eggs instead of toast if I was dealing with insulin resistance, or was starting my day at a higher number, or just wanted to mix it up.

For my lunches, about 50% of the time I eat a loaded veggie salad + protein source. The other 50% of the time I eat some sort of vegetables, protein, and small amount of starch. My snacks are usually homemade smoothies (plain yogurt/ milk/ frozen berries, or just plain yogurt and berries with nuts added sometimes), or one of the lower-carb Kind+ granola bars and/or a small piece of fruit.

Dinner is typically variable, but also not very high in carbs. Personally, I achieved great results eating anywhere from 60 to 120 grams of carbs daily during my pregnancy thus far, and sourcing my carbs to mostly come from vegetables and fibrous fruits, along with diligent pre-bolusing really helped keep any spikes to a minimum.

I could write a whole chapter of the benefits of pre-bolusing, but suffice it to say that doing so (for breakfast in particular) greatly improved my A1C and the CGM made me much more comfortable with doing that. The exercise consistency also plays a big part in my management. Many days at work, I would walk for 20 to 30 minutes after my morning snack, and it made the difference between a spike to 150 mg/dL and a spike to 120 mg/dL! Keeping sleep and stress levels as consistent as possible is also helpful, but can be easier said than done!

2. **DO NOT EAT UNTIL BLOOD SUGAR IS IN NORMAL RANGE**
This is a tough one at times, but made a huge difference for me. The amount of insulin it takes to get back to normal can vary depending on the level I correct from. Adding more variables like additional carbs and insulin into the mix when already high has not proven to be a good strategy for me. So if I can, I will wait to eat until my blood sugar is at or under 120 mg/dL, which I know will greatly minimize the amount of time that I spend above the normal range.

3. **KEEP IT STEADY OVERNIGHT**
The way I look at it is that if you have normal blood sugar overnight, you have won half of the battle. If the long-acting insulin dose (or rate of pumped insulin) is set well, one should be able to stop eating after 7 or 8 p.m. and flat-line for the following 10 to 12 hours before breakfast. If I found that I was correcting highs at night for several nights, it would mean I needed to increase my evening Levemir dose.

4. **DON'T BE AFRAID TO TAKE CHARGE AND MAKE ADJUSTMENTS**
Some patients see CDEs or communicate frequently with their medical team to make dosing changes. I personally follow my own trends very carefully and make changes if I see a pattern lasting for 2 to 3 days or

so. The way I look at it, at the end of the day I am the one living with diabetes, and I am the one who knows how to handle it best. By all means, you should do what works best for you!

A FEW MORE TIPS

- **DON'T BE AFRAID TO PAVE YOUR OWN PATH**
  I have to say that reading about the gazillions of doctor's appointments and low blood sugars that a type 1 pregnancy seemingly must entail made pregnancy sound very daunting to me. But that wasn't my experience! I opted out of any procedures I could opt out of without getting fired by my physician. I put in great efforts to maintain tight control of my blood sugar independently, explaining to my doctors that I was on top of it, and if I needed help I would ask for it! They seemed hesitant at first, but were quickly on board when they saw how well I was doing. This approach of managing my own diabetes allowed me to have a more normal pregnancy so far, and not one that revolves solely around doctor's appointments and feeling "high-risk" all the time. The doctors are there to help when you need, and it's very important to have a good medical team behind you, but as the patient, you can dictate what you want your experience to be. I plan to continue dictating my experience for the remainder of my pregnancy.

- **DON'T BEAT YOURSELF UP**
  It was hard not to feel guilty when I was above range for hours, or when I had a string of days (or a week!) of less than desirable blood sugars. But I did the best
  I could to make adjustments and move on. It's really all you can do!

- **ENJOY IT!**

Being pregnant is kind of a cool thing, and I feel lucky to be experiencing it. I wish I could worry less about what-ifs, because there are things we have no control over, and the things I do have control over, I am working hard at already. And that's all I can do!

HEATHER TUNISON'S STORY

GETTING PREGNANT WASN'T SO EASY

I always knew that I wanted to be a mother, even in my childhood I was called the baby whisperer and would gravitate toward children so there was no doubt in my mind that I wanted to have kids, but growing up with the shadow of diabetes over my head was something that always made me nervous with having children. In my teen years, I had complete burnout on diabetes and just stopped testing and stopped giving myself shots. I also was diagnosed with PCOS in my teen years and told that I had the possibility of struggles with conceiving. I worried that the combination of the previous high A1Cs from my past and the PCOS would make it to hard to actually have a baby. I was sure that somehow I had done too much damage to my body.

Before my husband and I even got married we talked about kids and both agreed that we wanted them. We had a plan to start trying a few years after getting married (I called it my 5 year plan). I am personally a crazy meticulous person. I met with the best group of high risk OB's in the area for a Pre-Conception Consultation months before hubby and I were ready to start trying.

The consultation was a great experience for a person like me who wants to plan everything as much as possible and feel in control. The OB sat down with me and we went through all of my numbers and my target ranges, we even talked about whether or not you can breastfeed while being a diabetic and what I should expect.

I met with my Endocrinologist and Ophthalmologist to make sure that we had baseline results prior to pregnancy and so that I knew what was expected of me with each doctor before I was even pregnant. I was aiming for an A1C in the low 6s and achieved an A1C of 5.7% before we actually got pregnant. I tightened up my CGM ranges and tested like crazy, always correcting even if my numbers were a little bit over the preferred range.

GETTING PREGNANT WASN'T SO EASY

I thought that getting pregnant was going to be easy. You go through all of these efforts trying to not get pregnant that you expect that once you prep your body and talk to all of the right doctors and do everything correctly that it should just happen, right? I had numerous friends that would just try, and within a few months they would get pregnant. I was hopeful that would be the case for me as well, but I was not that fortunate.

After meeting with my doctors and preparing my body as best I could for pregnancy, hubby and I started the fun of trying to have a baby. I tried not to over think things each month as my period time would approach, but I always got my hopes up. (Doesn't everyone?) As each month passed and I kept on taking pregnancy tests and getting negative results, I felt more and more crushed. I would pick myself up each time and put on a brave face, but inside I was just feeling like that was one more thing that my body couldn't do right. It couldn't produce insulin like it was supposed to, couldn't process wheat or gluten (Celiacs disease), and now it was failing at conceiving a baby. I went through periods of time feeling like a failure as a woman. I felt like my body wasn't doing the one thing that it was specifically made for: having a baby.

While dealing with the emotions of not getting pregnant I was trying to not over-react. I wanted to keep my A1C perfect for when my pregnancy would happen. I managed to stay in the high 5s throughout the entire process, but it was tough. After 6 months of trying, sometimes going through months of 6 weeks or more with no period because of PCOS, hormone level checks, negative pregnancy tests, and then the raging cycles that followed, my doctor decided that we should try fertility drugs. She said that they normally wait until someone has been trying for a year or more, but given the fact that I was a type 1 diabetic with perfect range A1C, not having normal cycles, and my hormones were not in the normal range, she decided to start with the fertility drugs sooner while my blood sugars were in the most optimal range.

I started Clomid first, and the side effects were not fun. From dizziness to headaches to random nausea, my body did not handle it well, but I was hopeful that it was all worth it and I would get my sweet baby. We did 4 rounds of Clomid unsuccessfully and then I started reaching out to the online community, asking people around me and reading everything that I could.

I read about Femara, and asked my doctor about it right away. It's a drug that is not FDA approved for fertility, but many doctors prescribe it. My first round of Femara, I had a positive pregnancy test and we were over the moon! I rushed off to get blood work to confirm the positive pregnancy test, and we told our parents. Unfortunately within a couple of weeks I had a miscarriage, my progesterone levels were not increasing enough to support a healthy pregnancy and that lead to the miscarriage. It was gut wrenching and happened right before Mother's Day. That was the hardest Mother's Day that I ever had. We released balloons to heaven to our lost baby and do that on the anniversary of the date every single year.

We did a 2nd round of Clomid once my body recovered from the miscarriage, and that's when I got pregnant with our beautiful baby girl. My doctors put me on progesterone right away to help my body sustain the pregnancy. One of the hardest things during the pregnancy was when they told me that it was okay to stop taking progesterone. I was so worried that my body was going to fail me once again and that the pregnancy wouldn't be sustained. Those 8.5 months of pregnancy were full of fears, concerns, doctor appointments, finger sticks, pump site changes, funny cravings, and so many firsts and even after all of that I would do it again in a heartbeat!

——————

JENNIFER BARRETT'S STORY

PRE-ECLAMPSIA & TYPE 1 DIABETES

My entire first pregnancy I felt, off. No, I felt like crap. I had morning sickness the entire pregnancy, which made day-to-day life a challenge. It also made recognizing any additional symptoms more difficult. When I reached the 7-month mark, I was in my best friends wedding party. When I look back at the pictures now I can see a significant weight-gain between being 6 months pregnant and 7 months. And the weight is everywhere but most obvious in my face.

I'd never been pregnant before so I didn't know what to expect, but as I got closer to 8 months, I started getting even more tired and weak. I remember going to Walmart with my mom one day to pick up some things for the baby, and suddenly, I could barely walk. I was out of breath, tired, dizzy, and I was having moments of vision loss. Everything would just go black and it would take a minute for it to slowly come back into focus.

Again, I just assumed this is what pregnancy was like for me.

I didn't have a headache and no one had mentioned my weight-gain at any of my pregnancy appointments, so I assumed I was gaining appropriately. While my blood pressure wasn't low (125/85), no one was saying anything about it either, and it had been staying consistent throughout my pregnancy. The night before one of my high-risk OB-GYN appointments, I remember telling my husband Tyler that I just didn't feel well. I wasn't sleeping at night very well, I had restless legs, and of course had to pee every hour. He suggested I go to bed early.

So I made a bowl of popcorn, and climbed the one flight of stairs up to our room to watch a movie and drift to sleep. I mention the stairs, because I specifically remember climbing them that night and thinking how anxious I was to have this pregnancy over with.

It took all of my energy and strength to climb those stairs and I was out of breath, exhausted, and I remember recognizing how swollen my feet and ankles were that night.

The next morning, even though I was only just over 35 weeks, I packed my hospital bag. I don't know what made me do it that morning, but I just thought I should.

My husband came home from work and drove me to my appointment. At the appointment, they took my blood pressure, it was 144/XX—I can't remember the second number. They asked me a bunch of questions about how I was feeling; did I have a headache that wouldn't go away: no. How was my vision: fine other than the times it would completely black out and come back a minute later. How was I feeling overall: like crap, and I had a pain in my upper right side (which I later found out was due to my liver starting to fail from a condition called HELLP).

I was told that if I was still working (which I wasn't as I own my own business and work for myself) that I should stop doing that and just rest. It was also decided, against my protest (I just mentally wasn't ready to have a baby), that I should spend the night for 24-hour observation.

I was checked into the hospital, grateful to have my own room, belly hooked up to a continuous non-stress test for the baby and compressors wrapped around my calves.

For the next 24 hours I just lay there, on partial bed rest, while they monitored my blood pressure and vitals every hour and kept an eye on the baby who was fine the entire time.

The next evening I was told that they wanted to keep me another night to watch what was happening. I, like the argumentative patient I was, didn't like this idea. I told them I literally could see my house from my hospital room (which was true) and I just wanted to go home for a bit. My doctor told me she would give me a pass to leave for a few hours as long as I came back sooner if I felt any worse. She left to start discharging me, and she never came back.

The next doctor that came in told me she hadn't passed this information along, but that I wasn't a prisoner and if I wanted to leave I could. Otherwise, if everything stayed the same, he'd let me go home in the morning for a few hours. It was Thursday night at this point, and they'd also decided that since my baby would be 36 weeks on Sunday, they would induce me then.

There was no point, for the sake of my health, for me to continue past that point. So, I stayed, and my husband spent the night with me at the hospital. The next morning, I knew they would let me go home for a few hours if I said I felt the same. Except I didn't feel the same, I felt much, much worse.

I had a pounding headache and my vision was much blurrier than normal. My blood pressure and my blood were tested, and they decided that while I had pre-eclampsia, I was also starting to show signs of HELLP. It was Friday and only two days before Sunday, so rather than wait, they wanted to induce me today.

I wasn't happy. I was scared, not ready.

But I felt horrible and just wanted to be done with it. It was deemed safe for me to attempt a vaginal birth, and so I was induced with a balloon catheter and hours after that, my water broke. I never went past 4 cm dilated, and so after 25 hours of labor, it was decided that an emergency C-section was necessary.

An hour after that, our daughter was born a day short of what we thought was 36 weeks, at 7lb 7oz. As she couldn't suck or swallow, she was sent to the NICU to be tube fed. She spent a total of 18 days there learning to suck and swallow before she was healthy enough for us to take her home.

Her name is Georgia-Mae and she is our blonde haired, blue-eyed beauty. She's two and a half now and completely healthy.

Unfortunately, during her stay at the NICU, it was decided between the NICU nurses, doctors and myself, that she was likely much younger than originally thought. As we all know, diabetes tends to make bigger babies and due, her due date had been adjusted to what they thought was correct. It turns out my guess of my due date, three weeks later based on my last period, was likely more accurate, and she was likely closer to 33 weeks when she was born rather than 36 weeks.

After Georgia-Mae was born, it took quite a while for me to heal and be released. In large part, this was due to the HELLP, but it also took quite a few days to bring my blood pressure back to normal.

My second pregnancy gave me no issues with pre-eclampsia/HELLP or my blood pressure thankfully. My biggest take from this: there's no such thing as paranoia in pregnancy. If you don't feel well, if you don't feel right, say something, get checked out, and fight for yourself and your baby. You might drive the hospital staff crazy, but better safe than sorry. You know your body better than they do and if it's your first pregnancy, and you don't know what it's supposed to "feel like," that's okay. You still know when you feel right or not, and it's still better to get checked out!

———

KELLEY KENT'S STORY

PREPARING FOR PREGNANCY & ALL THE REST

I started preparing for pregnancy about a year before my husband and I decided to start trying to get pregnant. My endocrinologist wanted my A1C below 7, but ideally below 6.5.

I had never had an A1C below 7 before, spending the majority of my adult life with an A1C in the 8's, so the task seemed daunting to me. The month that I decided to stop using my birth control, I had gotten my A1C to 7.1 and my doctor told me it wouldn't be the end of the world if I got pregnant but she wanted it lower. When I finally did get pregnant four months later, I had gotten my A1C down to 6.4!

I was able to lower my A1C by utilizing my CGM. When I downloaded my CGM data, I was able to see blood sugar trends and areas needing work. I found the biggest benefit of wearing a CGM to be the data, which showed how my blood sugars behaved overnight. In my 20+ years with type 1 diabetes, I was always afraid of lows, especially at night. Wearing a CGM overnight reduced my fear of lows because if I started to get low, my CGM would alert me and I would wake up and treat it. I believe that at least 75% of my lower A1C can be attributed to having lower blood sugars overnight, thanks to the CGM.

In the year leading up to our decision, I had also started running regularly for the first time in my life. My husband and I started off with the "Couch to 5K" program and then worked our way up to 5K's, 10K's and eventually two half marathons. I was in the best shape I've ever been in by the time we started trying. I completed a half marathon a month before getting pregnant so I think the exercise also helped me to lower and maintain my A1C.

When I first got my CGM (before pregnancy) my high alert was set-up at 240 mg/dL and my low alert was at 100 mg/dL. I had to drastically change my alerts for pregnancy. Gradually, I reduced my alerts to 140 mg/dL for high alerts, and 70 mg/dL for low alerts. I also set my target blood sugar to 90 mg/dL instead of 100 mg/dL to attack the highs a little more aggressively.

However, I wouldn't get a lot of sleep because of my CGM. Because my high and low settings were so tight, I would fall out of the target zone more often than if my alerts were higher. This was true especially overnight. At night, my blood sugar would hover around 90 mg/dL, but I would often dip down to the 60's, 70's or 80's, so my alert would go off.

It did take some getting used to when I adjusted my alert settings but over time it provided the best motivation to keep good blood sugars because I wouldn't want to hear the alerts going off!

I did still test my blood sugar frequently (12+ times per day) but the CGM provided comfort in between those checks.

THE STRESS & PRESSURE OF DIABETES DURING PREGNANCY

For me, diabetes added a lot of stress to my pregnancy. I was already stressed enough about making sure I was eating correctly, or that my heart rate didn't go too high when I was working out, or that I was drinking enough water, but then having diabetes to deal with on top of that added an entirely new level of stress and pressure.

Before I found out I was pregnant, I was going through a short-term diabetes burnout (for a couple weeks) because I didn't think I was going to be able to get pregnant so quickly, so I let my blood sugars get a little higher. Of course, a few weeks later, I found I was actually pregnant at the time! Once I got the big fat positive, I worried about how the higher blood sugars in those first few weeks were going to affect my son. After I found out I was pregnant, I would really stress anytime I saw a high blood sugar. If my post-meal blood sugar spiked too high I would feel guilty about not pre-bolusing sooner, or I would feel guilty about my food choices and maybe I didn't eat the right thing, causing the high.

I was also really stressed thinking about the labor and delivery of my son. I was so worried that I was going to have high blood sugars when I delivered him, and as a result, he would have low blood sugars when he was born. (He did have low blood sugars but they weren't too bad and he was able to stay in the room with me, not NICU).

Phew, I'm stressed just remembering how stressful the pregnancy was in dealing with d-management.

FEARS & CONCERNS WE'RE ALL GOING TO HAVE

BEING PREGNANT COMES WITH A LOT OF FEARS:

- Am I getting enough nutrients for the baby?
- Am I taking the right precautions to avoid listeria?
- Did the alcohol I had before I knew I was pregnant affect the baby?
- Am I drinking enough water?
- Have I remembered to take my pre-natal vitamins everyday?
- Is my heart rate below 140 bpm when I exercise?

- Will that high blood sugar affect my baby's health?
- Was my blood sugar too high for too long?
- How are all these low blood sugars affecting the baby?
- Is my A1C good enough?
- Will my baby be too big or too small?
- Will my baby make it to the full 40 weeks?
- Will I have to have a C-section and if so will I heal properly?
- Will my higher blood sugars before I found out I was pregnant affect my baby?
- Do I have a good medical team to support me and do they communicate well?
- Did I pre-bolus enough?
- Are my insulin-to-carb ratios, basal rates and correction factors accurate?

HOWEVER, THERE ARE TWO THINGS THAT SCARE/ WORRY ME THE MOST ABOUT BEING PREGNANT WITH TYPE 1 DIABETES:

1. What will I do when I can no longer use my stomach for my CGM and infusion set? I've only ever used my tummy in 17 years with a pump and 2 years with a CGM, I don't know anything else. I've slowly ventured more into the love handle region but I'm not quire there yet. My endo told me I could keep using my belly as long as the skin wasn't too tight but I'm getting there quickly! I'm absolutely dreading this day. (I did get to that point around the beginning of my third trimester and I moved my infusion set to my love handles and my CGM to my butt.)

2. Will I be able to keep my insulin pump and CGM on during delivery and who will monitor my blood sugar? I don't know if I will have a C-section or natural birth but I want to be able to keep my CGM and my pump on during delivery. The thought of having an insulin drip while delivering does not sound good to me. I've worked (and will continue to work) to have good basal rates that I want to have confidence going into delivery that my rates are the best possible for me. It's still too early to have this conversation with my doctors but I hope that I am able to keep them on.

I'm also worried about having a doctor being in control of my diabetes. I'm hoping I'll be able to but if not, I'm going to have to start training my hubby to take over for me. Fortunately, I was able to keep my CGM and infusion set on for delivery via C-section, so that worked out well! Phew!

FIRST TRIMESTER & D–MANAGEMENT

The first trimester was probably the hardest for me in terms of diabetes-management. I had to come to terms with the fact that my blood sugars needed to be a lot lower. My "d-team" (endo, CDE, high-risk OB) really emphasized that pre-meal blood sugars needed to be between 60 mg/dL and 90 mg/dL and post meal should be between 110 to 140 mg/dL. Before I became pregnant, I would treat a low blood sugar at 70 or 75 mg/dL, so trying to be comfortable with a blood sugar as low as 65 mg/dL sometimes was tough.

I found out I was pregnant pretty early on but I didn't start working with my CDE until I was 8 weeks pregnant so I had a lot of work to do to get in good shape before the first trimester ended. After getting pregnant, my A1C crept up to 6.8 from 6.4 so I needed to get serious about being comfortable with lower blood sugar ranges.

I didn't have low blood sugars too bad in the first trimester, if anything, my blood sugars were running a little higher so I had to make adjustments. I don't think I noticed insulin sensitivity until about week 8 or 9. Once I started working with a CDE, I did basal testing to really refine my basal and bolus rates. This proved to be a good foundation for the pregnancy so I could trust changes and tweaks I was making.

One thing that helped my d-management during the first trimester was that I didn't have any morning sickness, so I didn't need to worry about bolusing for a meal that wouldn't stay with me. I did, however, have really bad food aversions! I couldn't look at a green food (i.e. spinach, my usual go to food for lunch) without feeling nauseous. I also couldn't eat any meat. Not being able to eat meat or veggies made it harder to make good food choices. (I had no aversions to any carbs!) I had to get creative with meals those few weeks in the first trimester when my food aversions were at their worst.

I struggled to drink enough water so a strategy I implemented was putting 6 water bottles (16.9 fl oz. each) in the door of my fridge and I would make sure I drank all 6 bottles before I was done for the day. I am a self-proclaimed Diet Coke addict so I still drank caffeine while pregnant, but I limited myself to one 16.9 fl. oz. bottle per day.

SECOND TRIMESTER & D-MANAGEMENT

By the second trimester, I was feeling more comfortable with lows but I was having a lot more of them. In the beginning, I was making a lot of basal and bolus adjustments because I was becoming very insulin sensitive. As the second trimester progressed, I was making fewer changes as my blood sugars were becoming a little more stable. This was probably the best trimester for my diabetes (and in general in my 17 years with type 1).

Then around week 24, I started to become insulin resistant. The insulin resistance hit pretty hard between weeks 24 and 28 and I was making a lot of adjustments then, trying to prevent the high blood sugars.

THIRD TRIMESTER & D-MANAGEMENT

The third trimester started with increasing insulin resistance. Before pregnancy, I needed about 30 units of insulin a day but by the third trimester I was up to about 50 units. I do feel lucky though because insulin resistance didn't hit as bad as I was expecting. I had heard some people had a 1:2 or 1:1 breakfast insulin-to-carb ratio, and I was dreading that. I think the highest I:C ratio I had was 1:5.5 for my breakfast. Weeks 30 to 32 were tough and I was making weekly, sometimes daily (after noticing a 2-day trend), adjustments to my basal and bolus rates.

However, by week 34, I actually needed less insulin. I started having a lot of lows, especially overnight. My insulin sensitivity continued to increase until I delivered at week 38. I was worried that I was having placenta failure because of my decreased insulin needs but my doctors never seemed concerned.

SECOND TRIMESTER & D-MANAGEMENT

I had the worst spikes after breakfast. I ended up bolusing 45 minutes prior to eating. When I would wake up in the morning, first thing I did was test my blood sugar then bolus for breakfast. Then, I would get ready for the day, and by the time I was dressed and ready to get to work, it was time to eat breakfast. I ate two waffles with 20 carbs and a Danon Light and Fit Greek yogurt with 9 carbs for breakfast.

Per the advice of my CDE (Jenny Smith!), I would eat my waffles 45 minutes after bolusing and then I would eat my yogurt an hour after I ate the waffles. It seemed to work out well for me. Other meals didn't seem to create as big a spike as breakfast did but I still tried to pre-bolus by 10 minutes for each meal.

MY SON'S BIRTH STORY

My son's birth story was a bit of a roller coaster! He was born at 38 weeks and 4 days via C-section. He was scheduled to be delivered via C-section at 39+2 weeks (C-section due to his size), but the week before we hit a few bumps in the pregnancy.

At 37 weeks and 6 days, we went in for our weekly BPP test (biophysical profile) and he didn't pass the test. Of course, that day both my high-risk OB and my regular OB were on vacation. The substitute high-risk OB didn't know my history so he wanted to err on the side of caution. Since we failed the BPP, he wanted to take my son that day. My husband and I freaked out a little bit because we weren't expecting to deliver him then (it was also Halloween!). We hadn't even packed our hospital bag. Luckily, the doctor gave us the option to come back in the afternoon and try the BPP again. To our relief, my son passed that afternoon so we went home.

Over the weekend, I thought I noticed decreased movement (probably overly cautious after our scare the day before) so we went into the hospital, with our bags packed this time. However, he ended up passing the non-stress test when we got there so they sent us home.

The following Wednesday at 38+4 weeks, I had my regular OB appointment. Given all that had transpired the previous 5 days, my doctor decided she wanted to go ahead and deliver my son that day versus waiting until the following Monday (at 39+2 weeks) when I was originally planned to deliver. Of course my husband and I hadn't learned our lesson and we again didn't have our hospital bag with us! My husband rushed home and I headed towards Labor and Delivery.

My OB appointment was at 11 a.m., so I had eaten breakfast that morning. At the time, I had been struggling with post-breakfast lows, but I thought I had a few more days to get my rates corrected. When she told me we were going to deliver my son that day, she said that I couldn't eat or drink anything anymore. So off I went to Labor and Delivery (around 11:30 a.m.) and by noon, my blood sugar had dropped to 60 mg/dL and was still dropping. They hadn't admitted me back yet so I was waiting alone in the lobby to be admitted while my blood sugar continued to drop.

I was getting really nervous, but they finally took me back and set up an IV. By this point, I was breaking out in a bad sweat because I was getting so low. But the IV drip finally started to work and by 2:30 p.m., and my blood sugar had climbed to 187 mg/dL.

Once my blood sugar rose, I began to get nervous about being high because I had read that having high blood sugar when you deliver is bad for the baby because he will overcompensate for the extra sugar in the placenta and will have low blood sugar when he is born. I bolused for the high blood sugar and hoped I would come down before delivery. I think some of the high was from adrenaline—I was so nervous—because I dropped faster than I think the insulin could have accounted for. Around 3:30 p.m., they took me back to the operating room to deliver and my blood sugar had dropped to 86 mg/dL.

I had my son via C-section. My son was born 10 pounds, 14 ounces, a big boy but perfectly healthy. He received an 8 and a 9 on the APGAR test. He had low blood sugars the first 36 hours but he was able to stay with me, not in NICU. I breastfed him but also gave him formula to help bring his blood sugar up.

I was able to keep my infusion set and CGM on throughout the whole thing and manage my diabetes myself. I didn't immediately adjust my basal and bolus rates (to pre-pregnancy rates) like I should have so I spent the majority of my hospital stay drinking OJ and eating graham crackers to treat low blood sugars. We didn't get more than about an hour of sleep the three days we were at the hospital so when I finally got home, I was able to think a little more clearly (after catching up a little on sleep) and make the changes to my rates. I also was very nauseous and vomited so that complicated things a little bit when I was trying to treat my low blood sugars.

It wasn't quite the birth story I was planning on. I definitely wasn't planning to deliver that day, and I hadn't had a chance to properly prepare my blood sugars, but in the end I had a healthy baby boy and that's all that matters!

BREASTFEEDING & D-MANAGEMENT

I feel pretty lucky. My son latched-on well from the beginning and has not had a problem gaining weight. Surprisingly, when I was pregnant, I was more worried about being able to breastfeed than I was about giving birth. I really wanted to be able to breastfeed for a year and I was worried that having diabetes might inhibit my ability to produce milk. We are going on 8 months of breastfeeding exclusively (and introduced solids at month 6), and I feel really blessed.

The one surprising thing though about breastfeeding with diabetes is that I didn't really notice a change in my blood sugars from breastfeeding. I had heard that breastfeeding can cause you to go lower, but that hasn't been my experience. (I wish it was so my A1C would be better!)

I think the hardest part of breastfeeding with diabetes is that breastfeeding becomes the priority over my diabetes management, especially in the beginning when I was breastfeeding really often. If my son was formula-fed, my husband could help out more with the feedings but because we are exclusively breastfeeding, the responsibility lies solely with me. So I spend majority of my time stressing about his feeding schedule and less about my feeding schedule or my blood sugars. I love my time with my son while I'm breastfeeding though and I wouldn't have it any other way!

DIABETES MANAGEMENT... WITH A BABY TO CARE FOR!

I have actually found this to be the most difficult part of having a baby (more difficult than the pregnancy!). My son isn't a great sleeper. The nights I don't get much sleep, I am exhausted the next day and my blood sugars are usually elevated.

Also, my priority lies in making sure my son is fed when he needs to be, put down for sleep on time and is stimulated enough so he is learning and hitting his milestones on time. Because of all the energy focused on my son, I often let the focus on my health lapse. I don't upload my CGM data nearly as often as I should. I don't make adjustments when they are needed and as a result, my blood sugars have been climbing higher and higher and I'm becoming more comfortable higher than lower.

I also forget to put my CGM on some days and I haven't been changing my insulin pump infusion set sites as often as I should. I also grab prepackaged snack food for convenience instead of eating something healthier that I would have to weigh. It isn't all bad though! Because I am on a pretty structured schedule for my son (who is 8 months old), I find myself on a pretty structured schedule too so I'm able to test my blood sugars often.

I have had a hard time with postpartum depression. I felt fine the first few months but mainly because I had my husband helping with the baby a lot. Once he went back to work full-time it got a lot harder. I didn't have much support otherwise so I think the PPD hit me a little harder. At first, I thought it was just baby blues and having a hard time adjusting to a newborn but it continued on after a few months so I "self-diagnosed" myself with PPD. I mentioned it to my doctor, but it was a day that I was doing better so she told me she thought it was passing and I would be fine.

Relating to diabetes, I noticed that my PPD seemed to be worse when my blood sugar was high. They would also coincide with days I didn't get much sleep. I think the lack of sleep really had an effect on my PPD and blood sugars. Overtime, my symptoms improved—it just took patience and persistence.

READ MORE FROM KELLEY AT WWW.BELOW-SEVEN.COM

MEGAN HANSON'S STORY

PREGNANT WITH TWINS

I was 5 weeks pregnant, in my 2nd pregnancy, when we found out we were having identical twins. We were in absolute shock. The first thought I remember having was something diabetes related: Pregnancy is difficult for anyone. Adding multiple births to pregnancy with type 1 diabetes was scary. I was sure it would be near impossible!

Surprisingly, the overall pregnancy with tins mirrored my first pregnancy with one baby in almost all ways, just a few more appointments. So many appointments!

When the twins arrived, they had to spend a few days in the special care nursery for feeding but once we left, they were both nursing (tandem) and continued with great success for a year. I also had an 18 month old at home so diabetes management definitely took a back seat for the first few months.

If I could go back and do this part again, I would make sure I had a plan to make sure I had time to see my endocrinologist regularly. I would make sure I made it to that first appointment and didn't reschedule it over and over. I would figure out a better plan ahead of time on how to make time to check my blood sugar more often. I would make a point to keep my CGM on during this time period, too. Instead, it was so full of chaos, just with taking care of three little ones on my own all day, I was constantly trying to take care of low blood sugars, eat enough calories to feed two babies, etc. I was just trying to keep everybody taken care of as best I could.

WHEN MY TWIN BOYS WERE DIAGNOSED WITH TYPE 1 DIABETES

I was diagnosed with type 1 diabetes when I was 11 years old. I was old enough to remember life without it, but young enough that it helped form me into the person I am today. I have always known that I want children. I was determined to learn as much as I could about my likelihood of having a child with type 1 diabetes and I was going to do whatever it took to make sure I did everything I could to lessen that likelihood. I worked incredibly hard to keep my A1Cs in the 5s during pregnancy, I nursed all four of my boys for a year—anything that I had heard or read could reduce the chance of my children developing type 1 diabetes, I tried.

My twins were my second pregnancy, and I was even more determined since having twins was such a scary thing in the first place. With all of my boys, anytime they were excessively thirsty or went to the bathroom often, I immediately tested their blood sugars. I always knew it would come up with a normal blood sugar, but I just wanted to do it so I wouldn't have to worry. I never actually thought it would come back high. It was just for peace of mind that I had checked everything that I could. Test them and move on. Ease my worries.

So, on average, I'd estimate that I tested my boys' blood sugars once every couple months. This time, my twins were just one day shy of turning 1 year old. It was Halloween day, right before lunchtime. I had just finished taking pictures of my three boys in their dragon costumes. Lincoln had a heavy diaper, we had a busy day full of festivities and trick-or-treating to look forward to so before putting them down for naps, I thought, "I'll just test really quick so we can enjoy the day."

I remember testing him and seeing the 568 number blink back at me. I've never felt so frantic, heartbroken, scared, or sad as I did in that split second. I tested his other hand, then I tested both of his feet. I called my husband and I remember calling his doctor and they couldn't understand what I was saying because I was crying so hard. I knew what he was in for.

I knew what was coming.

I knew the millions of ways this day would forever change the rest of his life. The doctor wanted to see him so we headed there first. She thought maybe I just forgot to wipe some sugar off his finger before testing. Psh! Please!

So from there we dropped my 2 year-old off with his aunt, and we headed to the Children's hospital, where we stayed for four days, mostly getting set-up with an insulin pump.

His A1C was only up to 6.2 percent, so he was pretty much acting and feeling like his normal self, and since I had a pretty good handle on all things type 1 diabetes related (carb-counting, injections, etc.) it was a pretty quiet time.

We celebrated his 1st birthday in the hospital. His twin brother wasn't there to celebrate it with him. I couldn't be with both of my babies on their first birthday. I felt so sad. I felt so guilty. I felt like this was entirely my fault. I was so scared of the fact that he was just a baby. He wasn't even walking yet. He was only breastfed at this point.

How do you carb-count for breast-milk? How can I tell if he is low? I'm never going to sleep again! I have enough of a time figuring my own diabetes out, how can I manage his too?

I felt so lucky that I wasn't one of the other parents on that floor getting this diagnosis for their child. I'm constantly in awe of parents who know nothing about type 1 diabetes, and they have all these facts and scary things thrown at them when their child is diagnosed—not knowing what their future holds. I feel so grateful that I had such a short learning curve. I felt grateful that I knew the adequate amount of fear to feel.

I've met parents of newly diagnosed children, and they are a wreck. They are terrified. Too scared to give their child a carbohydrate, too scared to let them run, too scared of what this means for their children's lives. I'm grateful that I can recognize the severity but know that my children will lead happy normal lives.

Since my twins are identical, we were told that Leland had a 60% of also developing type 1 diabetes. Within 10 weeks of Lincoln's diagnosis, I noticed Leland's diapers were also heavy. I tested him as well. I remember so much less of the precise feelings and facts of his diagnosis day. I remember feeling defeated, heartbroken. But, I felt much more prepared this time.

I mentally tried to prepare myself for this over the past many months since Lincoln's diagnosis. When I called the doctor, instead of having me bring him in, she sent us right to the hospital. I guess I was an expert now. We had all the same nurses, stayed for the same 4 days, got set-up on an insulin pump again, etc. When we returned home, it was almost easier having to keep them both on the same routine. I obviously would never wish this on anyone, but if they have to have it, I am so grateful they have each other—facing diabetes together every day.

MAKING MY DIABETES MANAGEMENT A PRIORITY... AND AN EXAMPLE FOR MY BOYS

I have always known I wanted to have children. I have never seen type 1 diabetes as a reason not to have them. I've let myself feel guilty about that decision from time to time, but I try really hard to see the big picture. My life is a good, full life. I've lived with type 1 diabetes since I was 11 years old. If my mom, who also has type 1 diabetes, decided she didn't want to risk having a child with type 1 diabetes and didn't conceive me, then what a life I would have missed out on!

Everyone has a struggle in life, and this is mine. I prayed that it wouldn't be my children's struggle but, so far, for two out of my four boys, it will also be one of their struggles.

I love being a mom. It is the most challenging, rewarding, heartwarming, magical, time of my life. I would have missed out on so much in choosing not to have babies. And they would have missed out too. I'm a really good mom (at least I really try to be) and I get to try my hardest every day with my boys. Diabetes doesn't change that.

Pursuing motherhood since my twins' diagnosis has changed somewhat. I now place so much more emphasis on what we are all eating, how active we are, how diligent I am with my own type 1 diabetes care. I have two little boys looking up to me, and I will forever be their gauge. If I was a slacker in my care and then I ended up with complications, I could have a direct impact on how they live their own lives with type 1 diabetes.

If I take the best care of myself that I can, and continue doing really well—no complications, no visible downsides to having type 1 diabetes other than the daily work—then I think that shows them they can do anything in their lives, too.

RECIPES & PRODUCTS WE LOVE

In the next few pages you'll find a few of the recipes and products that we personally love! These recipes and products are all made of at least mostly whole ingredients, if not completely. They are a combination of low-carb and moderate-carb quantities.

For recipes that are not our own, we've listed the title and the website to search for that title. For the products, we've listed the product name along with either the store or website where it can most easily be purchased.

Everything on this list is gluten-free. Some items are very low-carb. Some items are moderate in carb-quantity, and others are as carb-full as brown rice pasta. The goal during pregnancy is not to eliminate carbs entirely. Instead, we aim for some of our choices to be lower in carbs and others are higher.

Nothing on this list is "sponsored" by a website or manufacturer—it is a simply a list of recipes and products we genuinely use and love!

PRODUCTS

The following is a list of a few products we love that can help make healthy eating during pregnancy easier.

- [ ] **LOW-CARB, GRAIN-FREE PIZZA**
  REALGOODFOODS.COM

- [ ] **ROASTED BROAD BEAN TRAIL MIX**
  EATENLIGHTENED.COM

- [ ] **BRAZI BITES**
  WHOLE FOODS

- [ ] **KIRKLAND TURKEY BURGER PATTIES**
  COSTCO

- [ ] **KIRKLAND FROZEN STIR-FRY VEGETABLES**
  COSTCO

- [ ] **KIRKLAND FROZEN ORGANIC NORMANDY VEGETABLES**
  COSTCO

- [ ] **ORGAIN VEGAN PROTEIN POWDER**
  COSTCO

- [ ] **JAY ROBB EGG OR WHEY PROTEIN POWDER**
  AMAZON

- [ ] **BOUNCE PROTEIN BARS**
  TRADER JOE'S

- [ ] **BROWN RICE PASTA**
  TRADER JOE'S

- [ ] **EXPLORE ASIAN BLACK BEAN SPAGHETTI**
  AMAZON

RECIPES

The following 14 recipes can be found online by searching the listed title at the listed website:

1 **FLAXSEED MUFFIN IN A MUG**
DIABETESDAILY.COM

2 **ALMOND FLOUR BROWNIES**
KINGARTHURFLOUR.COM

3 **MUM'S LOW-CARB BREAD**
THELONDONER.ME

4 **LOW-CARB ZUCCHINI BREAD**
LOWCARBYUM.COM

5 **MULTI-PURPOSE LOW-CARB BREAD**
ALLDAYIDREAMABOUTFOOD.COM

6 **GINGER'S HOMEMADE CHILI**
DIABETESDAILY.COM

7 **GINGER'S MULTI-GRAIN, LOW-CARB MUFFINS**
DIABETESDAILY.COM

8 **GINGER'S LOW-CARB BLUEBERRY MUFFINS**
DIABETESDAILY.COM

9 **RICE & LEEK GINGER STIR-FRY**
DIEPLICIOUS.COM

10 **TOFU LASAGNA WITH ZUCCHINI NOODLES**
EATINGBIRDFOOD.COM

11 **PINTO BEAN-DIP**
FOOD.COM

12 **SESAME CRUSTED TOFU**
LOVEANDOLIVEOIL.COM

13 **COCONUT CURRY THAI CHICKEN**
FOODNETWORK.COM

14 **CLASSIC OVERNIGHT OATS**
BACKTOHERROOTS.COM

JENNY'S FAVORITE RECIPES

The following recipes are a few of Jenny's personal favorites!

PUMPKIN COCONUT FLOUR PANCAKES

INGREDIENTS

- 1/2 cup coconut flour
- 1/4 cup whey protein powder (vanilla is nice)
- 1/4 cup Coconut syrup
- 1 tsp baking powder
- 1 tsp cinnamon
- 1/2 tsp salt
- 1/2 tsp ginger
- 1/4 tsp cloves (ground)

- 6 large eggs
- 1/2 cup pumpkin puree (canned without sugar— not the pumpkin pie puree)
- 3 tbsp coconut oil, melted
- 1/2 to 3/4 cup unsweetened almond milk (or regular milk of choice)
- 1/2 tsp vanilla extract
- Coconut oil for the pan

INSTRUCTIONS

1. Preheat oven to 200F.

2. In a large bowl, whisk together coconut flour, protein powder, sweetener, baking powder, cinnamon, salt, ginger, and cloves.

3. In a medium bowl, whisk together eggs, pumpkin puree, melted coconut oil, 1/2 cup almond milk and vanilla extract.

4. Add the egg mixture to the coconut flour mixture and stir well to combine. Add more almond milk if batter is very thick. It should not be runny.

5. Heat a large skillet over medium high heat and add a little coconut oil. Once oil is melted, scoop two heaping tablespoons of batter onto skillet and spread into a 4 inch circle. Repeat until you can't fit any more pancakes into the skillet (you should be able to get 3 or 4 in).

6. Cook until bottom is golden brown and top is set around the edges. Flip carefully and continue to cook until second side is golden brown. Remove from pan and keep warm on plate or baking sheet in oven, while repeating with remaining batter.

NUTRITION
SERVINGS: 6
PER SERVING: 14 GRAMS OF CARBS AND 8 GRAMS OF FIBER

ALMOND MEAL CINNAMON PANCAKES

INGREDIENTS

- 1 cup almond meal (almond flour)
- 2 eggs
- 1/4 cup water (for fluffier pancakes, you can use sparkling water)
- 2 tbsp coconut oil (melted)
- 1 tsp vanilla extract
- 1/4 teaspoon salt
- 1 tsp cinnamon
- 1 tbsp sweetener of choice (stevia, coconut syrup, honey, etc)

INSTRUCTIONS

1. Mix ingredients together and cook as you would other pancakes. Use a nonstick pan with a little oil. The only real difference is that they won't "bubble" on top the same way as regular pancakes. Flip them when the underside is brown. Serve with sliced berries.

NUTRITION

SERVINGS: SIX 4-INCH PANCAKES
PER SERVING: 5 GRAMS CARBOHYDRATE

PROTEIN PANCAKES

INGREDIENTS FOR ONE SERVING OF 3 PANCAKES

- 1 egg
- ¼ cup ricotta-full or low fat
- 2 tbsp ground flax seed meal
- ½ tsp baking powder
- dash of salt
- sweetener to taste (recommended: 2 packets of Stevia)
- optional: 1 tsp cinnamon and a pinch of nutmeg
- ½ tsp vanilla extract

INGREDIENTS FOR A FAMILY SIZE BATCH OF 12 PANCAKES

- 4 eggs
- 1 cup ricotta (full or low fat)
- ½ cup ground flax-seed meal
- 2 tsp baking powder
- ⅛ tsp salt
- sweetener to taste (6 packets of Stevia)
- 1½ tsp vanilla
- optional: 1 tbsp cinnamon and ½ tsp nutmeg

INSTRUCTIONS

1. Add ingredients to bowl in order listed.

2. Blend with a fork until well mixed.

3. Warm skillet or griddle over medium to medium low heat.

4. Melt butter if you like crispy edges.

5. ASpread a single serving recipe into 3 equal pancakes, about 4-5 inches in diameter.

6. Cook slowly until they are firm enough to flip.

7. Turn and cook on opposite side.

8. AServe immediately, with your choice of toppings. Greek Yogurt with coconut syrup or berries or all fruit jam (like Polaner all fruit).

NUTRITION

PER SERVING OF 3 PANCAKES: 4 GRAMS CARBOHYDRATE

NOTE: THE PANCAKES FREEZE WELL, SEPARATED BY A LAYER OF PAPER TOWEL OR PARCHMENT. THEY REHEAT QUICKLY IN THE OVEN, DIRECTLY ON THE RACK, OR IN A TOASTER OR FRYING PAN

COCONUT
FLOUR PANCAKES

INGREDIENTS

- 2 tbsp extra virgin coconut oil
- 1 tbsp raw honey
- 3 large eggs
- 1/4 cup coconut milk
- 1/2 tsp vanilla extract

- 1/4 cup coconut flour, sifted
- 1/4 tsp cream of tartar
- 1/8 tsp baking soda
- 1/8 tsp sea salt.

INSTRUCTIONS

1. Cream together the coconut oil and honey.
   Add the eggs one at a time.

2. Add coconut milk and vanilla. Mix until smooth.

3. Add coconut flour. Mix until smooth.

4. Lastly add cream of tartar, baking soda and salt.

5. Do not overmix. Overmixing will result in the baking agents (cream of tartar & baking soda) not working.

6. Use a ladle and pour small amount of batter into a crepe pan with ghee/butter etc on medium heat.

7. Flip once the bottom is light brown. The pancakes will not bubble as much as "regular" pancakes.

8. Serve immediately with a drizzle of maple syrup.

NUTRITION

SERVINGS: 8–10 SMALL PANCAKES
PER SERVING: 24 GRAMS IN ENTIRE RECIPE

HIGH-PROTEIN OAT WAFFLE

INGREDIENTS

- 2 ¼ cups water
- 1 can (15oz) cannellini beans (drained and rinsed)
- 1 ¾ cups uncooked old fashioned rolled oats (gluten free—Bob's Red Mill is a good brand)
- ½ cup pumpkin puree
- 2 tbsp ground flax seed(flaxmeal)
- 1 tsp cinnamon (or more to your flavor preference)
- 1 tbsp sugar or honey
- 1 full dropper of liquid vanilla stevia or 2 packets of stevia powder
- 1 tsp vanilla extract
- 1 tsp almond extract
- 1 tbsp baking powder
- 1 tsp salt

INSTRUCTIONS

1. 1Place water into blender. Add all ingredients to the blender. Blend until batter consistency

2. In an 8" waffle maker pour ½ cup batter, close and allow to cook for 6-7 minutes each (these take a bit longer to cook than other waffles due to the beans and oats).

** IF making pancakes, use ¼ cup batter for each pancake

NUTRITION
PER WAFFLE: 20 GRAMS CARBOHYDRATE

BERRY SCONES

- 2 cups + 2 tbsp Organic Coconut Flour
- 1/2 cup Almond Meal/Flour
- 2 tsp Baking Powder
- 3/4 tsp Baking Soda
- 1/2 tsp Sea Salt
- 4 eggs, lightly beaten
- 1-1/4 cups Almond Milk
- 3/4 cup coconut sugar
- 1/3 cup Coconut Oil or Butter (room temperature)
- 1 tsp liquid vanilla stevia drops
- 1 tbsp Apple Cider Vinegar
- 1 tbsp Vanilla Extract
- 1 tsp Almond Extract
- 3/4 cup Blackberries, raspberries or blueberries

INSTRUCTIONS

1. Preheat oven to 350°F and cover a cookie sheet with parchment paper (or use a baking stone).

2. In a large mixing bowl, combine all dry ingredients with a fork or whisk. With a pastry cutter, or a fork, cut in the butter or coconut oil into the dry ingredients to get a crumbly mixture .

3. In a separate bowl, combine all wet ingredients (everything left, except the blackberries).

4. Thoroughly combine the wet and dry ingredients. When batter is homogeneous, gently stir in blackberries and form the batter into balls evenly spaced on the parchment paper.

5. Bake for 18–20 minutes or until lightly browned.

6. Allow to cool for 10 minutes before eating.

7. Allow to completely cool before storage—allow the scones to actually dry out a bit. In storage they will get a bit moist—they still taste great, but will not be as dry/crumbly as when first baked.

NUTRITION

SERVINGS: 12 SCONES
PER SERVING: 16 GRAMS CARBOHYDRATE

NO-BAKE CHOCOLATE PEANUT BUTTER QUINOA COOKIES

YIELDS: 20-25 SMALL COOKIES

INGREDIENTS

- 1/4 cup coconut oil
- 1/2 cup maple syrup
- 1/4 cup unsweetened cocoa powder
- 1/2 cup creamy peanut butter
- 1/2 tsp vanilla extract

- 1/4 tsp kosher salt
- 3 cups cooked quinoa (from about 1 cup uncooked quinoa)
- mini chocolate chips for decorating (optional)

INSTRUCTIONS

1. Line a baking sheet with parchment paper and clear a space in your fridge or freezer for it. Set aside.

2. Combine coconut oil, maple syrup, and cocoa powder in a small saucepan. Bring to a boil over medium heat, stirring to combine. Let boil for about one minute, then remove from heat. Stir in peanut butter, vanilla and salt. Mix in quinoa. Make sure to taste test!

3. Drop batter in small scoops onto the parchment paper. If desired, top with a few mini chocolate chips.

4. Place trays in fridge or freezer to set, which will take at least an hour. The cookies are ready once they are completely firm. For best results, store in the fridge.

NUTRITION
SERVINGS: 20-25
PER SERVING: 8 GRAMS CARBOHYDRATE

FLAX-MEAL PIZZA CRUST

INGREDIENTS

- 1/4 cup ground flax-seed meal
- 1/4 tsp baking powder
- 1/4 tsp Nu-salt
- 1 tbsp italian seasoning
- 1 tbsp parmesan cheese (grated)
- 1/8 tsp sugar substitute of choice OR 1 tsp regular sugar
- 1 egg
- 2 tsp water
- 2 tsp olive oilingredients

INSTRUCTIONS

1. Preheat oven to 375 degrees.

2. Mix dry ingredients, then add egg, water, and oil.

3. Spread batter on a silicone baking mat on a cookie sheet.

4. Bake 8 minutes or until top is dry and bottom is crispy. Flip crust over and bake an additional 5 minutes or so.

5. Crust can be made even more crispy by heating in a pan on the stovetop after baking.

6. Transfer to cookie sheet (minus silicone mat).

7. Top crust with sauce, cheese, and favorite toppings.

8. Bake until cheese is melted. Broil to brown cheese and crisp pepperoni.ingredients

NUTRITION
SERVINGS: ONE 10-INCH PIZZA
ENTIRE PIZZA CRUST (WITHOUT TOPPINGS): 8 GRAMS CARBOHYDRATE

OAT/BANANA COOKIES

INGREDIENTS

- 1 cup uncooked Old Fashioned oats
- ½ cup walnuts
- 2 very ripe bananas
- 2 packets stevia OR alternative sweetener of choice (I use 1 tsp vanilla stevia liquid)
- 1 tsp vanilla extract
- 2 tsp cinnamon
- 1 pinch salt
- ¼ cup mini-chocolate chips

INSTRUCTIONS

1. Blend oats, walnuts, stevia and cinnamon in food processor until ground (not all the oats need to be ground, but finer than just the whole oat). Place in a bowl and mix in the mashed bananas, and all (except chocolate chips) other ingredients.

2. Mix in mini-chocolate chips at the end.

3. Drop by rounded tablespoonful onto a baking pan and flatten a bit with back of the spoon.

4. Bake at 350 for 12-15 minutes.

5. Store in the refrigerator (they will mold on the counter).

NUTRITION

SERVINGS: 15 TO 20 COOKIES
PER SERVING: APPROXIMATELY 9 GRAMS CARBOHYDRATE PER COOKIE

SOURCES & REFERENCES

AMERICAN JOURNAL OF MEDICINE AND ENDOCRINE PRACTICE

JOURNAL OF THE AMERICAN MEDICAL ASSOCIATION

INTEGRATED DIABETES SERVICES (INTEGRATEDDIABETES.COM)

Made in the USA
Monee, IL
09 May 2021